Feyza Küçük
Serap Özdemir
Editors

Evidence-Based Care Practices in Pediatric Nursing

nova
Medicine & Health
New York

DOI: https://doi.org/10.52305/KKWR1517

Library of Congress Cataloging-in-Publication Data

ISBN: 979-8-89530-304-7 (Hardcover)
ISBN: 979-8-89530-358-0 (eBook)

Published by Nova Science Publishers, Inc. † New York

Contents

Preface v

Chapter 1 **Evidence-Based Nursing Practices: Transition to Oral Feeding in Preterm Infants** 1
Şerife Tutar, PhD

Chapter 2 **Evidence-Based Nursing Practices in Preterm Newborn Baths** 13
Hande Özgörü, MSc and Şerife Tutar, PhD

Chapter 3 **Evidence-Based Care for Nipple Problems While Breastfeeding** 27
Zeynem Yildirim Balkan, PhD and Serap Balcı, PhD

Chapter 4 **Evidence-Based Nursing Practices in Newborn Hyperbilirubinemia** 39
Maksude Yıldırım, PhD

Chapter 5 **Evidence-Based Nursing Practices in Newborn Skin Care** 51
Serap Özdemir, PhD

Chapter 6 **Evidence-Based Nursing Practices in Diaper Dermatitis** 65
Esin Keskin, PhD and Büşra Gül, MSc

Chapter 7 **Evidence-Based Nursing Practices in Umbilical Cord Care** 85
Esra Cumur Baskır, MSc and Zeynem Yildirim Balkan, PhD

Chapter 8 **Evidence-Based Nursing Practices in Relieving Colic Infants** 93
Aylin Kurt, PhD

Chapter 9 **Evidence-Based Nursing Practices for Newborn Sleep** 103
Mehmet Emin Düken, PhD and Fatma Bozdağ, PhD

Chapter 10 **Evidence-Based Nursing Practices for Mother-Baby Attachment** 115
Fatma Bozdağ, PhD and Mehmet Emin Düken, PhD

Chapter 11 **Evidence-Based Nursing Practices in Children Suffering from Asthma** 129
Emine Gunes San, MSc

Chapter 12 **Evidence-Based Nursing Practices in Type 1 Diabetes Mellitus** 143
Emine Çubukcu, MSc

Chapter 13 **Evidence-Based Nursing Practices in Epilepsy Management** 153
Zeynep Erkut, PhD and Zeynep Aközlü, MSc

Chapter 14 **Evidence-Based Multidisciplinary Approaches in Childhood Obesity** 165
Meltem Catalbas, PhD

Chapter 15 **Evidence-Based Nursing Practices in Oncological Pediatric Palliative Care** 175
Sümeyye Yıldız, PhD

Chapter 16 **Evidence-Based Practices for Energy Therapies Used in Pain Management in Pediatric Oncology** 189
Duygu Demir, PhD

Chapter 17 **Evidence-Based Nursing Practices for Nausea and Vomiting in Pediatric Oncology** 199
Fatma Dinç, PhD

Chapter 18 **Evidence-Based Nursing Practices in Mucositis in Pediatric Oncology** 213
Aysel Topan, PhD and Betül Akkoç, MSc

Chapter 19 **Evidence-Based Nursing Practices in Non-Pharmacological Procedural Pain Management in Children** 225
Selver Mete İzci, PhD

Chapter 20 **Evidence-Based Nursing Practices to Prevent Home Accidents in Children** 239
Feyza Küçük, PhD

Chapter 21 **Evidence-Based Nursing Practices Involving Yoga in Children** 251
Pelin Gökoğlu Gürer, MSc

Chapter 22 **Evidence-Based Serious Games in Pediatric Care** 263
Hilal Parlak Sert, PhD

Chapter 23 **Evidence-Based Nursing Practices in Wearable Technologies in Children** 277
Aylin Akca Sumengen, PhD and Damla Ozcevik Subasi, PhD

Index 293

Preface

Pediatric nursing is one of the most critical professional fields in protecting and improving the health of children. Effective, safe and scientifically based nursing practices directly affect the health outcomes of both pediatric patients and their families. In this context, our book titled "Evidence-Based Care Practices in Pediatric Nursing" aims to base nursing practices on scientific foundations by bringing together the most up-to-date and reliable information in the field of pediatric diseases and health services.

Our book is a study that emphasizes the importance of evidence-based care practices in pediatric nursing and provides a comprehensive guide on how research results can be reflected in the clinic. In the light of scientific research and clinical experience, strategies, methods and best practices for improving children's health and care processes are discussed in detail. In each chapter, various aspects of pediatric nursing practice are explained based on current research and clinical guidelines, and evidence-based information is presented to contribute to nurses' decision-making processes. The content of the book can be used as a resource in nursing education and is designed as a reference source for professionals in the field.

While preparing this book, we believe that the information created with the contributions of competent academicians and clinician nurses will play an important role in increasing the quality of nursing practice and improving child health. We are happy to share this book with you, considering the importance of constantly staying up-to-date and bringing together scientific and clinical information in order to cope with the problems encountered in the field of pediatric nursing, to improve the quality of care and care results, and to make a difference in clinical practice and patient care results.

We hope that our book will contribute to pediatric nursing practice and enable nurses to develop their knowledge and skills; we would like to thank our authors who contributed to this process and Nova Science Publishers, who worked devotedly to make the book reach its readers.

Best regards,

Feyza Küçük
Assistant Professor
Uşak University
Uşak, 2024

Serap Özdemir
Assistant Professor
Gaziantep University
Gaziantep, 2024

Chapter 1

Evidence-Based Nursing Practices: Transition to Oral Feeding in Preterm Infants

Şerife Tutar*, PhD
Assistant Professor, Department of Nursing, Faculty of Health Sciences, Süleyman Demirel University, Isparta, Türkiye

Abstract

Technological developments experienced in recent years in the field of neonate intensive care have increased the survival rates of preterm infants. These infants, who leave the intrauterine environment without acquiring physiological and neurological maturity, encounter countless problems. One of the most significant problems faced by these infants, whose developmental processes are ongoing in the neonate intensive care unit environment, is the transition process to oral feeding. Transition to oral feeding is a multidimensional process in preterm infants. Oral feeding requires the coordination of respiration, sucking, and swallowing that are related to the musculoskeletal, cardiorespiratory, gastrointestinal, and neurological systems. Furthermore, intraoral and pharyngeal senses should be present. Therefore, for preterm infants to be fed orally, both sensory and motor systems must reach a certain functional level. As respiration and feeding take place in different anatomical structures, the synchronization of these functions is rather important in the feeding of preterm infants. Insufficiency in these functions can lead to apnea, bradycardia, a decrease in oxygen saturation, and aspirations during feeding. Therefore, in the transition to oral feeding, oral motor therapy, which facilitates both sensory inputs and environmental stimulants for the development of the brain and the establishment of synaptic connections in the brain as well as supporting neurological development, is required. When the literature is reviewed, it is seen that there are various applications that support the transition to oral feeding in preterm infants. The most significant responsibility in the transition to oral feeding in the early period falls on the shoulders of neonate intensive care nurses. Neonate intensive care nurses should evaluate the readiness levels of preterm infants for oral feeding and use evidence-based practices in this regard. In this section, it was aimed to evaluate evidence-based practices applied in the transition to oral feeding in preterm infants.

Keywords: neonatal intensive care, neonatal nursing, preterm birth, preterm oral feeding

* Corresponding Author's Email: serifeguven@sdu.edu.tr.

In: Evidence-Based Care Practices in Pediatric Nursing
Editors: Feyza Küçük and Serap Özdemir
ISBN: 979-8-89530-304-7

Introduction

With technological advances in neonatal care, the survival rates of premature infants in neonatal intensive care units have notably improved in recent years. Despite the increase in survival rates, many challenges are encountered in nutrition and the transition to oral feeding in premature infants (weak oral feeding ability is one of the most apparent developmental problems) (Bertoncelli et al., 2012; Vizzari et al., 2023). Oral feeding is a crucial step for optimal growth and development in preterm infants, and the first months of neonatal intensive care are a period with high nutrient requirements for optimal growth. During this period, infants have high energy needs and face physiological complications that can negatively affect growth. Various physiological and environmental factors influence oral feeding skills in preterm infants. Metabolic imbalances and incomplete maturation of all organs and systems, especially the gastrointestinal system, make nutrition a vital urgency for preterms from the first hours after birth (Türkyılmaz, 2018). Additionally, the nutritional needs of preterm infants vary with the infant's gestational age, the degree of growth retardation, the postnatal age, and existing diseases. Various complications caused by immaturities, such as respiratory distress syndrome, intracranial hemorrhage, and bronchopulmonary dysplasia, are among the physiological factors (Astuti, Rustina & Wanda, 2022; Chen et al., 2021; Bedroni, 2023), which affect the neurological system regulating the development of feeding skills (Chen et al., 2021; Astuti, Rustina & Wanda, 2022). During treatment in the intensive care environment, procedures such as intubation, aspiration, removal of plasters around the mouth, and placement of a gastrostomy tube can pose a negative experience for preterm infants regarding oral feeding (Kamity et al., 2021; Astuti, Rustina & Wanda, 2022).

Before transitioning to enteral feeding, many preterm infants may require total parenteral nutrition due to organ immaturity and complications arising from premature birth. However, prolonged total parenteral nutrition, particularly in small preterms, is associated with various short- and long-term complications, including atrophy of the gastrointestinal system, which can adversely affect the success of enteral nutrition (Türkyılmaz, 2018).

Neonatal intensive care unit nurses face numerous challenges in achieving the nutritional goals for preterm infants and also in deciding on the most appropriate method of nutrition according to the developmental stage of the infant. One of the most significant problems encountered by these infants, who are undergoing developmental processes in the NICU environment, is the transition to oral feeding. The transition to oral feeding in preterm infants is a multifaceted process. Oral feeding requires the coordination of respiratory, sucking, and swallowing functions, which are related to the musculoskeletal, cardiorespiratory, gastrointestinal, and neurological systems. Since respiration and feeding occur in the same anatomical structures, the synchronization of these functions is of great importance in the nutrition of the preterm infant. Therefore, the transition to oral feeding necessitates not only sensory input and environmental stimuli for brain development but also oral motor therapy, which assists in the establishment of synaptic connections in the brain and supports neurological development.

In the early transition to oral feeding in preterm infants, the primary responsibility falls upon neonatal intensive care unit nurses. NICU nurses must assess the readiness of premature infants for feeding and use evidence-based practices in this regard. A review of the literature reveals that these practices include cue-based feeding, interventions for the development of oral motor functions, non-nutritive sucking, and interventions related to the oral feeding position. This section aims to evaluate evidence-based practices applied in the transition to oral feeding in preterm infants, according to literature.

Cue-Based Feeding

In recent years, cue-based feeding has emerged as a leading intervention to support the transition to oral feeding in preterm infants. Cue-based feeding is a feeding method where the infant's physiological and behavioral cues are taken as criteria for initiating and continuing oral feeding (Gözen & Girgin, 2017; Whetten, 2016; Lubbe, 2018). The review of the literature indicates that for successful and safe oral feeding, it is necessary to transition from the traditional feeding model, which is based on gestational age, body weight, and amount of food, to the cue-based feeding model, which prioritizes infant behaviors (Fry et al., 2018; Thomas et al., 2021; Spagnoli et al., 2023).

In the traditional feeding method, the infant's weight and gestational age are considered, and the amount of milk consumed is monitored at specific intervals. This method focuses on feeding times rather than evaluating the infant's readiness for feeding based on the overall condition. In this model, the transition to oral feeding is made without regard to the infant's physiological and behavioral signs. In this feeding model, nurses use bottle nipples that promote fast flow to encourage the infant to finish the meal and use oral stimuli such as rotating the nipple inside the mouth and moving it back and forth, trying to ensure that the infant consumes the entire prescribed amount of food. This can lead to increased signs of stress in the infant and slow the successful transition to oral feeding. Therefore, in recent years, it has been recommended to move away from the traditional feeding approach in neonatal intensive care units (Ludwig & Waitzman, 2007; Gözen & Girgin, 2017; Giannì et al., 2017).

Contrary to the traditional feeding method, cue-based feeding progresses based on each infant's developmental cues and signs of readiness for feeding. This model focuses on enhancing the infant's oral feeding skills regardless of the amount of intake. Cue-based feeding is a component of standard care managed by the neonatal intensive care unit nurse. The nurse assesses the infant's readiness signs before feeding, including physiological stability (thermoregulation, maintenance of alertness, cardiorespiratory stability, coordination of sucking-swallowing and breathing functions), the infant's response to oral stimuli, tolerance to full enteral feeding, the opening of the mouth, licking lips with the tongue, sucking motions, moving hands around the face and mouth area, turning the face towards the bedsheet and hands, among other behaviors (Kirk et al., 2007; Ludwig & Waitzman, 2007).

During the initiation of oral feeding, the nurse should continue to observe all of the infant's physiological and behavioral signs. Signs of stress that may occur during feeding include attempting to push the nipple away, arching the back, turning the head, lifting the eyelids, increased respiratory effort, splaying the fingers, grimacing, hiccupping, spilling milk from the bottle, changes in color, apnea, bradycardia, and a drop in oxygen saturation. If the nurse observes these stress signs during feeding, they should apply the cue-based feeding approach by facilitating the infant's external rest and pausing the feeding according to the severity of the stress signs (Gözen & Girgin, 2017; Ross & Philbin, 2011; Thoyre et al., 2012; Thoyre et al., 2013).

Table 1. Evidence for Cue-Based Feeding in Preterm Infants

Benefits of cue-based feeding	Evidence
Earlier transition to oral feeding	Kirk et al., 2007 Pickler et al., 2015 Samane et al., 2022 Thomas et al., 2021 Fry et al., 2018 Spagnoli et al., 2023 Gentle et al., 2022 Kamran et al., 2020
Improved weight gain	Samane et al., 2022 Fry et al., 2018
Improved physiological outcome	Thoyre et al., 2016 Samane et al., 2022
Shorter length of stay in hospital	Puckett et al., 2008 Pickler et al., 2015 Thomas et al., 2021 Fry et al., 2018 Spagnoli et al., 2023 Gentle et al., 2022 Kamran et al., 2020
Fewer adverse events	Puckett et al., 2008
Increased parents' involvement in the feeding process	Thomas et al., 2021
Cost savings for the institution	Thomas et al., 2021

External pacing is a technique utilized when an infant is unable to coordinate sucking, swallowing, and breathing functions during feeding. In this technique, the nurse decreases the angle of the bottle to support the infant's breathing and slows the flow of milk from the bottle. This allows the infant to swallow more effectively and reduces the volume of fluid intake, thereby preventing the risk of aspiration. This technique is named external pacing because it involves the nurse carefully observing the infant to balance respiratory and swallowing functions and support the infant's physiological state during feeding (Gözen & Girgin, 2017).

Cue-based feeding in preterm infants offers numerous benefits. The early transition to oral feeding can lead to accelerated weight gain, stabilization of physiological parameters, decreased hospital stay, prevention of potential adverse effects, inclusion of the parent in the feeding process, and reduced cost of patient care (Table 1). Furthermore, some studies indicate that cue-based feeding training for nurses also accelerates the transition to full oral feeding in the early period (Beissel et al., 2022; Astuti et al., 2023).

Interventions for Supporting Oral Motor Functions in Oral Feeding

Oral feeding is a complex process that necessitates the coordination of sucking, swallowing, and respiratory functions (Dietrich & Blanco, 2022; Greene et al., 2023). Although non-nutritive sucking is thought to occur as early as the 12th week of gestation, the integration of respiratory function for successful oral feeding is not expected before 33-34 weeks of pregnancy. Therefore, preterm infants are a sensitive group to the development of oral feeding skills due to the immaturity associated with premature birth (Dietrich & Blanco, 2022; da Rosa Pereira et al., 2020; Pados et al., 2021). Consequently, oral motor stimulation techniques are implemented to enhance feeding skills in preterm infants (Rodriguez Gonzalez et al., 2021; Atay et al., 2023; Sasmal et al., 2023).

Oral motor stimulation is defined as the tactile stimulation of the lips, jaws, tongue, and soft palate to activate the oropharyngeal mechanism. The primary goal of these stimuli is to strengthen the structures of the neuronal and musculoskeletal systems that play a role in coordinating sucking, swallowing, and breathing (Dietrich & Blanco, 2022). The literature indicates the use of various oral motor stimulation techniques to improve oral feeding skills in preterm infants, with the Fucile technique and the Preterm Infant Oral Motor Intervention (PIOMI) among the standardized techniques frequently used (Shokri et al., 2023).

- *Fucile Technique*: This method consists of two steps, oral motor stimulation, and non-nutritive sucking, carried out over a total of 15 minutes-7 minutes of tactile stimulation to the cheeks, lips, and jaw; 5 minutes of intraoral stimulation to the gums and tongue; followed by 3 minutes of non-nutritive sucking. Circular movements massage the cheeks, while the fingertips perform anteroposterior massage on the lips, gums, and the vestibular area of the tongue (Fucile & Gisel, 2010; Fucile et al., 2021).
- *PIOMI (Preterm Infant Oral Motor Intervention):* This technique involves an 8-step, 5-minute application, including stimulating the cheeks (30 seconds twice), stimulating the lips (30 seconds once), puckering the lips (30 seconds once), gum stimulation (30 seconds twice), stimulating the lateral regions of the tongue and cheek (15 seconds once), stimulating the medial septum of the tongue and palate (30 seconds twice), placing a finger along the midline of the palate to elicit a sucking reflex with light stimuli (15 seconds), and non-nutritive sucking (2 minutes) (Lessen, 2011).

In preterm infants, the development of oral feeding skills incorporates the combined application of oral motor stimulation and non-nutritive sucking. These practices, especially non-nutritive sucking and aspects of swallowing physiology, have been found to be effective in facilitating oral feeding skills. However, preterm infants also experience pharyngeal swallowing issues alongside sucking problems. Interventions of oral motor stimulation and non-nutritive sucking in these infants are not designed to address pharyngeal swallowing deficiencies (Huang et al., 2024). Therefore, considering the insufficient movement of the tongue and submandibular muscles and clinical signs of aspiration during bottle feeding in preterm infants, Lau and Smith developed a new "swallowing exercise" to enhance neurobehavioral organization. This exercise involves placing 0.05-0.2 ml of milk directly onto the posterior midline of the infant's tongue, thereby facilitating a swallowing action. The foundation of this exercise developed by Lau and Smith is based on the theory that applied interventions can accelerate the normal development of physiological functions. Lau and Smith (2012) compared this swallowing exercise with standard care in the neonatal intensive care unit, finding that preterm infants undergoing swallowing exercise transitioned to oral feeding more rapidly. A study by Ostadi et al. (2021) observed that preterm infants who received both non-nutritive sucking and swallowing exercises were more likely to be discharged from tube feeding (Ostadi et al., 2021).

Non-Nutritive Sucking

Non-nutritive Sucking (NNS) is a fundamental skill necessary for oral feeding and self-regulation in the postnatal period. NNS begins very early, as soon as 12-15 weeks after conception, and is observed throughout intrauterine life. At 20 weeks, rhythmical NNS has been reported, characterized by the fetus opening and closing the mouth at regular intervals, in organized bursts with pauses between compressions. The development of NNS continues throughout pregnancy and plays a critical role in the feeding of a term infant (Pineda et al., 2019). NNS holds significant importance in early oral feeding in preterm infants by facilitating the coordination of sucking and swallowing and establishing a normal sucking pattern. When applied alongside tube feeding, it supports the infant in associating sucking with satiety and encourages sucking behavior. Additionally, NNS during invasive procedures in preterm infants results in reduced pain levels and easier relaxation. Its calming effect decreases the infant's energy expenditure, contributing to growth, development, and weight gain. NNS through oral motor movements also stimulates the stomach, facilitating faster digestion of ingested milk (Giannì et al., 2017; Bedroni, 2023).

The literature distinguishes between two types of NNS (Fucile et al., 2021): one involving sucking on an empty maternal breast and the other using a pacifier. The optimal method to initiate oral feeding in preterm infants is breastfeeding (Girgin et al., 2018). In this initial breastfeeding, milk is expressed from the mother's breast, and then the empty breast is sucked. The requirement for mothers to be present multiple times for breastfeeding in the intensive care setting complicates the application of this method. An alternative method involves bottle-feeding expressed breast milk. During bottle feeding, the infant should be positioned as close as possible to the breastfeeding position in the mother's arms, ideally in a semi-elevated side-lying position (Girgin et al., 2018; Bedroni, 2023). If the infant cannot complete feeding orally, the remainder is provided through a feeding tube. The transition to full oral feeding is a crucial factor in determining the duration of the infant's hospital stay. The interventions applied during the transition to oral feeding can result in either positive or negative outcomes for preterm infants, influencing the success of the transition to full oral feeding (Lubbe 2018; Brun et al., 2020; Bedroni, 2023). In a study by Fucile et al. (2021), two non-nutritive sucking methods (bottle and emptied maternal breast) were compared. It was found that the infants in the group using the emptied maternal breast had a higher rate of exclusive breastfeeding at discharge compared to those fed by bottle, though no significant difference was found between the groups regarding the transition to full oral feeding and hospital stay duration.

Oral Feeding Position

Enhancing the quality and safety of oral feeding is a significant care responsibility in the neonatal intensive care unit. Due to the immaturity of the neurological, respiratory, muscular, and digestive systems in preterm infants, and their limited abilities to adapt to extrauterine life, support during oral feeding is crucial. Particularly, infants born ≤34 weeks of gestation often undergo tube feeding, which is gradually transitioned to oral feeding (Raczyńska et al., 2022; Hockenberry et al., 2023).

The transition to full oral feeding can lead to issues such as decreased oxygen saturation, bradycardia, and aspiration in infants. This situation usually arises from the inability to coordinate sucking, swallowing, and breathing during feeding in preterm infants. All of these events can stress the infant and negatively impact the immature neurological system. Additionally, this situation can create feelings of inadequacy in parents and increase their anxiety regarding infant care. Therefore, interventions aimed at ensuring adequate respiration and maintaining physiological stabilization during oral feeding in preterm infants are necessary (Zelkowitz et al., 2009; Gross & Trapani-Hanasewych, 2017).

The position given to a preterm infant during oral feeding is a significant factor in supporting respiration and physiological stabilization during feeding. However, different positions are applied in the oral feeding of preterm infants. These include the cradle hold, side-lying, semi-elevated supine, and semi-elevated side-lying positions.

In the cradle hold position, the infant is positioned semi-recumbent on the nurse's arm, with the infant's head supported in the crook of the nurse's elbow. Since the infant's head is on the arm of the mother/nurse, it remains in flexion. This means that in this position, the infant's head and neck are not in a neutral plane similar to the breastfeeding position in a mother's lap, so it is not considered a position that supports the infant's respiration. In this position, the infant's head can tilt backward, and retroflexion of the neck can be observed. Therefore, feeding problems related to respiratory issues can occur in infants (Dawson et al., 2013).

In the side-lying position, a pillow is placed under the nurse's arm to support the infant, and the infant is laid on its side facing the nurse (Dawson et al., 2013). In a study comparing the side-lying and semi-elevated positions in the oral feeding of preterm infants, it was stated that the side-lying position, compared to the semi-elevated position, was safer in terms of the infant's choking episodes and resulted in a higher milk consumption (Raczyńska & Gulczyńska, 2019; Raczyńska et al., 2022). Conversely, a systematic review by Park et al. (2018) indicates that there is no strong and consistent evidence that the side-lying position improves outcomes related to oral feeding in preterm infants.

In the semi-elevated supine position, the nurse supports the infant's head and neck on the same plane with one hand, while holding the bottle with the other hand to feed the infant (Dawson et al., 2013). This position offers benefits such as maintaining the infant's head and neck on the same plane, enabling eye contact during feeding, and allowing better observation of the infant's responses. However, the effect of gravity, along with the retraction of the tongue and soft palate, can lead to closure of the upper airway, disrupting respiratory functions during feeding. Additionally, in this position, the hydrostatic pressure created by inverting the bottle due to gravity causes a large amount of milk to flow into the infant's mouth, making it difficult for the infant to control the intake of milk, leading to swallowing difficulties, aspiration, and apnea (Gözen & Girgin, 2017; Clark et al., 2007).

In the semi-elevated side-lying position, the infant lies on the nurse's lap in a side-lying position with the head elevated at a 45-60 degree angle. During feeding, the nurse keeps the infant's head and neck in flexion, on the same plane as the body. This position resembles the "breastfeeding at the mother's breast" position, allowing preterm infants to benefit from the advantages of breastfeeding during feeding. Since the bottle is raised at a smaller angle in this position, the milk flows with less hydrostatic pressure and more slowly. The reduced flow rate of milk helps the infant to better control the intake. Moreover, the semi-elevated side-lying position prevents the anatomical retraction of the tongue and soft palate due to gravity, maintaining airway patency (Park et al., 2014; Gözen & Girgin, 2017; Aktaş et al., 2022). In a study comparing right and left semi-elevated side-lying positions by Aktaş et al. (2022), no difference was found between the positions in terms of the percentage and volume of intake and feeding duration.

Conclusion

Oral feeding in preterm infants is a critical indicator for achieving optimal growth and development and for early hospital discharge. However, due to the physiological and neurological immaturity associated with premature birth, preterm infants lack the necessary coordination of sucking-swallowing and breathing for oral feeding. As a result, preterm infants may experience apnea, bradycardia, drops in oxygen saturation, and aspiration during feeding, highlighting the need for the development of oral feeding skills in this population (da Rosa Pereira et al., 2020; Kamran et al., 2021; Dietrich & Blanco, 2022).

The enhancement of oral feeding skills in preterm infants is a significant concern for nurses and parents, with approximately 40% of preterm infants experiencing difficulties in transitioning from enteral to oral feeding (da Rosa Pereira et al., 2020). Insufficient nutrition, particularly in infants born between 34-37 weeks, is a common reason for rehospitalization within the first two weeks after discharge from the neonatal intensive care unit. These late preterm infants are more susceptible to inadequate oral feeding due to medical issues such as respiratory distress, jaundice, hypoglycemia, and thermal instability (Lubbe, 2018).

The term "oral feeding skill" is frequently used in multidisciplinary clinical practices, encompassing concepts such as feeding success, intolerance, infant response to feeding, readiness for oral feeding, performance, behavior, and adequacy (Azuma & Maron, 2020). The diversity of these concepts indicates a lack of consensus in expressing oral feeding skills (Brantes et al., 2021; Samane et al., 2022; Girgin et al., 2021; Sasmal & Shetty, 2021). Additionally, many healthcare professionals employ a developmental approach to describe oral feeding skills, defining them in terms of regulation and stabilization of physiological and behavioral states (Kamran et al., 2021; Dietrich & Blanco, 2022). The absence of a common language to evaluate oral feeding skills can lead to improper assessment of infants at discharge and subsequent rehospitalizations due to nutrition-related complications. Furthermore, the use of inappropriate terms in research can result in measurement errors in the infant's oral feeding skill variable (Girgin et al., 2021).

Various practices are used to enhance oral feeding skills in preterm infants, focusing largely on the development of oral motor skills. However, pharyngeal swallowing deficiencies are also observed due to physiological immaturity in preterm infants (Lau & Smith, 2012). Therefore, enhancing oral feeding skills in preterm infants is a multifaceted process. Interventions should consider multiple factors, such as ensuring appropriate positioning and developing oral motor and pharyngeal swallowing skills. The initiation and maintenance of the transition process to oral feeding, according to atraumatic care principles, are fundamental care responsibilities of neonatal intensive care nurses. Consequently, neonatal intensive care nurses must establish a common language and continue evidence-based care approaches during the transition process of preterm infants to oral feeding.

Disclaimer

None.

References

Aktaş, E., Aykanat Girgin, B., Gözen, D., Ergün, K., Pekyiğit, A., & Çetınkaya, M. (2022). Effect of left and right semi-elevated side-lying positions on feeding performance of preterm infants. *Journal of Obstetric, Gynecologic, and Neonatal Nursing: JOGNN, 51*(1), 65–72. https://doi.org/10.1016/j.jogn.2021.09.006.

Astuti, D. D., Rohsiswatmo, R., Wanda, D., & Utari, D. M. (2023). Experiences of Indonesian nurses in improving preterm oral feeding readiness in special care units: A qualitative descriptive study. *Belitung Nursing Journal, 9*(5), 478–488. https://doi.org/10.33546/bnj.2772.

Astuti, D. D., Rustina, Y., & Wanda, D. (2022). Oral feeding skills in premature infants: A concept analysis. *Belitung Nursing Journal, 8*(4), 280–286. https://doi.org/10.33546/bnj.2107.

Atay, F. Y., Ciftci, H. B., Sahin, O., Guran, O., Colak, D., Gok, N. R., Erdem, B. K., & Akin, I. M. (2023). Evaluation of the effect of oral motor stimulation exercises on feeding skills in premature infants. *Sisli Etfal Hastanesi Tip Bulteni, 57*(2), 189–194. https://doi.org/10.14744/SEMB.2022.96562.

Azuma, D., & Maron, J. L. (2020). Individualizing oral feeding assessment and therapies in the newborn. *Research and Reports in Neonatology*, 23-30.

Bedroni, M. (2023). Breastfeeding preterm infants as the initial oral feeding: An integrative review. *Journal of Neonatal Nursing, 29*(2), 267-272.

Beissel, A., Denis, A., Laborie, S., Pillet, F., Gauthier-Moulinier, H., Hommey, S., Tume, L. N., Butin, M., & Touzet, S. (2022). Impact of a nurse education programme on oral feeding in a neonatal unit. *Nursing in Critical Care.* Advance online publication. https://doi.org/10.1111/nicc.12840.

Bertoncelli, N., Cuomo, G., Cattani, S., Mazzi, C., Pugliese, M., Coccolini, E., Zagni, P., Mordini, B., & Ferrari, F. (2012). Oral feeding competences of healthy preterm infants: A review. *International Journal of Pediatrics, 2012*, 896257. https://doi.org/10.1155/2012/896257.

Brantes, A. L. G., dos Santos Curado, M. A., & Cruz, I. R. (2021). Feeding methods in promoting the oral motor skills of the Preterm Newborn: A Scoping Review. *Enfermería Global, 20*(1), 521-535.

Brun, G., Fischer Fumeaux, C. J., Giannoni, E., & Bickle Graz, M. (2020). Factors associated with postmenstrual age at full oral feeding in very preterm infants. *PloS one, 15*(11), e0241769. https://doi.org/10.1371/journal.pone.0241769.

Chen, D., Yang, Z., Chen, C., & Wang, P. (2021). Effect of oral motor intervention on oral feeding in preterm infants: A systematic review and meta-analysis. *American Journal of Speech-Language Pathology, 30*(5), 2318-2328.

Clark, L., Kennedy, G., Pring, T., & Hird, M. (2007). Improving bottle feeding in preterm infants: Investigating the elevated side-lying position. *Infant, 3*(4), 154-158.

da Rosa Pereira, K., Levy, D. S., Procianoy, R. S., & Silveira, R. C. (2020). Impact of a pre-feeding oral stimulation program on first feed attempt in preterm infants: Double-blind controlled clinical trial. *PloS One, 15*(9), e0237915.

Dawson, J. A., Myers, L. R., Moorhead, A., Jacobs, S. E., Ong, K., Salo, F., Murray, S., Donath, S., & Davis, P. G. (2013). A randomised trial of two techniques for bottle feeding preterm infants. *Journal of Paediatrics and Child Health, 49*(6), 462–466. https://doi.org/10.1111/jpc.12208.

Dietrich, L. A. J., & Blanco, C. (2022). Oral feeding of preterm infants in the NICU: interventions and outcomes. *Newborn, 1*(1), 104-108.

Fry, T. J., Marfurt, S., & Wengier, S. (2018). Systematic Review of Quality Improvement Initiatives Related to Cue-Based Feeding in Preterm Infants. *Nursing for Women's Health, 22*(5), 401–410. https://doi.org/10.1016/j.nwh.2018.07.006.

Fucile, S., & Gisel, E. G. (2010). Sensorimotor interventions improve growth and motor function in preterm infants. *Neonatal Network: NN, 29*(6), 359–366. https://doi.org/10.1891/0730-0832.29.6.359.

Fucile, S., Wener, E., & Dow, K. (2021). Enhancing breastfeeding establishment in preterm infants: A randomized clinical trial of two non-nutritive sucking approaches. *Early Human Development, 156*, 105347. https://doi.org/10.1016/j.earlhumdev.2021.105347.

Gentle, S. J., Meads, C., Ganus, S., Barnette, E., Munkus, K., Carlo, W. A., & Salas, A. A. (2022). Improving Time to Independent Oral Feeding to Expedite Hospital Discharge in Preterm Infants. *Pediatrics, 149*(3), e2021052023. https://doi.org/10.1542/peds.2021-052023.

Giannì, M. L., Sannino, P., Bezze, E., Plevani, L., Esposito, C., Muscolo, S., Roggero, P., & Mosca, F. (2017). Usefulness of the Infant Driven Scale in the early identification of preterm infants at risk for delayed oral feeding independency. *Early Human Development, 115*, 18–22. https://doi.org/10.1016/j.earlhumdev.
2017.08.008.

Girgin, B. A., Gözen, D., & Karatekin, G. (2018). Effects of two different feeding positions on physiological characteristics and feeding performance of preterm infants: A randomized controlled trial. *Journal for Specialists in Pediatric Nursing: JSPN, 23*(2), e12214. https://doi.org/10.1111/jspn.12214.

Girgin, B. A., Gözen, D., Uslubaş, R., & Bilgin, L. (2021). The evaluation of oral feeding in preterm infants: Turkish validation of the Early Feeding Skills Assessment tool. *Turkish Archives of Pediatrics, 56*(5), 440.

Gözen, D., & Girgin, B. A. (2017). Preterm bebeklerde oral beslenmeyi destekleyici kanıta dayalı girişimler [Evidence-based interventions to support oral feeding in preterm infants]. *Clinical and Experimental Health Sciences, 7*(4), 171-174.

Greene, Z., O'Donnell, C. P., & Walshe, M. (2023). Oral stimulation for promoting oral feeding in preterm infants. *The Cochrane Database of Systematic Reviews, 6*(6), CD009720. https://doi.org/10.1002/14651858.CD009720.pub3.

Gross, R. D., & Trapani-Hanasewych, M. (2017). Breathing and Swallowing: The Next Frontier. *Seminars in Speech and Language, 38*(2), 87–95. https://doi.org/10.1055/s-0037-1599106.

Hockenberry, M. J., Bryant, R., & Hellsten, M. B. (2023). *Wong's Clinical Manual of Pediatric Nursing E-Book*. Elsevier Health Sciences.

Huang, C. C., Hwang, Y. S., Lin, Y. C., & Huang, M. C. (2024). Effects of oral stimulation on feeding readiness of preterm infants: A randomized controlled study. *Journal of Neonatal Nursing, 30*, 160-164.

Kamity, R., Kapavarapu, P. K., & Chandel, A. (2021). Feeding Problems and Long-Term Outcomes in Preterm Infants-A Systematic Approach to Evaluation and Management. *Children (Basel, Switzerland), 8*(12), 1158. https://doi.org/10.3390/children8121158.

Kamran, F., Khatoonabadi, A. R., Aghajanzadeh, M., Ebadi, A., Faryadras, Y., & Sagheb, S. (2020). Effectiveness of cue-based feeding versus scheduled feeding in preterm infants using comprehensive feeding assessment scales: A randomized clinical trial. *Iranian Journal of Pediatrics, 30*(6), e107475.

Kamran, F., Sagheb, S., Khatoonabadi, S. A., Ebadi, A., Faryadras, Y., & Aghajanzadeh, M. (2021). The validity and reliability of early feeding skills assessment and cue-based feeding scales for preterm infants. *Middle East Journal of Rehabilitation and Health Studies, 8*(3).

Kirk, A. T., Alder, S. C., & King, J. D. (2007). Cue-based oral feeding clinical pathway results in earlier attainment of full oral feeding in premature infants. *Journal of Perinatology: Official Journal of the California Perinatal Association, 27*(9), 572–578. https://doi.org/10.1038/sj.jp.7211791.

Lau, C., & Smith, E. O. (2012). Interventions to improve the oral feeding performance of preterm infants. *Acta Paediatrica (Oslo, Norway: 1992), 101*(7), e269–e274. https://doi.org/10.1111/j.1651-2227.2012.02662.x.

Lessen, B. S. (2011). Effect of the premature infant oral motor intervention on feeding progression and length of stay in preterm infants. *Advances in Neonatal Care: Official Journal of the National Association of Neonatal Nurses, 11*(2), 129–139. https://doi.org/10.1097/ANC.0b013e3182115a2a.

Lubbe, W. (2018). Clinicians guide for cue-based transition to oral feeding in preterm infants: An easy-to-use clinical guide. *Journal of Evaluation in Clinical Practice, 24*(1), 80–88. https://doi.org/10.1111/jep.12721.

Ludwig, S. M., & Waitzman, K. A. (2007). Changing feeding documentation to reflect infant-driven feeding practice. *Newborn and Infant Nursing Reviews, 7*(3), 155-160.

Ostadi, M., Jokar, F., Armanian, A. M., Namnabati, M., Kazemi, Y., & Poorjavad, M. (2021). The effects of swallowing exercise and non-nutritive sucking exercise on oral feeding readiness in preterm infants: A randomized controlled trial. *International Journal of Pediatric Otorhinolaryngology, 142*, 110602. https://doi.org/10.1016/j.ijporl.2020.110602.

Pados, B. F., Hill, R. R., Yamasaki, J. T., Litt, J. S., & Lee, C. S. (2021). Prevalence of problematic feeding in young children born prematurely: A meta-analysis. *BMC Pediatrics, 21*, 1-15.

Park, J., Pados, B. F., & Thoyre, S. M. (2018). Systematic Review: What Is the Evidence for the Side-Lying Position for Feeding Preterm Infants? *Advances in Neonatal Care: Official Journal of the National Association of Neonatal Nurses, 18*(4), 285–294. https://doi.org/10.1097/ANC.0000000000000529.

Park, J., Thoyre, S., Knafl, G. J., Hodges, E. A., & Nix, W. B. (2014). Efficacy of semielevated side-lying positioning during bottle-feeding of very preterm infants: A pilot study. *The Journal of Perinatal & Neonatal Nursing, 28*(1), 69–79. https://doi.org/10.1097/JPN.0000000000000004.

Pickler, R. H., Wetzel, P. A., Meinzen-Derr, J., Tubbs-Cooley, H. L., & Moore, M. (2015). Patterned feeding experience for preterm infants: Study protocol for a randomized controlled trial. *Trials, 16*, 255. https://doi.org/10.1186/s13063-015-0781-3.

Pineda, R., Dewey, K., Jacobsen, A., & Smith, J. (2019). Non-Nutritive Sucking in the Preterm Infant. *American Journal of Perinatology, 36*(3), 268–276. https://doi.org/10.1055/s-0038-1667289.

Puckett, B., Grover, V. K., Holt, T., & Sankaran, K. (2008). Cue-based feeding for preterm infants: A prospective trial. *American Journal of Perinatology*, 623-628.

Raczyńska, A., & Gulczyńska, E. (2019). The impact of positioning on bottle-feeding in preterm infants (≤ 34 GA). A comparative study of the semi-elevated and the side-lying position-a pilot study. *Developmental Period Medicine, 23*(2), 117–124. https://doi.org/10.34763/devperiodmed.20192302.117124.

Raczyńska, A., Gulczyńska, E., & Talar, T. (2022). Advantages of side-lying position. A comparative study of positioning during bottle-feeding in preterm infants (≤34 weeks GA). *Journal of Mother and Child, 25*(4), 269–276. https://doi.org/10.34763/jmotherandchild.20212504.d-22-00008.

Rodriguez Gonzalez, P., Perez-Cabezas, V., Chamorro-Moriana, G., Ruiz Molinero, C., Vazquez-Casares, A. M., & Gonzalez-Medina, G. (2021). Effectiveness of oral sensory-motor stimulation in premature infants in the neonatal intensive care unit (NICU): Systematic Review. *Children (Basel, Switzerland), 8*(9), 758. https://doi.org/10.3390/children8090758.

Ross, E. S., & Philbin, M. K. (2011). Supporting oral feeding in fragile infants: an evidence-based method for quality bottle-feedings of preterm, ill, and fragile infants. *The Journal of Perinatal & Neonatal Nursing, 25*(4), 349–359. https://doi.org/10.1097/JPN.0b013e318234ac7a.

Samane, S., Yadollah, Z. P., Marzieh, H., Karimollah, H. T., Reza, Z. M., Afsaneh, A., & Als, H. (2022). Cue-based feeding and short-term health outcomes of premature infants in newborn intensive care units: A non-randomized trial. *BMC Pediatrics, 22*(1), 23. https://doi.org/10.1186/s12887-021-03077-1.

Sasmal, S., & Shetty, A. P. (2021). Systematic review protocol examining the effect of prefeeding oromotor stimulation on preterm neonate's feeding outcomes. *Manipal Journal of Nursing and Health Sciences, 7*(1), 3.

Sasmal, S., Shetty, A. P., Saha, B., Knoll, B., & Mukherjee, S. (2023). Effect of prefeeding oromotor stimulation on oral feeding performance of preterm neonates during hospitalization and at corrected one month of age at a tertiary neonatal care unit of India: A randomized controlled trial. *Journal of Neonatology, 37*(2), 149-158.

Shokri, E., Zarifian, T., Soleimani, F., Knoll, B. L., Mosayebi, Z., Noroozi, M., ... & Pascoe, M. (2023). Effect of premature infant oral motor intervention [PIOMI] combined with music therapy on feeding progression of preterm infants: A randomized control trial. *European Journal of Pediatrics, 182*(12), 5681-5692.

Spagnoli, J., Dhanireddy, R., Gannon, E., & Chilakala, S. (2023). Effect of cue-based feeding on time to nipple feed and time to discharge in very low birth weight infants. *Scientific Reports, 13*(1), 9509. https://doi.org/
10.1038/s41598-023-36634-y.

Thomas, T., Goodman, R., Jacob, A., & Grabher, D. (2021). Implementation of Cue-Based Feeding to Improve Preterm Infant Feeding Outcomes and Promote Parents' Involvement. *Journal of Obstetric, Gynecologic, and Neonatal Nursing: JOGNN, 50*(3), 328–339. https://doi.org/10.1016/j.jogn.2021.02.002.

Thoyre, S. M., Holditch-Davis, D., Schwartz, T. A., Melendez Roman, C. R., & Nix, W. (2012). Coregulated approach to feeding preterm infants with lung disease: Effects during feeding. *Nursing Research, 61*(4), 242–251. https://doi.org/10.1097/NNR.0b013e31824b02ad.

Thoyre, S. M., Hubbard, C., Park, J., Pridham, K., & McKechnie, A. (2016). Implementing co-regulated feeding with mothers of preterm infants. *MCN. The American Journal of Maternal Child Nursing, 41*(4), 204.

Thoyre, S., Park, J., Pados, B., & Hubbard, C. (2013). Developing a co-regulated, cue-based feeding practice: The critical role of assessment and reflection. *Journal of Neonatal Nursing: JNN, 19*(4), 139–148. https://doi.org/10.1016/j.jnn.2013.01.002.

Türkyılmaz, C. (2018). Prematüre Bebeklerin Enteral Beslenmesi. İçinden: Yenidoğan Yoğun Bakım Hemşireliği Esaslar ve Uygulamalar [Enteral Feeding of Premature Infants. In: Neonatal Intensive Care Nursing Basics and Practices] (Eds: Özek, E., Bilgen, H. S.). Güneş Tıp Kitabevleri, ss: 159-172.

Vizzari, G., Morniroli, D., D'Auria, A., Travella, P., Bezze, E., Sannino, P., ... & Giannì, M. L. (2023). Feeding difficulties in late preterm infants and their impact on maternal mental health and the mother–infant relationship: A literature review. *Nutrients, 15*(9), 2180.

Whetten, C. H. (2016). Cue-based feeding in the NICU. *Nursing for Women's Health, 20*(5), 507–510. https://doi.org/10.1016/j.nwh.2016.08.006.

Zelkowitz, P., Papageorgiou, A., Bardin, C., & Wang, T. (2009). Persistent maternal anxiety affects the interaction between mothers and their very low birthweight children at 24 months. *Early Human Development, 85*(1), 51–58. https://doi.org/10.1016/j.earlhumdev.2008.06.010.

Chapter 2

Evidence-Based Nursing Practices in Preterm Newborn Baths

Hande Özgörü[1], MSc
and Şerife Tutar[2,*], PhD
[1]Egirdir Vocational School of Health Services, Süleyman Demirel University, Isparta, Türkiye
[2]Department of Nursing, Faculty of Health Sciences, Süleyman Demirel University, Isparta, Türkiye

Abstract

Approximately 15 million preterm births occur annually across the world. Along with the transition from intrauterine life to extrauterine life, in addition to separation from their mothers, these infants are faced with various stressors, such as painful interventions, inability to fall asleep, a noisy environment, exposure to bright lights, and nursing care/treatment in the neonate intensive care unit. These stressors negatively affect the neurodevelopmental processes of these infants in the long term. One of the nursing care interventions commonly applied in neonate intensive care units is infant bathing. Bathing has many benefits for the infants such as providing comfort for the infant, preventing infections, and removing meconium and blood residues away from the baby. When interventions regarding bathing application in preterm neonates are examined, it is seen that different bathing methods such as bathtubs, submerging, sponges, and swaddling. In implementing the bathing application, which is among the routine nursing care, when the appropriate bathing method and timing are not determined, stress and traumas can develop in infants. This elevated level of stress in infants can result in physiological instabilities such as hypothermia, dyspnea, and tachycardia. Physiological instability can bring along complications such as acidosis, pulmonary failure, intracranial hemorrhage, and hypoglycemia. Hence, determining the appropriate bathing frequency and bathing method to be preferred is significant in terms of ensuring neuroprotective and atraumatic care. In this context, neonate intensive care unit nurses have important responsibilities. It is important that these nurses, who are responsible for the primary care of the neonates, make use of evidence-based current approaches in their practices. In this section, it was aimed to evaluate evidence-based bathing methods and the appropriate bathing frequency in preterm neonates.

* Corresponding Author's Email: serifeguven@sdu.edu.tr.

In: Evidence-Based Care Practices in Pediatric Nursing
Editors: Feyza Küçük and Serap Özdemir
ISBN: 979-8-89530-304-7

Keywords: preterm bath, neonatal nursing care, evidence-based care

Introduction

Approximately 15 million preterm births occur every year in the world. With the transition from intrauterine life to extrauterine life, these babies face many stressors such as separation from the mother, as well as painful interventions in the neonatal intensive care environment, inability to fall asleep, noisy environment, exposure to bright light, and nursing care/treatment. These stressors negatively affect the neurodevelopmental processes of babies in the long term. One of the nursing cares commonly applied in neonatal intensive care units is baby bathing (Gözen et al., 2019; Warren et al., 2020). Baby bathing is an important stressor in preterm babies. In preterm babies, bathing practices can cause a deterioration of physiological stabilization due to the immaturity of the neurological system, the thin stratum corneum layer of the skin, and the lack of subcutaneous fat tissue (Sun et al., 2023). For this reason, research to determine the appropriate bathing method for preterm babies is still ongoing.

When interventions regarding bathing in preterm newborns are examined, it is seen that different bathing methods such as traditional bathtub, immersion, sponge, and swaddling are used (Taşdemir & Efe, 2019; Freitas et al., 2014; Loring et al., 2012; Çaka & Gözen, 2018). When the correct bathing method and the appropriate timing are not determined during bathing, which is in routine nursing care, babies can develop stress and trauma.

Hence, determining the appropriate bathing frequency and bathing method to be preferred is significant in terms of ensuring neuroprotective and atraumatic care. In this context, neonate intensive care unit nurses have important responsibilities. It is important that these nurses, who are responsible for the primary care of the neonates, make use of evidence-based current approaches in their practices. In this section, it was aimed to evaluate evidence-based bathing methods and appropriate bathing frequency in preterm neonates (Roychoudhury & Yusuf, 2017).

Clinical Characteristics of Preterm Neonatal Skin

The dermis layer of the skin provides resilience and elasticity to the skin, thanks to its collagen and elastin fibers, while the stratum corneum layer serves as a protective barrier against external factors and plays a significant role in the functions of the skin barrier. The skin barrier serves as a crucial defense mechanism for the human body against trauma, pathogens, and infections. Skin not only acts as a protective barrier but also plays a crucial role in thermoregulation, vitamin synthesis, and immunity regulation, as well as in controlling transepidermal water loss and electrolyte balance (Aredes et al., 2017; Bişgin et al., 2022). However, the skin barrier and its functions in preterm neonates differ significantly from those of term neonates and adults. The skin development and function of preterm neonates are suboptimal. This situation complicates the skin care provided to preterm infants (Lawn et al., 2013; Aredes et al., 2017; Kaur et al., 2021).

When the skin characteristics of preterm neonates are examined; (Lawn et al., 2013; Aredes et al., 2017; Gözen et al., 2019; Aşut & Gözen 2020; Kaur et al., 2021; Bişgin et al., 2022),

- The stratum corneum layer is found to be thin.
- Due to the thinner stratum corneum layer and lower sweat gland activity, the skin's ability to retain moisture is more limited.
- There is a reduced presence of collagen and elastin fibers between the layers. Hence, the risks of injury are higher.
- The skin and its appendages (integumentary system) are immature, and the hypodermis has undergone atrophy.
- The skin is highly sensitive, thin, and fragile.
- The cells are thinner and less densely packed and have superficial blood vessels.
- The permeability of the skin is high, and due to incomplete maturation, its protective function is weak.
- The skin pH of preterm infants becomes acidic later compared to term infants. Because the acid barrier protects against pathogens, preterm infants are more susceptible to infections.
- Applied substances are absorbed more quickly, leading to a higher risk of colonization and associated infections.
- The effects of global warming have begun to be observed in our country, as is the case worldwide.
- In the early years, the development of the skin's structure and functions continues.
- The body surface areas are extensive, and adipose tissues are less abundant.
- The absence or scarcity of brown adipose tissue increases the susceptibility of preterm infants to hypothermia. Brown adipose tissue supports thermoregulation by releasing heat through the oxidation of fatty acids.

Evidence-Based Current Bathing Recommendations for Preterm Neonatal Skin Care

Globally, inconsistencies have been found in many research studies and hospital practices regarding newborn bathing methods. It is known that bathing practices vary between countries and institutions (Lund, 2016). The most common reasons for bathing newborns are cultural rituals, aesthetics, and reducing the risk of infection. These practices may vary in hospitals due to policies and cultural differences. In modern times, some hospitals prefer to bathe newborns with water only as part of daily care, while others may prefer to use mild cleansers. Additionally, bathing methods to be implemented in many different countries are generally left to the preference of nurses (Ar & Gözen, 2018). The Association of Women's Health, Obstetric and Neonatal Nurses (AWHONN) recommends bathing preterm infants 2-3 times per week as a routine. However, it has been expressed that for preterm infants receiving treatment in level 3 neonatal intensive care units, the recommended bathing frequency can be very stressful and painful. There is no established procedure for bathing time in international neonatal intensive care units (AWHONN, 2018).

Preterm infants are often subjected to rapid cold stress during bathing as they are typically shaken and cry vigorously. As a result, the risk of hypoglycemia and hypoxemia increases in preterm infants receiving treatment in level 3 neonatal intensive care units. The stress experienced has a negative impact on the development of preterm infants. During bathing, the baby will have expended all its energy to maintain body temperature, so nurses typically prefer to feed the babies after bathing (Johnson, 2021).

Recommended Bathing Methods for Preterm Infants

There are many studies comparing the effects of bathing methods on vital signs, skin colonization, crying, and stress levels of preterm infants (Ar & Gözen, 2018). When examining bathing practices in preterm infants, it is observed that different bathing methods are used, such as traditional bath, immersion, sponge, swaddling, and underbody water bath (Kuller, 2014; Aşut & Gözen, 2020). It is recommended that the room temperature be 27 C during bathing (Kuller, 2014). It is stated that immediately taking the towel the baby is first dried with after the bath, wrapping the baby in a newly warmed dry towel, and putting a hat on the baby's head will reduce the risk of hypothermia in preterm infants (Gözen et al., 2019; Warren et al., 2020). Additionally, it is recommended that the bathing duration be planned not to exceed 5 minutes (Kuller, 2014; AWHONN, 2018).

Traditional Tub Bathing Method

Newborns bathed in a tub should never be left alone. Because they can drown in the bathwater if left unattended in the tub. Before undressing the newborn for the bath, all necessary items should be ready and available by the tub. The water temperature in the tub should be adjusted to approximately 38 °C. In a tub bath, after removing the baby's clothes, they should be immediately placed in the tub to prevent them from getting cold. In the tub bathing method, except for the baby's head and neck, the entire body should be immersed in warm water (Kuller, 2014; AAP, 2023). The nurse should always support the baby's head with one hand. Occasionally, warm water can be gently poured over their bodies. The soap used during the bath can dry out the newborn's skin. Therefore, if soap is to be used, gentle, neutral pH, and additive-free soaps should be preferred. If a brush is to be used to wash the baby's head, a soft-bristled brush should be used. The towels used during the bath should be soft, and the baby's skin should be gently massaged. If foam gets into the newborn's eye, it should be wiped with a soap-free cloth dampened with warm water. In the tub bathing method, since the newborn's body is immersed in warm water, there is an even distribution of temperature on the skin compared to the sponge bathing method, and heat loss through evaporation is less (AAP, 2023). Taşdemir and Efe (2019) found that in the tub bathing method applied to late preterm infants, there was less heat loss compared to the sponge bathing method (Taşdemir & Efe, 2019).

Immersion Bathing Method

It is noted that traditional bathing methods applied in neonatal intensive care units can lead to increased stress and pain levels in preterm infants. It is mentioned that the increase in stress and pain levels in these infants adversely affects the developmental and physiological parameters. To provide a positive bathing experience for newborns and parents and eliminate these negative outcomes, immersion bathing is recommended instead of traditional bathing practices (AWHONN, 2013; Warren et al., 2020; Johnson, 2021).

The immersion bathing method is commonly used in neonatal services in Brazil. After the immersion bathing method, the sponge bathing method is often applied, especially in the incubator. During the immersion bathing method, the newborn can be submerged in water with the diaper on and wrapped in a towel (Freitas et al., 2014). The immersion bathing method, which is superior in terms of development, supports newborns to be calmer, increases parental satisfaction, and ensures thermoregulation control (Kuller, 2014). Loring et al. (2012) found in their study with late preterm infants after postnatal 24 hours that heat loss was less in the immersion bathing method compared to the traditional sponge bathing method (Loring et al., 2012).

Sponge Bathing Method

In the sponge bathing method, the newborn is not directly submerged in water. Before the bath, all materials (a basin of water, a moist cloth soaked in unscented water, a dry towel, etc.) should be prepared and readily available. Prior to the bath application, the baby should be laid on a comfortable flat surface. If the baby is to be bathed on an elevated surface, necessary safety precautions should be taken to prevent falls (Kuller, 2014). If the surface where the baby is laid is hard, a soft towel or blanket should be placed underneath the baby. The temperature of the bathwater should be checked again before the baby is undressed. The washing begins with the baby's face using the previously prepared moistened cloth. Care should be taken to prevent water from entering the baby's eyes and mouth while washing the face. Then dip it in the basin of water before washing the rest of their body and, finally, the diaper area. In sponge bathings, special attention should be given to areas such as the baby's armpits, behind the ears, and the genital area, ensuring they are thoroughly cleaned (AAP, 2023).

The first bathing of preterm newborns should be completed with gentle movements and in a short time (AAP, 2023). Preterm infants undergoing the sponge bath method may experience heat loss due to crying and agitation along with cold stress, as they wait on the surface with their clothing removed. Additionally, during sponge bath, situations such as desaturation and tachycardia may occur. Therefore, routine sponge bath application is not recommended for preterm infants (Kuller, 2014). However, the sponge bath method is recommended by the American Academy of Pediatrics until the umbilical cord falls off in the early postnatal period. It has been noted that the sponge bath method can be applied inside the incubator as adverse environmental conditions can be prevented within the incubator (AAP, 2023). In a study conducted by Freitas et al. (2014), it was found that the sponge bath method applied to late preterm infants resulted in a greater decrease in body temperature compared to the immersion bath method. In Indonesia, it is noted that the most commonly used bathing method is the sponge bath method due to its simplicity and its ability to reduce the workload of nurses (Tambunan & Mediani, 2019). In Turkey, it is stated that the most commonly used bathing methods are the tub bath, sponge bath, and underflowing water bath methods (Taşdemir & Efe, 2019).

Swaddling Bathing Method

In this method, the baby is immersed in warm water, but unlike the tub bathing method, the baby's body is covered to help reduce fluctuations in body temperature (Johnson, 2021). Swaddling should be done flexibly with a soft, thin blanket or towel. Swaddling the newborn simulates the intrauterine position, increasing the newborn's comfort level and reducing heat loss (Kaur et al., 2021). Because swaddling reduces the newborn's uncontrolled motor movements, it helps them feel safe (Kuller, 2014). For swaddling bath application to be performed in preterm newborns, they need to be at ≥32 weeks of gestation or have a body weight of more than 1500 grams. Additionally, they should be able to maintain thermal and cardiorespiratory stability for more than 10 minutes away from the monitor and mechanical ventilator. The immersion method should not be applied to preterm infants in the presence of peripheral and arterial routes such as umbilical catheters. Considering these criteria , the swaddling bath method can be safely chosen for preterm infants. Furthermore, teaching parents the swaddling bath method will support nursing care, family-centered care, and parental satisfaction. The swaddling bath method is supported by AWHONN as an evidence-based best practice for bathing (AWHONN, 2018). In the conducted studies, it has been indicated that infants subjected to the swaddling bath method maintain their body temperature better and exhibit reduced behavioral stress symptoms compared to infants subjected to traditional bathing methods (Çaka & Gözen, 2018; Edraki et al., 2014; Paran et al., 2016; Swanpa et al., 2017; Sun et al., 2023). Ceylan and Bolışık (2018) stated in their study of preterm infants that the swaddling bath method has a positive effect on physiological parameters, duration of crying, stress, and pain levels compared to the sponge bath method (Ceylan & Bolışık, 2018). In the systematic review conducted by Tambunan and Mediani (2019), it is stated that the swaddling bath method is the best and safest bathing method for preterm infants in a hospital setting, and the infants are more stable in terms of physiological and behavioral symptoms (Tambunan & Mediani, 2019).

Bathing Under Running Water

In Turkey, the traditional bathing method commonly practiced for newborns is bathing under running water (Ar & Gözen, 2018). However, bathing newborns under running water from the tap is generally not recommended. The reason is that maintaining a constant temperature of the water is difficult, which can lead to skin burns in newborns. Therefore, instead of bathing newborns under running water, the bathtub bathing method is safer and easier to control heat loss for newborns (Meredith, 2016).

The First Bath Application in Preterm Newborns

In the literature, while the optimal timing of the first bath for newborns is not clear, there are more recommendations to delay the first bath for preterm newborns. It is stated that bathing shortly after birth is safe for stable term newborns compared to preterm infants, as stable term newborns better maintain their thermoregulation (Lund, 2016). One of the most important reasons for delaying the first bath in preterm infants is that the vernix caseosa, present on their skin, remains for a longer period, contributing to the strengthening of the newborn's skin barrier. At the same time, the goal is to reduce the risk of hypothermia and hypoglycemia (Brogan & Rapkin, 2017).

It is known that bathing practices vary among countries and institutions. In recent years, some institutions have begun to delay the first bath, while others still bathe newborns within 1-2 hours after birth, according to the AAP guidelines (AAP, 2023). In a study conducted in Japan, newborns bathed 2-5 minutes after birth were found to have higher rectal temperatures compared to those who were not bathed, whereas in a study conducted in Uganda, most newborns bathed within 1 hour after birth experienced hypothermia (Brogan & Rapkin, 2017). Additionally, some hospitals may conduct the first bath for newborns early to remove pathogens, primarily transmitted through the bloodstream, from the skin (Kuller, 2014). Some studies have shown that giving baths to newborns shortly after birth to clean meconium, maternal blood, and body secretions can increase the risk of hypothermia, increased oxygen consumption, and various respiratory problems (Brogan & Rapkin, 2017; Lund, 2016; Çaka & Gözen, 2018). Therefore, based on research and recommendations of AWHONN, it is suggested that newborns should be bathed at least 2-4 hours after birth when their body temperature (36.5-36.8°C) and vital signs are stable (Lund, 2016; Çaka & Gözen, 2018; AWHONN, 2018).

The World Health Organization recommends delaying the first bath of the newborn until 24 hours after birthor, if not possible due to cultural reasons, waiting at least 6 hours after birth. The World Health Organization also emphasizes that physiological parameters of newborns should be stable during bathing procedures (AAP, 2023). During the first bath, the physiological parameters of the newborns should be stable for at least 4-6 hours, and bathing should be performed by nurses considering the hygiene status of the baby and the environmental conditions (Ceylan & Bolışık, 2018). In a study conducted by Gupta et al. (2023), they recommended that the first bath for newborns in hospitals should be performed 6-24 hours after birth to provide evidence-based guidance on neonatal skin care practices for healthcare workers from birth to discharge, ensuring thermal stabilization (Gupta et al., 2023). In the study conducted by Gözen et al. (2019), newborns bathed after 48 hours postnatally were found to have higher body temperatures compared to those bathed after 24 hours postnatally. Furthermore, delaying the first bath has been shown to increase newborns' skin moisture, thereby supporting skin development (Gözen et al., 2019).

The Benefits of Delaying the First Bath in Preterm Neonates

Preservation of Vernix Caseosa

Although the timing of bathing in the literature remains unclear, delaying the first bath facilitates the absorption of vernix from the newborn's skin. Vernix caseosa in the newborn provides various benefits, including protection against infections, reduction of skin permeability, prevention of transepidermal water loss, moisturizing the skin, supporting thermoregulation control, maintaining appropriate pH levels, and aiding in wound healing (Visscher & Narendran, 2014; Kuller, 2014). The American Academy of Pediatrics (AAP) recommends allowing vernix caseosa to remain on the skin of newborns for a period of time due to the sensitivity of newborn skin and their susceptibility to skin dryness, which can lead to the formation of wounds. As a result, the moisture of the newborn's skin will be supported, and the skin barrier will be protected by the antibacterial properties of vernix. For this reason, postponing the first bath for newborns will contribute to skin care (AAP, 2023). Leaving vernix on the skin, unless mechanically removed, not only provides skin cleansing, but also contributes to the development of the acidic barrier on the skin. Therefore, the World Health Organization recommends leaving vernix on the skin of preterm infants even if bathing is performed (Kuller, 2014).

Initiating Breastfeeding

Preterm infants expend considerable energy to mitigate heat loss induced by cold stress during and after bathing, potentially leading to respiratory distress. This condition may adversely affect the infant's suckling activity. Therefore, delaying the first bath increases the likelihood of the newborn initiating breastfeeding. In a study, newborns bathed within the first few hours were compared to newborns whose first bath was delayed by 12 hours, and it was determined that delaying the first bath increased the breastfeeding success of newborns (AAP, 2023).

Control of Thermoregulation and Encouragement of Parental Involvement

The timing of the first bath and the selection of the appropriate method help to protect newborns from hypothermia. The cold stress caused by bathing in the first hours after birth increases the likelihood of hypoglycemia in newborns (AAP, 2023). Loring et al. (2012) found that preterm infants bathed in the bathtub method better maintained body temperature compared to infants bathed in the sponge bath method (Loring et al., 2012). Delaying the first bath also allows for interaction between mothers and newborns. Because early bathing can interrupt skin-to-skin contact and the development of the mother-infant bond (AWHONN, 2013; AAP, 2023). In the study by Brogan and Rapkin (2017), it was observed that neonates who underwent delayed immersion baths as much as possible had a lower incidence of hypothermia compared to neonates who underwent sponge baths shortly after birth. Furthermore, parents expressed enjoyment in participating in their infants' immersion baths and feeling prepared to bathe their infants at home (Brogan & Rapkin, 2017). Parents should be informed, especially for preterm infants, that bathing every day is not necessary. Because preterm infants sweat less and have more sensitive skin compared to term infants. The control of thermoregulation is more challenging in preterm infants compared to term infants (AAP, 2023). The frequency and timing of bathing are equally important in newborn care. Because the stratum corneum layer of the skin in preterm newborns is thin, and its thickness is inversely proportional to the skin permeability. Therefore, newborns experience more easily transepidermal water loss. Frequent bathing, especially in newborns, will reduce skin moisture and increase transepidermal water loss due to the weakening of the epidermal barrier (Gözen et al., 2023).

Umbilical Cord Separation

The World Health Organization recommends dry umbilical cord care until the cord stump falls off, emphasizing that it should not be kept wet, and the diaper should be folded below the cord to prevent soiling (Kaur et al., 2021). Therefore, sponge baths are recommended for newborns until the umbilical cord stump falls off. If other bathing methods are preferred instead of sponge baths, it is essential to ensure that the umbilical cord is kept dry (AAP, 2023). Some studies have shown that the first bath of preterm newborns using either sponge or immersion bathing method does not increase the risk of umbilical cord infection (Loring et al., 2012; Meredith, 2016).

In conclusion, the first bath for preterm newborns can be given using either the sponge or immersion bathing method. The crucial aspect is to ensure that the umbilical cord is completely dried after the bath (Meredith, 2016). There is no internationally accepted evidence-based clinical procedure for bathing practices. Therefore, the appropriate bathing method for newborns is often determined based on guidelines from the current literature and can vary depending on the clinical decision of the nurse (AAP, 2023).

The Positive Aspects of Bathing Practices in Preterm Neonates

In recent years, the recommended care practice for newborns has been individualized care. In individualized developmental care, the aim is to reduce environmental stressors that newborns may encounter in the neonatal intensive care unit, initiate early mother-infant bonding, and support the neurobehavioral maturation of the infant. Many studies have investigated the effects of bathing methods on newborn physiological parameters and comfort, including vital signs, skin colonization, stress, and crying (Lund, 2016).

In preterm newborns, bathing practices contribute to various positive outcomes, including ensuring skin cleanliness, increasing muscle tone and well-being, stimulating blood circulation, enhancing comfort through its soothing effect, removing meconium and blood residues from the baby, preventing infection, promoting relaxation, and strengthening the bond between the mother and the baby (Aşut & Gözen, 2020). Post-bath, newborns typically become calmer, facilitating mother-infant interaction, and parents experience less stress (Ar & Gözen, 2018). Involvement in caring for their baby instills a sense of parenting competence and reduces the stress level of the mother, which also supports her milk production. However, for bath procedures to positively affect preterm infants, it is crucial to make appropriate decisions regarding the frequency of bathing and to select the appropriate bathing method. AWHONN recommends individualizing the frequency of bathing based on the newborn's needs. It is stated that bathing newborns more than 2-3 times a week, except for situations such as vomiting or extensive meconium soiling, would be an unnecessary practice. Ensuring control over the frequency of bathing helps minimize excessive stress in preterm newborns (Meredith, 2016; AWHONN, 2018; Johnson, 2021). In the study conducted by Lee et al. (2018), no difference was found in terms of skin condition and axillary skin colonization between preterm newborns bathed every two days and those bathed every four days. Therefore, reducing the frequency of baths in preterm infants will positively affect their growth and development, along with their physiological parameters (Lee et al., 2018). It is stated that using only warm water for bathing during the first week after birth is sufficient for preterm infants with a gestational age of <32 weeks (Kuller, 2014). However, if soap is used, especially for late preterm infants with excessive blood and meconium on their skin, it is recommended to prefer hypoallergenic, gentle, neutral pH, and additive-free soaps (Meredith, 2016).

Potential Complications Arising from Improperly Implemented Bathing Procedures

Preterm infants are at risk of various complications, including hypothermia, if they do not bathe under appropriate environmental conditions and if their body temperatures are not regulated after bathing (Ar & Gözen, 2018). Following hypothermia, symptoms such as increased oxygen consumption, desaturation, decreased peak heart rate, and inadequate nutrition can occur (Freitas et al., 2014; Ar & Gözen, 2018). Washing preterm infants daily can disrupt the pH balance of the skin and lead to skin irritation. Therefore, it is suggested that bathing them every three days on average would be sufficient (Aşut & Gözen 2020; Johnson, 2021).

When the correct bathing method and the appropriate timing are not determined in routine nursing care such as bathing, newborns may experience pain, stress, and trauma. The increased stress in newborns can result in physiological instability such as hypothermia, hypoxia, dyspnea, and tachycardia. Physiological instability can lead to complications such as acidosis, pulmonary insufficiency, intracranial hemorrhage, and hypoglycemia. Because cold stress increases the rate of metabolism in newborns, leading to increased glucose and oxygen consumption. This condition can result in hypoglycemia and hypoxemia (Brogan & Rapkin, 2017; Warren et al., 2020), and it can also prolong the length of stay in the hospital for babies, thereby increasing healthcare costs (Johnson, 2021).

The ineffective implementation of a bath in preterm infants, due to their immature central nervous system, can lead to cold stress, which can adversely affect the neurosensorial development of newborns (Paran et al., 2016). Therefore, determining the appropriate frequency of bathing and the preferred bathing method in preterm infants is essential to provide neuroprotective and non-traumatic care. In this context, neonatal intensive care nurses bear significant responsibilities (Tambunan & Mediani, 2019). It is crucial for nurses responsible for the primary care of preterm infants to use current evidence-based approaches in their practices. Bathing practice also serves as a supportive factor in the development of parenting skills and the bonding between the mother and the infant. It has been observed that parents who do not participate in bathing experience higher levels of stress (Ar & Gözen, 2018).

Points That Nurses Should Pay Attention to when Bathing Preterm Infants

According to the 2019 data from the Centers for Disease Control and Prevention (CDC), it is reported that 1 out of every 10 births in the United States occurs in less than 37 gestational weeks. Many preterm newborns, if not all, need to be admitted to Neonatal Intensive Care Units (NICUs) to receive appropriate treatment that will accelerate their growth and development. Because the prenatal period has been shortened due to various medical reasons, the physiological structures and organs of preterm infants have been interrupted in their maturation. Therefore, many unavoidable procedures, including simple actions such as bathing, applied to preterm infants can be a source of stress (Johnson, 2021).

According to the World Health Organization (WHO), skin care for newborns constitutes an integral part of essential newborn care. Skin care practices in newborns can affect skin integrity, acid mantle, skin microbiome diversity, immunomodulation, and infection prevention (Gupta et al., 2023). Therefore, neonatal nurses are the primary caregivers responsible for skin care in preterm infants. Additionally, nurses have many responsibilities including maintaining skin integrity, preventing the absorption of toxic substances from the skin, ensuring hygiene and comfort, controlling moisture and environmental lighting, performing invasive procedures, administering medication and dressings, providing repositioning, infection control, and health education for parents (Bişgin et al., 2022).

Nursing care aimed at maintaining and preserving skin integrity in preterm neonates begins with practices to preserve body temperature in the delivery room and neonatal intensive care unit (Smith et al., 2013; Aredes et al., 2017). Exposure to numerous invasive procedures and incomplete skin maturation in the neonatal intensive care unit makes the skin of preterm neonates more susceptible to infections, necessitating careful skin care practices (Aşut & Gözen, 2020; Bişgin et al., 2022). Therefore, nursing care practices targeting the skin of preterm infants in the neonatal intensive care unit are of critical importance. These applications are as follows; (Fontenele et al., 2012).

- Preserving thermoregulation
- Protecting babies from unnecessary invasive procedures
- The use of incubators (humidity control)
- Bathroom applications
- The use of topical products applied to the skin
- The controlled removal of skin adhesives.

Preterm infants are at high risk for morbidity and mortality. Effective skin care is an approach that can reduce complications in preterm infants. Additionally, skin injuries and dryness can occur due to the use of skin adhesives or devices. Therefore, ensuring skin moisture in preterm infants is a critical component of neonatal care (Kaur et al., 2021). In the study by Gözen et al. (2023), waiting 10 minutes after bathing before applying moisturizer has been shown to positively affect the skin moisture and body temperature of newborns.

Table 1. Mistakes Made by Nurses when Bathing Preterm Newborns

Mistakes made in bathroom application	**Complications that may develop**
Bathing newborns whose physiological parameters are unstable	Deterioration of the general situation
Bathing a newborn during a continuous night shift	Delaying the development of newborn-parent attachment and decreasing parental satisfaction
Delaying drying after bathing and laying the baby on a cold surface	Delay in thermoregulation and the initiation of breastfeeding
Keeping the newborn in the towel on which she/he dried herself/himself after bathing	Increased risk of hypothermia
Early application of moisturizer after bathing	Shortening the time the skin stays moist
Taking baths more than 2-3 times a week without necessity	Increased stress level, Negatively affects the developmental and physiological parameters of preterm babies Causes skin problems

Conclusion

The timing, method, and frequency of bathing are factors that affect the thermoregulatory control of preterm newborns (Loring et al., 2012; Meredith, 2016). AWHONN recommends that the first bath for newborns should be performed between 2 to 4 hours after vital signs and body temperature have stabilized (AWHONN, 2018). The World Health Organization (WHO) recommends delaying the first bath until 24 hours after birth, or if cultural reasons make waiting a full day not possible, then at least waiting 6 hours (AAP, 2023). Most studies have shown that increasing the frequency of bathing in preterm infants does not alter skin colonization (Meredith, 2016; Lee et al., 2018). AWHONN also recommends individualizing the frequency of bathing based on the needs of the newborn. It is recommended that newborns should not be bathed more than 2-3 times a week unless they experience situations such as vomiting or widespread meconium soiling. Regulating the frequency of baths helps minimize excessive stress in preterm newborns (AWHONN, 2018; Johnson, 2021). While AWHONN recommends a routine bathing frequency of 2-3 times per week for preterm neonates, it has been suggested that this frequency may be too stressful and painful for preterm infants receiving care in a level 3 NICU. There is no internationally accepted standard procedure for bathing time in neonatal intensive care units (NICUs), as AWHONN in 2018.

Nurses are recommended to plan the bathing procedure not to exceed 5 minutes (Kuller, 2014; AWHONN, 2018). The use of the swaddle bath method has been indicated in various current evidence as the safest bathing approach for enhancing neurodevelopmental care in premature infants through an atraumatic care approach (AWHONN, 2018; Tambunan & Mediani, 2019). Instead of traditional bathing practices such as sponge baths, tub baths, or baths under running water, immersion bathing is recommended (AWHONN, 2013; Warren et al., 2020; Johnson, 2021). In developed countries like Brazil and the United States, developmentally superior bathing methods are mostly preferred, while in developing or underdeveloped countries like Indonesia and Turkey, traditional bathing practices are more commonly preferred, as seen in the current literature. Evidence-based recommendations for bathing practices in premature newborns will particularly help improve the quality of skin care administered by nurses. Many of the interventions are cost-effective and can be easily implemented in the neonatal intensive care unit. When bathed properly and using the correct method, bathing preterm infants helps minimize the adverse effects on the baby's physiological and behavioral systems.

Disclaimer

None.

References

American Academy of Pediatrics-AAP (2023). Bathing Your Baby. Date of Access: 02.25.2024, Retrieved from: https://www.healthychildren.org/English/ages-stages/baby/bathing-skin-care/Pages/Bathing-Your-Newborn.aspx.

Ar, I., & Gözen, D. (2018). Effects of underrunning water bathing and immersion tub bathing on vital signs of newborn infants: A comparative analysis. *Advances in Neonatal Care: Official Journal of the National Association of Neonatal Nurses,* 18(6), E3–E12. https://doi.org/10.1097/ANC.0000000000000484.

Aredes, N. D. A., Santos, R. C. D. A., & Fonseca, L. M. M. (2017). Skin care of premature newborns: Integrative review. *Rev Eletr Enf, 19*, a59.

Association of Women's Health, Obstetric, and Neonatal Nurses. (2018). *Neonatal skin care: Evidence-based clinical practice guideline* (4th ed.).

Association of Women's Health, Obstetric and Neonatal Nurses (AWHONN). (2013). *Evidence based clinical practice guideline. Neonatal skin care* (pp. 14-22). Washington: Association of Women's Health, Obstetric and Neonatal Nurses, 2007.

Aşut, G., & Gözen, D. (2020). Annelerin süt çocuğu dönemindeki bebeklerine banyo yaptırma alışkanlıklarının belirlenmesi. *Black Sea Journal of Health Science Open Access Journal*, 3(1), 1-7.

Bişgin, B., Taplak, A. Ş. & Polat, S. (2022). Determination of neonatal unit nurses' practices for newborn skin care: A cross-sectional study. *Journal of Neonatal Nursing,* 28(3), 182-187.

Brogan, J., & Rapkin, G. (2017). Implementing evidence-based neonatal skin care with parent-performed, delayed immersion baths. *Nursing for Women's Health,* 21(6), 442-450.

Ceylan, S. S., & Bolışık B. (2018). Effects of swaddled and sponge bathing methods on signs of stress and pain in premature newborns: Implications for evidence-based practice. *Worldviews on Evidence-Based Nursing,* 15(4), 296-303.

Çaka, S. Y., & Gözen, D. (2018). Effects of swaddled and traditional tub bathing methods on crying and physiological responses of newborns. *Journal for Specialists in Pediatric Nursing: JSPN,* 23(1), 10.1111/jspn.12202. https://doi.org/10.1111/jspn.12202.

Edraki, M., Paran, M., Montaseri, S., Nejad, M. R., & Montaseri, Z. (2014). Comparing the effects of swaddled and conventional bathing methods on body temperature and crying duration in premature infants: a randomized clinical trial. *Journal of Caring Sciences*, *3*(2), 83.

Fontenele, F. C., Pagliuca, L. M. F., & Cardoso, M. V. L. M. L. (2012). Cuidados com a pele do recém-nascido: análise de conceito. *Escola Anna Nery*, *16*, 480-485.

Freitas, P. D., Marques, S. R., Alves, T. B., Takahashi, J., & Kimura, A. F. (2014). Changes in physiological and behavioral parameters of preterm infants undergoing body hygiene: A systematic review. *Revista da Escola de Enfermagem da USP*, *48*, 178-183.

Gözen, D., Akarsu, Ö., Dur, Ş. & Akça, B. (2023). Timing of post-bath skin moisturizer application to newborn infants: A randomized controlled study. *Advances in Skin & Wound Care*, *36*(1), 1-8.

Gözen, D., Çaka, S. Y., Beşirik, S. A., & Perk, Y. (2019). First bathing time of newborn infants after birth: A comparative analysis. *Journal for Specialists in Pediatric Nursing*, *24*(2), e12239.

Gupta, P., Nagesh, K., Garg, P., Thomas, J., Suryawanshi, P., Sethuraman, G., ... & Pandita, A. (2023). Evidence-based consensus recommendations for skin care in healthy, full-term neonates in India. *Pediatric Health, Medicine and Therapeutics*, 249-265.

Johnson, K. (2021). "Implementation of an evidence based quality improvement project to improve bathing practices in the neonatal intensive care unit." Doctor of Nursing Practice Papers. Paper 98. Retrieved from https://ir.library.louisville.edu/dnp/98.

Kaur, S., & Sidhu, N. S. (2021). Evidence based skin care in preterm neonates-a short review. *Int. J. Res. Rev*, *8*(7), 381-385.

Kuller, J. M. (2014). Update on newborn bathing. *Newborn and Infant Nursing Reviews*, *14*(4), 166-170.

Lawn, J. E., Davidge, R., Paul, V. K., Xylander, S. V., de Graft Johnson, J., Costello, A., ... & Molyneux, L. (2013). Born too soon: care for the preterm baby. *Reproductive Health*, *10*(1), 1-19.

Lee, J. C., Lee, Y., & Park, H. R. (2018). Effects of bathing interval on skin condition and axillary bacterial colonization in preterm infants. *Applied Nursing Research*, *40*, 34-38.

Loring, C., Gregory, K., Gargan, B., LeBlanc, V., Lundgren, D., Reilly, J., ... & Zaya, C. (2012). Tub bathing improves thermoregulation of the late preterm infant. *Journal of Obstetric, Gynecologic & Neonatal Nursing*, *41*(2), 171-179.

Lund, C. (2016). Bathing and beyond: current bathing controversies for newborn infants. *Advances in Neonatal Care*, *16*, S13-S20.

Meredith, E. L. (2016). Neonatal Skin Care Evidence Based Practice Project A Manuscript for Publication (Doctoral dissertation, Chapman University).

Paran, M., Edraki, M., Montaseri, S., & Nejad, M. R. (2016). Comparing the effects of swaddle and conventional bathing methods on behavioral responses in preterm neonates. *Iranian Journal of Neonatology*, *7*(4).

Roychoudhury, S., & Yusuf, K. (2017). Thermoregulation: Advances in preterm infants. *NeoReviews*, 18(12), e692-e702.

Smith, J., Alcock, G., & Usher, K. (2013). Temperature measurement in the preterm and term neonate: a review of the literature. *Neonatal Network*, *32*(1), 16-25.

Sun, X., Xu, J., Zhou, R., Liu, B., & Gu, Z. (2023). Effectiveness of different bathing methods on physiological indexes and behavioral status of preterm infants: a systematic review and meta-analysis. *BMC Pediatrics*, *23*(1), 507. https://doi.org/10.1186/s12887-023-04280-y.

Tambunan, D. M., & Mediani, H. S. (2019). Bathing Method for Preterm Infants: A Systematic Review. *KnE Life Sciences*, 1-11.

Taşdemir, H. İ. & Efe, E. (2019). The effect of tub bathing and sponge bathing on neonatal comfort and physiological parameters in late preterm infants: A randomized controlled trial. *International Journal of Nursing Studies*, *99*, 103377.

Visscher, M., & Narendran, V. (2014). Vernix caseosa: Formation and functions. *Newborn and Infant Nursing Reviews*, *14*(4), 142-146.

Warren, S., Midodzi, W. K., Allwood Newhook, L. A., Murphy, P., & Twells, L. (2020). Effects of Delayed Newborn Bathing on Breastfeeding, Hypothermia, and Hypoglycemia. *Journal of Obstetric, Gynecologic, and Neonatal Nursing: JOGNN*, 49(2), 181–189. https://doi.org/10.1016/j.jogn.2019.12.004.

Chapter 3

Evidence-Based Care for Nipple Problems While Breastfeeding

Zeynem Yildirim Balkan[1,*], PhD and Serap Balcı[2], PhD

[1]Department of Nursing, Faculty of Health Sciences, Tekirdag Namık Kemal University, Tekirdag, Türkiye
[2]Department of Child Health and Disease Nursing, Florence Nightingale Faculty of Nursing, Istanbul University Cerrahpaşa, Istanbul, Türkiye

Abstract

Breast milk is the most suitable and nutritious food for babies and contains all the nutrients needed for healthy growth and development. It is recommended that breast milk is given within the first hour after birth and that exclusive breastfeeding is continued for the first 6 months. Breastfeeding is the easiest way to give breast milk to the baby. Breastfeeding is defined as feeding the baby with breast milk directly from the breast. However, breastfeeding can be interrupted by problems caused by the mother or the baby. Common nipple problems that interfere with breastfeeding are painful, fissure/wound, and flat/inverted nipples. While flat/inverted nipples are usually congenital, painful, fissure, or wound nipples can occur later. As a result, the baby may be prevented from receiving breast milk. To ensure babies' uninterrupted access to breast milk, nipple problems must be eliminated through planned and effective breastfeeding management. Mothers should be encouraged to breastfeed, and breastfeeding should be initiated and maintained in a healthy way. Appropriate and individualized nursing approaches should be planned. In this section, evidence-based practices for nipple problems which prevent breast milk intake and cause breastfeeding problems will be discussed in the light of the literature.

Keywords: nipple problems, cracked nipples, painful nipples, flat or inverted nipples, breastfeeding

* Corresponding Author's Email: zyildirim@nku.edu.tr.

In: Evidence-Based Care Practices in Pediatric Nursing
Editors: Feyza Küçük and Serap Özdemir
ISBN: 979-8-89530-304-7

Introduction

Breast milk alone contains all the nutrients required for the healthy growth and development of babies. It also protects the baby against microorganisms (bacteria, viruses, etc.) (WHO 2017). It is the best food that each mother produces specifically for her own baby, and it is easy to access, free, clean, and fresh. Direct access to breast milk is the right of every baby born (Soylu, 2018; Tiryaki & Altınkaynak 2021). The easiest way to give breast milk, which is essential for the baby, to the baby is by breastfeeding. Breastfeeding is the ability of the baby to receive breast milk directly from the breast without any barrier (WHO 2017). However, breastfeeding may sometimes be interrupted due to problems caused by the baby and sometimes by the mother. As a result, the baby may be prevented from receiving breast milk (Şahin et al. 2013; Karaçam and Sağlık 2018; Kavle et al. 2017). In a study, one out of every three mothers reported that they experienced one or more problems related to breastfeeding (Bossert et al., 2001). When the research are examined, the most common breastfeeding problems can be listed as insufficient milk anxiety, fullness/engorgement, obstructed milk duct, mastitis, hyperlactation, flat/ collapsed nipple, redness/cracks/wounds/bleeding on the nipple, etc. (Şahin et al., 2013; Karaçam & Sağlık, 2018; Kavle et al., 2017). Nipple-specific problems that interfere with breastfeeding are often painful, cracked/injured, and flat/inverted nipples. Although flat/inverted nipples are usually congenital, painful, cracked, or injured nipple problems may occur later (Karkee et al., 2014; Borstlap et al., 2016; Dash, 2017). Health professionals have important responsibilities in maintaining breastfeeding (Soylu, 2018; Tiryaki and Altınkaynak 2021). With planned and effective management of breastfeeding, measures can be taken before nipple problems occur. However, the problems that occur can also be eliminated quickly (Balcı et al. 2012; Soylu, 2018; Tiryaki and Altınkaynak 2021). In this review, nipple problems that prevent breast milk intake and breastfeeding will be discussed and nursing practices will be discussed in light of the literature.

Research

Nipple problems that prevent the baby from receiving breast milk and breastfeeding: often painful, cracked/injured, and flat/inverted nipples (Karkee et al. 2014; Borstlap et al. 2016; Dash, 2017). In the following section, care practices for these problems will be examined and discussed based on the literature, and reliable practices that can be used in care will be determined.

Painful Nipples

One of the reasons why mothers stop breastfeeding early after birth is nipple pain (Buck et al. 2014; Puapornpong et al. 2017; Spencer 2020). In a study conducted by Watkins et al. (2011) with 2586 women, it was reported that the rate of depression doubled in women who experienced severe pain on the first day of breastfeeding in the second month after birth (Watkins et al., 2011). In another study, it was reported that 28.1% of 1649 newborn breastfeeding women had nipple pain, and 9.6% of women had persistent pain at the end of the first week (Puapornpong et al., 2017). Although nipple pain is divided into two as transient/sensitive and persistent pain, they should be distinguished from each other (Spencer, 2020). Temporary nipple pain or tenderness is mild in intensity. It usually occurs within a few minutes at the beginning of breastfeeding and decreases as breastfeeding continues. It also usually resolves completely after birth when the baby is about one week old (Kara et al., 2016; Puapornpong et al., 2017; Örs, 2018; Spencer 2020; Boran 2020). Although it improves over time, transient nipple pain/sensitivity should be evaluated. However, nursing care for the solution of this problem can be listed as follows:

- Explaining to mothers that this sensitivity usually disappears after the first few sucklings of feeding and stops after the first week or two of breastfeeding (Spencer, 2020).
- If they find the sensation uncomfortable, they should take prescribed painkillers (Spencer, 2020).

There are many causes of persistent nipple pain. If this pain is ignored, serious complications such as duct obstruction, mastitis, and breast abscess can occur (Puapornpong et al. 2017; Spencer, 2020). Early diagnosis and active management including treatment and care for the cause of nipple pain allows mothers to recover within 2 weeks (Puapornpong et al., 2017). There are many causes of persistent nipple pain. These are generally: Raynaud syndrome, nipple vasoconstriction/vasospasm, infections (fungal, viral and bacterial), diseases, maternal causes, and infant causes (Buck et al., 2014; Berens, 2015; Puapornpong et al., 2017; Spencer, 2020).

Raynaud's syndrome is the sudden contraction of the blood vessels in the nipple, not allowing enough blood to pass through and depriving the cells here of oxygen (Boran, 2020; Onat, 2021). Raynaud's phenomenon is a white-blue-red discoloration of the nipple accompanied by pain in the nipple (Onat, 2021). In a study in which 22 women who were thought to have Raynaud's syndrome were evaluated, it was reported that in 21 cases that started in the first 6 weeks postpartum, 91% were accompanied by sensitivity to cold or discoloration in the hands and feet, and 64% had discoloration in the nipple (Boran, 2020). If there is a color change in the nipple at the time of pain, other possible causes of pain may be excluded (Onat, 2021). Nipple vasoconstriction/vasospasm as well is the sudden contraction of the blood vessels in the nipple, not allowing enough blood to pass through and depriving the cells here of oxygen (Spencer, 2020; Onat, 2021). Vasoconstriction may be caused by raynoud femonene (Onat, 2021). The way to distinguish pain caused by vasoconstriction from other causes is that vasoconstriction is affected by cold, while other causes of pain are not triggered by cold. Nursing care that can be performed in a situation where Raynaoud's phenomenon or vasospasm develops can be listed as follows:

- Mothers should wear warm and thick clothes (Spencer, 2020; Onat, 2021; Berens, 2015; Boran, 2020),
- Taking a hot shower before breastfeeding (Boran, 2020; Onat, 2021),
- Breastfeeding should be done in warm environments and not exposed to cold (Spencer, 2020; Poli and Yao, 2021),

- It is recommended that the mother should avoid nicotine, caffeine, and vasoconstricting drugs (Boran 2020; Spencer, 2020).

One of the causes of pain in the breast is breast/nipple infections (Spencer, 2020; Onat, 2021; Puapornpong et al., 2017; Buck et al., 2014; Berens, 2015; Boran, 2020).

If the cause of infection is fungal, moderate pain is detected. It is felt intensely while the baby settles on the breast and continues during breastfeeding. The pain is seen as burning from the breast to the chest wall and decreases within 1-3 days after the start of treatment (Boran, 2020). It is also possible to have symptoms such as a flaky or shiny appearance on the affected breast, a thrush or fungal rash in the mouth in the baby, and a history of vaginal fungus in the mother (Spencer, 2020; Amir & Committee, 2016; Ovalı, 2018). In a situation where a fungal infection develops in the nipple, the nursing care that can be done can be listed as follows:

- Mother and baby taking prescribed antifungal agents (Spencer, 2020; Amir & Committee, 2016; Ovalı, 2018),
- Maintenance of breastfeeding (Poli and Yao, 2021),
- Especially in order to prevent excessive drug use by breastfeeding mothers and infants, nipple trauma should be prevented by ensuring that the baby holds on to the breast in the correct position while breastfeeding (Douglas, 2021; Betts et al., 2020).
- If the infection is due to a viral cause, the region should be diagnosed by a dermatologist (Berens, 2015). Nursing care for viral infections can be listed as follows:
- Taking the prescribed antiviral agent (Berens, 2020; Poli and Yao, 2021),
- Not breastfeeding directly from the lesioned breast (Berens, 2020; Poli and Yao, 2021),
- Teaching hygiene rules to mothers (Berens, 2015).

It is thought to occur when bacteria, especially Staphyloccocus aureus, enter the breast through a terminal duct in the nipple and can develop in a lactose-rich environment (Poli and Yao, 2021). In a study, it was reported that giving a single daily dose of probiotics (lactobacilli) in the postnatal period reduced the rate of staphylococcal bacteria in the milk of mothers (Bond et al., 2017). If the cause of the infection is bacterial, the nursing care that can be done can be listed as follows:

- Taking prescribed antibiotics (Poli & Yao, 2021; Amir & Committee, 2016; Berens, 2015; Pustotina, 2016; Spencer, 2020),
- Resting the mother (Amir & Committee, 2016; Ovalı, 2018),
- Pain control (Poli & Yao, 2021; Spencer, 2020; Amir & Committee, 2016; Berens, 2015),
- If the mother is unable to breastfeed due to pain, milking the breasts with different methods such as pumps and manual methods (Berens, 2015; Amir & Committee, 2016),
- Milking the breast to relieve the breast after breastfeeding (Amir & Committee, 2016; Berens, 2015),

- Cold compress to reduce pain and edema after breastfeeding (Spencer, 2020; Amir & Committee, 2016; Pustotina, 2016),
- Boiling breastfeeding apparatus such as pump parts to avoid contamination (Yurtsal et al., 2018),
- Taking probiotics (Berens, 2015; Bond, Morris, & Nassar, 2017),
- Antibiotic treatment that does not provide improvement within 48 hours or referral for culture in recurrent attacks (Poli and Yao, 2021; Berens, 2015).

Skin disorders affecting the nipple (such as dermatitis, eczema, or psoriasis) should first be diagnosed by a dermatologist (Spencer, 2020; Onat, 2021; Berens, 2015; Boran, 2020). Nursing care for skin disorders in the nipple can be listed as follows:

- If there is dermatitis in the breast, use of the prescribed topical steroid (Poli and Yao, 2021; Betts et al., 2021; Berens, 2015).
- If there is eczema in the breast, the agent that triggers eczema is identified and its use is removed (Poli and Yao, 2021; Betts et al., 2021; Berens, 2015).

Infant-related causes of nipple pain;

- Torticollis, which makes it difficult for the baby to bend the neck (Spencer, 2020),
- Ankyloglossia (tongue tie) and birth defects in the mouth that make it difficult for the baby to move, grasp, and suck the tongue (Spencer, 2020; Onat, 2021; Puapornpong et al., 2017; Buck et al., 2014; Berens, 2015),
- Weak sucking and nipple compression (Puapornpong et al., 2017; Buck et al., 2014; Berens, 2015),
- It is the uncoordinated sucking of the baby, which cannot move the tongue in the correct rhythm to extract the milk (Spencer, 2020).

Mother-related causes of nipple pain:

- Inappropriate placement of the baby on the breast and incorrect breastfeeding position (Spencer, 2020; Puapornpong et al., 2017; Boran, 2020),
- Engorjman (Spencer, 2020),
- Blocked milk ducts (Spencer, 2020; Onat, 2021),
- Hyperlactation (Spencer, 2020; Puapornpong et al., 2017; Berens, 2015),
- Skin disorders affecting the nipple, such as dermatitis, eczema, or psoriasis (Spencer, 2020; Boran, 2020; Berens, 2015),
- Nipple and breast infections (Spencer, 2020; Onat, 2021; Puapornpong et al., 2017; Buck et al., 2014; Berens, 2015; Boran, 2020),
- Nipple vasoconstriction/vasospasm and raynaus syndrome (Spencer, 2020; Onat, 2021; Puapornpong et al., 2017; Berens, 2015; Buck et al., 2014; Boran, 2020),
- Nipple crack/wound (Spencer, 2020; Onat, 2021; Berens, 2015; Boran, 2020).

The nursing care that can be provided in these situations can be listed as follows:

- A breastfeeding specialist observes and evaluates the baby and mother in terms of breastfeeding behaviors (Spencer, 2020),
- Demonstrating the correct breastfeeding positions and technique to the mother (Spencer, 2020),
- Explaining the importance that the baby should hold the breast, not the nipple (Spencer, 2020),
- Teaching the appropriate separation technique of the baby from the breast (Zeliha Burcu Yurtsal et al., 2018),
- Furthermore, non-pharmacological lanolin creams (Dennis C.L. et al., 2014; Brent et al., 1998), jojoba fruit lotion (Shahrahmani et al., 2016), purslane cream (Niazi et al., 2018), breast milk (Kirlek and Akdolun-Balkaya, 2013), hydrogel dressings and nipple shields (Kirlek and Akdolun-Balkaya, 2013; Dennis et al., 2012). In addition, pharmacological treatments (antiviral, antibacterial, anti-fungal, and cortisol creams) are recommended.

Another cause of nipple pain is nipple crack/injury (Spencer, 2020; Onat, 2021; Berens, 2015; Boran, 2020). This problem will be discussed in detail in the following section.

Cracked/Injured Nipples

Cracked/injured nipples are among the nipple problems that change the way the baby cannot receive breast milk and change the way of feeding (Durmuş & Gürkan, 2020). Cracked/injured nipples can occur for many reasons. Generally, the baby's inability to grasp the breast correctly (grasping only the nipple), poor position, the baby biting the breast, ankyloglossia (tongue tie) that makes it difficult to suck, intraoral asymmetry, and birth defects in the mouth. Incorrect breastfeeding technique of the mother, trying to separate the baby from the breast by "pulling", or using a pressurized pump. Furthermore, a frequent wetting-drying cycle of the nipples due to frequent breastfeeding, humidity, and heat caused by breastfeeding, harsh cleaning of the breast, and the use of irritating products and candida infection can also be added (Türkyilmaz 2016; Thompson et al. 2016; Kara et al. 2016; Örs 2018; Spencer 2020). If the cracked/injured nipple is not treated, it is usually accompanied by pain. Additionally, it may cause bleeding, perception of milk insufficiency, mastitis, and infections (Durmuş and Gürkan, 2020; Kent et al., 2015; Jakson and Dennis, 2017). Cracked/ injured nipples should also be taken care of for the cause (Kara et al., 2016; Örs, 2018). Nursing care that can be done in this case can be listed as follows:

- Since the main reason is that the baby grasps the breast incorrectly, the problem cannot be corrected unless the grasp is corrected. For this reason, the baby's grasp of the breast should be corrected first (Türkyilmaz, 2016),
- Explaining to the mother that this situation will improve and can be prevented (Kara et al., 2016; Örs, 2018),
- Providing education and support for the correct breastfeeding technique in the prenatal and early postnatal period and supporting the mother (Spencer, 2020; Kirlek and Akdolun-Balkaya, 2013),

- Placing the baby correctly on the breast and giving the correct position (Kara et al., 2016; Örs, 2018),
- Changing the ongoing breastfeeding technique/position in the mother (Thompson et al., 2016),
- Ensuring breastfeeding by leaning back, as the baby grasps the areola on its own (World Health Organization, 2011),
- Taking prescribed painkillers before starting breastfeeding (Spencer, 2020),
- Starting breastfeeding from the breast without cracks/injuries (Spencer, 2020),
- If nipple pain prevents breastfeeding, expressing by hand or with a pump and giving the expressed breast milk to the baby (Spencer, 2020),
- Saying "no" every time the baby bites during breastfeeding by inserting the finger into the baby's mouth (Spencer, 2020),
- The baby does not pull away from the breast (Onat 2021; Yurtsal et al., 2018),
- If the baby has a tongue tie, referral for frenotomy (Spencer, 2020),
- Keeping the nipple clean and dry (Spencer, 2020),
- Applying breast milk to the nipple after breastfeeding and moisturizing the tissue (Boran, 2020; Spencer, 2020), Abou-Dakn, et al., 2011),
- Application of hot tea compress and hot moist compress (Abd-Elselam et al., 2011),
- Applying mint juice/gel (Ismail et al., 2019; Masoudin, 2016; Thabet et al., 2013),
- Application of olive oil (Pezeshki et al., 2020; Nageeb et al., 2018; Eshgizade et al., 2016; Cordero et al., 2015; Kirlek and Akdolun-Balkaya, 2013),
- Hydrogel dressing (Shanazi et al., 2015),
- Application of dexpanthenol cream (Shanazi et al., 2015; Masoudin, 2016),
- Application of aloe vera gel (Pezeshki et al., 2020; Eshgizade et al., 2016; Saeidi et al., 2015; Alamolhoda et al., 2014; Tafazoli et al., 2010),
- Nipple care with Vernix caseosa (Merih et al., 2021),
- Not using plastic-based and airtight breast pads (Spencer, 2020),
- Application of purslane cream (Niazi et al., 2018),
- Application of menthol essence (Akbari, Alamolhoda, Baghban, & Mirabi, 2014),
- Application of a silver cap (Marrazzu et al., 2015),
- Application of gum tree ointment (As'adi et al., 2017),
- Application of therapeutic honey Apicar ointment (Essa & Ebrahim, 2013),
- Application of lanolin (Spencer, 2020; Shanazi et al., 2015; Masoudin, 2016; Dennis et al., 2012),
- If candida is present, administering the prescribed antifungal medication to both mother and baby, as well as cleaning the nipple with carbonated water and keeping the nipple dry (Spencer, 2020; Amir & Committee, 2016),
- Not applying ice to the nipple (Spencer, 2020).
- Not applying irritating harsh soaps and cleaners after breastfeeding (Spencer, 2020).

Flat/Inverted Nipples

Another problem related to the nipple that prevents breastfeeding is flat/inverted nipples, which are usually congenital (Karkee et al., 2014; Borstlap et al., 2016; Dash, 2017). The frequency of flat/inverted nipples can be seen between 9% and 34.9% in the literature (Maastrup et al., 2019; Karkee et al., 2014; Kent et al., 2015; Sarper 2015; Sohag and Memon, 2011; Alexander and Campbell 1997). Although it is stated in the literature that the nipple is not required for the baby to suck and that it is sufficient for the baby to fully grasp the areola, it has been reported that the baby has difficulty sucking (Association, 2019; Bulbuli et al., 2018; Bagal et al., 2017; Sahin et al., 2013; Suzuki et al., 2015; Puapornpong et al., 2013; Chakrabarti & Basu, 2011). Nursing care for mothers with flat/inverted nipples can be listed as follows:

- Informing, educating, and supporting mothers by a breastfeeding specialist due to the difficulty of infants' grasping (Ashby et al., 2021; Mangel et al., 2019; Borstlap et al., 2016b¸ Association, 2019),
- During the first few days (when colostrum is being made), the mother's breasts are softer, making it easier for babies to latch on. If the breasts are full, to make it easier for the baby to latch on to the breast, milking with very little hand or softening the area around the nipple with a slight reverse pressure, making it easier for the baby to grasp (Association, 2019),
- Attempting to remove the nipple by hand or pump before breastfeeding (Association, 2019)
- Use of the nipple injector method (Bagal et al., 2017; Arsenault, 1997; Kesaree et al., 1993),
- Application of the simple rubberband method to the nipple (Dash, 2017; Chakrabarti & Basu, 2011),
- The recommendation of high-powered suction by women's husbands (Jain et al., 2013).
- Use of silicone nipple protectors and extractors (Maastrup et al., 2019; Association, 2019; Dash, 2017; Kronborg et al., 2016; Bouchet-Horwitz, 2011; Eglash et al., 2010),
- Use of the breast shield (Chanprapaph et al., 2013),
- Performing Hoffman exercises after birth (Youssef and Fouad, 2021; Bulbuli et al., 2018; Padmavathi, 2015),
- If it is necessary to give breast milk or formula, it should be given with a bottle or syringe (Association, 2019).

Conclusion

In a meta-analysis study in which nearly thirty thousand mothers and babies were evaluated, it was proved that the duration of breastfeeding was prolonged with the support given to the mother, regardless of how (Birtton et al., 2007). In the process of initiating, encouraging, and maintaining breastfeeding, it is one of the important duties of nurses/midwives to educate and support breastfeeding mothers and to provide care for nipple problems. In this chapter, the practices developed by health professionals for painful, cracked/wounded, and flat/ collapsed nipple problems are discussed and summarized. However, more interventional research is needed.

Disclaimer

The authors declare that they have no competing interests.

References

Abd-Elsalam, S., Hamido, S., & Abd el Hameed, H. (2011). Effect of using pharmacological versus alternative therapy on traumatic nipples for lactating mothers. *J Am Sci, 7*(11), 485-96.

Abou-Dakn, M., Fluhr, J. W., Gensch, M., & Woeckel, A. (2010). Positive effect of HPA lanolin versus expressed breastmilk on painful and damaged nipples during lactation. *Skin Pharmacology and Physiology, 24*(1), 27-35.

Akbari, S. A. A., Alamolhoda, S. H., Baghban, A. A., & Mirabi, P. (2014). Effects of menthol essence and breast milk on the improvement of nipple fissures in breastfeeding women. *Journal of Research in Medical Sciences: The Official Journal of Isfahan University of Medical Sciences, 19*(7), 629.

Alamolhoda, S. H., AmirAliAkbari, S., Baghban, A. A., & Esmaili, S. (2014). Effects of Aloe vera gel on breast fissures in breastfeeding women. *Pajoohandeh Journal, 19*(1), 13-17.

Amir, L. H., & Committee, A. o. B. M. P. (2016). ABM clinical protocol #4: Mastitis. *Breastfeeding Medicine, 9*(5), 840-844.

Arsenault, G. (1997). Using a disposable syringe to treat inverted nipples. *Canadian Family Physician, 43*, 1517.

As'adi, N., Kariman, N., Mojab, F., & Pourhoseingholi, M. A. (2017). The effect of Saqez (Pistacia atlantica) ointment on the treatment of nipple fissure and nipple pain in breastfeeding women. *Electron Physician, 9*(8), 4952-4960. https://doi.org/10.19082/4952.

Ashby, N., Coombs, C., Bevan, S., & Savoie-Roskos, M. R. (2021). Breastfeeding: Tools for Success.

Association, A. B. (2019). Inverted and flat nipples.

Bagal, S. U., Salunkhe, A., Salunkhe, H., Kakade, V., & Mohite, R. (2017). A comparative study to assess the problem of inverted nipple and its relationship to successful breastfeeding among antenatal mothers. *International Journal of Health Sciences & Research, 7*(4), 280-288.

Balcı, E., Kondolot, M., Horoz, D., Elmalı, F., Çiçek, B., & Demirtaş, T. (2012). Factors affecting the duration of breastfeeding: A cross-sectional study from Kayseri province in Turkey. *Archives of Turkish Paediatrics, 47*(2), 99-103.

Berens, P. D. (2015). Breast pain: Engorgement, nipple pain, and mastitis. *Clinical Obstetrics and Gynecology, 58*(4), 902-914.

Betts, R. C., Johnson, H. M., Eglash, A., & Mitchell, K. B. (2021). It's not yeast: Retrospective cohort study of lactating women with persistent nipple and breast pain. *Breastfeeding Medicine, 16*(4), 318-324.

Bond, D. M., Morris, J. M., & Nassar, N. (2017). Study protocol: Evaluation of the probiotic Lactobacillus Fermentum CECT5716 for the prevention of mastitis in breastfeeding women: A randomized controlled trial. *BMC Pregnancy and Childbirth, 17*(1), 1-8.

Boran, P. (2020). Emzirme sorunlarına kanıta dayalı yaklaşım [Evidence-based approach to breastfeeding problems]. *Osmangazi Tıp Dergisi*, 35-40.

Borstlap, C., Du Bruyn, W., Leech, R., & Yazbek, M. (2016). Do pregnant women know how to correct inverted nipples? *African Journal for Physical Activity and Health Sciences (AJPHES), 22*(31), 692-700.

Bossert, R., Rayburn, W. F., Stanley, J. R., Coleman, F., & Mirabile, J. C. (2001). Early postpartum discharge at a university hospital. Outcome analysis. *The Journal of Reproductive Medicine, 46*(1), 39-43.

Brent, N., Rudy, S. J., Redd, B., Rudy, T. E., & Roth, L. A. (1998). Sore nipples in breastfeeding women: A clinical trial of wound dressings vs conventional care. *Archives of Pediatrics & Adolescent Medicine, 152*(11), 1077-1082.

Britton, C., McCormick, F. M., Renfrew, M. J., Wade, A., & King, S. E. (2007). Support for breastfeeding mothers. *Cochrane Database of Systematic Reviews* (1).

Buck, M. L., Amir, L. H., Cullinane, M., Donath, S. M., & Team, C. S. (2014). Nipple pain, damage, and vasospasm in the first 8 weeks postpartum. *Breastfeeding Medicine, 9*(2), 56-62.

Bulbuli, A., Fernandes, S., & Shelke, S. (2018). Effect of Hoffman's exercises on flat or inverted nipples in immediate postpartum mothers–A randomized control trial. *Executive Editor, 12*(3), 88.

Chakrabarti, K., & Basu, S. (2011). Management of flat or inverted nipples with simple rubber bands. *Breastfeeding Medicine, 6*(4), 215-219. https://doi.org/10.1089/bfm.2010.0028.

Chanprapaph, P., Luttarapakul, J., Siribariruck, S., & Boonyawanichkul, S. (2013). Outcome of non-protractile nipple correction with breast cups in pregnant women: A randomized controlled trial. *Breastfeeding Medicine, 8*(4), 408-412. https://doi.org/10.1089/bfm.2012.0118..

Cordero, M. J. A., Villar, N. M., Barrilao, R. G., Cortés, M. E. C., & López, A. M. S. (2015). Application of extra virgin olive oil to prevent nipple cracking in lactating women. *Worldviews on Evidence-Based Nursing, 12*(6), 364-369.

Dash, M. (2017). Intervention strategies for successful breastfeeding: Randomized clinical trial. *Academic Journal of Pediatrics & Neonatology*.

Dennis, C.-L., Schottle, N., Hodnett, E., & McQueen, K. (2012). An all-purpose nipple ointment versus lanolin in treating painful damaged nipples in breastfeeding women: A randomized controlled trial. *Breastfeeding Medicine, 7*(6), 473-479.

Douglas, P. (2021). Overdiagnosis and overtreatment of nipple and breast candidiasis: A review of the relationship between diagnoses of mammary candidiasis and Candida albicans in breastfeeding women. *Women's Health, 17*, 17455065211031480.

Durmuş, A., & Gürkan, Ö. C. (2020). Evidence-based complementary and supportive care practices in early postpartum breast problems. *Ordu University Journal of Nursing Studies, 3*(2), 185-192.

Eglash, A., Ziemer, A. L., & McKechnie, A. C. (2010). Health professionals' attitudes and use of nipple shields for breastfeeding women. *Breastfeeding Medicine, 5*(4), 147-151.

Eshgizade, M., Basiri, M. M., Mohammadzadeh, M. H., Mahmoudian, A., & Mesbah, M. (2016). Comparison of the effect of olive oil, aloe vera extract and breast milk on healing of breast fissure in lactating mothers: A randomized clinical trial. *Tehran University Medical Journal, 67*(10).

Essa, R. M., & Ebrahim, E. M. (2013). Effect of breast milk versus therapeutic honey (Apicare) on cracked nipples' healing. *Life Sci J, 10*(1), 2137-2147.

Jackson, K. T., & Dennis, C. L. (2017). Lanolin for the treatment of nipple pain in breastfeeding women: A randomized controlled trial. *Maternal & Child Nutrition, 13*(3), e12357.

Jain, S., Jain, A., Singh, A. K., Goswami, D., Upadhyay, A. N., & Negi, N. (2013). Newer innovations in treatment of retracted nipple. *The Indian Journal of Pediatrics, 80*(6), 483-487.

Kara, M., Caner, İ. & Tekgündüz, K., Ş. (2016). Common problems in neonatal nutrition. *Journal of Clinical Medicine Paediatrics, 8*(2), 14-18.

Karaçam, Z., & Sağlık, M. (2018). Breastfeeding problems and interventions related to problems: A systematic review based on studies conducted in Turkey. *Turkish Pediatrics Archive/Turkish Pediatrics Archives, 53*(3).

Karkee, R., Lee, A. H., Khanal, V., & Binns, C. W. (2014). A community-based prospective cohort study of exclusive breastfeeding in central Nepal. *BMC Public Health, 14*(1), 927.

Kavle, J. A., LaCroix, E., Dau, H., & Engmann, C. (2017). Addressing barriers to exclusive breastfeeding in low- and middle-income countries: A systematic review and programmatic implications. *Public Health Nutrition, 20*(17), 3120-3134. https://doi.org/10.1017/S1368980017002531.

Kent, J. C., Ashton, E., Hardwick, C. M., Rowan, M. K., Chia, E. S., Fairclough, K. A., ... Geddes, D. T. (2015). Nipple pain in breastfeeding mothers: Incidence, causes, and treatments. *International Journal of Environmental Research and Public Health, 12*(10), 12247-12263. https://doi.org/10.3390/ijerph121012247.

Kirlek, F., & Akdolun-Balkaya, N. (2013). The effect of breast milk and olive oil on prevention of nipple pain and cracks in early postpartum period. *Turkish Journal of Research & Development in Nursing, 15*(2).

Kronborg, H., Foverskov, E., Nilsson, I., & Maastrup, R. (2017). Why do mothers use nipple shields and how does this influence duration of exclusive breastfeeding? *Maternal & Child Nutrition, 13*(1), e12251.

Mangel, L., Mimouni, F. B., Mandel, D., Mordechaev, N., & Marom, R. (2019). Breastfeeding difficulties, breastfeeding duration, maternal body mass index, and breast anatomy: Are they related? *Breastfeeding Medicine, 14*(5), 342-346.

Marrazzu, A., Sanna, M. G., Dessole, F., Capobianco, G., Piga, M. D., & Dessole, S. (2015). Evaluation of the effectiveness of a silver-impregnated medical cap for topical treatment of nipple fissure of breastfeeding mothers. *Breastfeeding Medicine, 10*(5), 232-238.

Masoudin, K. (2016). Comparison of the effects of lanolin, peppermint, and dexpanthenol creams on treatment of traumatic nipples in breastfeeding mothers in Sanandaj: A randomized clinical trial. Tabriz University of Medical Sciences, School of Nursing and Midwifery.

Melli, M. S., Rashidi, M.-R., Nokhoodchi, A., Tagavi, S., Farzadi, L., Sadaghat, K., ... Sheshvan, M. K. (2007). A randomized trial of peppermint gel, lanolin ointment, and placebo gel to prevent nipple crack in primiparous breastfeeding women. *Medical Science Monitor, 13*(9), CR406-CR411.

Merih, Y. D., Alioğulları, A., & Potur, D. C. (2021). The effect of vernix caseosa in preventing nipple problems among early postpartum women: A randomized-controlled single-blind clinical trial. *Complementary Therapies in Clinical Practice, 45*, 101475.

Nageeb, H., Fadel, E., & Hassan, N. (2018). Olive oil on nipple trauma among lactating mothers. *Mansoura Nursing Journal, 5*(3), 159-170.

Niazi, A., Yousefzadeh, S., Rakhshandeh, H., & Esmaeili, H. (2018). Comparison of purslane cream and lanolin on nipple pain among breastfeeding women: A randomized clinical trial. *The Iranian Journal of Obstetrics, Gynecology and Infertility, 20*(12), 77-85.

Onat, G. (2021). *Breastfeeding with Awareness Milk Increase and Birth*. Akademisyen Kitabevi.

Organization, W. H. (2011). *World Health Statistics 2011*.

Organization, W. H. (2017). *Guideline: Protecting, Promoting and Supporting Breastfeeding in Facilities Providing Maternity and Newborn Services*. Retrieved from

Ovalı, F. (2018). One day of a breastfeeding mother: Tips for breastfeeding and solutions to problems. *Journal of Clinical Medicine Paediatrics, 10*(4), 1-6.

Örs, R. (2018). Approach to the newborn who cannot gain weight. *Journal of Clinical Medicine Paediatrics, 10*(4), 30-34.

Padmavathi, P. (2015). Effectiveness of Hoffman's exercise on successful breastfeeding among primipara mothers with flat and retracted nipples. *International Journal of Nursing Education and Research, 3*(2), 124-126.

Pezeshki, B., Pouredalati, M., Zolala, S., Moeindarbary, S., Kazemi, K., Rakhsha, M., ... Razmjouei, P. (2020). Comparison of the effect of aloe vera extract, breast milk, calendit-E, curcumin, lanolin, olive oil, and purslane on healing of breast fissure in lactating mothers: A systematic review. *International Journal of Pediatrics, 8*(2), 10853-10863.

Poli, E., & Yao, K. (2021). Review of the diagnosis and management of benign breast issues during pregnancy and lactation. *Annals of Breast Surgery, 5*.

Puapornpong, P., Paritakul, P., Suksamarnwong, M., Srisuwan, S., & Ketsuwan, S. (2017). Nipple pain incidence, the predisposing factors, the recovery period after care management, and the exclusive breastfeeding outcome. *Breastfeeding Medicine, 12*(3), 169-173.

Puapornpong, P., Raungrongmorakot, K., Paritakul, P., Ketsuwan, S., & Wongin, S. (2013). Nipple length and its relation to success in breastfeeding. *J Med Assoc Thai, 96*(Suppl 1), S1-4.

Pustotina, O. (2016). Management of mastitis and breast engorgement in breastfeeding women. *The Journal of Maternal-Fetal & Neonatal Medicine, 29*(19), 3121-3125.

Saeidi, R., Tafazoli, M., Gholami, M., & Mazlom, R. (2015). New treatment for nipple soreness in breastfeeding mothers: A clinical trial study.

Sahin, H., Yilmaz, M., Aykut, M., Balci, E., Sagiroglu, M., & Ozturk, A. (2013). Risk factors for breastfeeding problems in mothers who presented to two public healthcare centers in Kayseri province. *Turk Pediatri Arsiv, 48*, 145-147.

Shahrahmani, N., Amir Ali Akbari, S., Mojab, F., Mirzai, M., & Shahrahmani, H. (2016). The effect of Zizyphus jujuba fruit lotion on improvement of nipple fissure pain in breastfeeding primipara women. *The Iranian Journal of Obstetrics, Gynecology and Infertility, 19*(35), 13-21.

Shanazi, M., Khalili, A. F., Kamalifard, M., Jafarabadi, M. A., Masoudin, K., & Esmaeli, F. (2015). Comparison of the effects of lanolin, peppermint, and dexpanthenol creams on treatment of traumatic nipples in breastfeeding mothers. *Journal of Caring Sciences, 4*(4), 297.

Soylu, H. (2018). Nutrition of the newborn and infants in the first months of life. *Clinical Medicine Family Medicine, 10*(4).

Spencer, J. (2020). Patient education: Common breastfeeding problems (Beyond the basics).

Suzuki, S., Kotake, M., Fujikawa, A., Kasahara, Y., Nishikawa, M., Wada, Y., & Kanai, S. (2015). Outcomes of breastfeeding in Japanese women with flat or inverted nipples. *Journal of Clinical Gynecology and Obstetrics, 4*(2), 235-236.

Tafazoli, M., Saeedi, R., Gholami Robatsangi, M., & Mazloom, R. (2010). Aloe vera gel vs. lanolin ointment in the treatment of nipple sore: A randomized clinical trial. *Tehran University Medical Journal, 67*(10).

Thabet, H. A., Mourad, M. A., Alahadal, A. M., Alsenany, S., & Alsaif, A. (2013). Prevention of nipple cracks with peppermint water versus breast milk in lactating primiparous women. *Life Science J, 10*(4), 2010-2017.

Tiryaki, Ö., & Altinkaynak, S. (2021). The role of the nurse in breastfeeding counselling. *Journal of Continuing Medical Education, 30*(3).

Thompson, R., Kruske, S., Barclay, L., Linden, K., Gao, Y., & Kildea, S. (2016). Potential predictors of nipple trauma from an in-home breastfeeding programme: A cross-sectional study. *Women and Birth, 29*(4), 336-344.

Türkyilmaz, C. (2016). Breastfeeding counselling and problems encountered in breastfeeding. *Journal of Clinical Medicine Paediatrics, 8*(2), 19-33.

Watkins, S., Meltzer-Brody, S., Zolnoun, D., & Stuebe, A. (2011). Early breastfeeding experiences and postpartum depression. *Obstetrics & Gynecology, 118*(2), 214-221.

Youssef Ahmed Abd-Ella, N., & Fouad Mohammed, S. (2021). Effectiveness of Hoffman's exercise on the level of breastfeeding among primiparous women with inverted nipple. *Egyptian Journal of Health Care, 12*(1), 607-624.

Yurtsal, Z. B., Kaya, N., Şahin, S. A., & Eroğlu, V. (2018). *Evidence-based practices in breast milk and breastfeeding.* Elazig: Anadolu Nobel Medical Bookstores.

Chapter 4

Evidence-Based Nursing Practices in Newborn Hyperbilirubinemia

Maksude Yıldırım*, PhD
Department of Child Health and Disease Nursing, Faculty of Health Sciences, Adıyaman University, Adıyaman, Türkiye

Abstract

Hyperbilirubinemia, defined as an elevated level of total serum bilirubin in the blood, is observed in approximately 60% of term infants and around 80% of preterm infants. In neonates, hyperbilirubinemia results from the breakdown of hemoglobin, leading to yellow discoloration of the skin and sclera. While hyperbilirubinemia generally follows a benign and transient course, it can occasionally lead to irreversible brain damage in some newborns. Therefore, interventions aimed at reducing serum bilirubin levels to within the normal range are crucial the elimination of bilirubin from the body requires its binding to albumin for transport to the liver, where it is then converted into direct bilirubin. It is known that albumin concentration is low, and the liver is immature in neonates. Hence, non-pharmacological interventions used to treat hyperbilirubinemia are valuable as they do not impose additional burdens on the liver. Review of the literature indicates that adjunctive non-pharmacological methods such as foot reflexology, massage, tub bathing, sponge bathing, and home-based phototherapy have been reported to be effective in reducing bilirubin levels in neonates. These methods, which have positive effects on bilirubin levels, could be recommended to maintain bilirubin levels within normal limits without burdening the liver. Additionally, limited, or conflicting results from studies exist regarding the effects of applying prebiotics or probiotics to newborns, changing positions during phototherapy, and the duration of umbilical cord clamping on hyperbilirubinemia. More comprehensive studies on these methods are recommended.

Keywords: evidence-based practice, hyperbilirubinemia, nursing

* Corresponding Author's Email: maksudeyildirim@adiyaman.edu.tr.

In: Evidence-Based Care Practices in Pediatric Nursing
Editors: Feyza Küçük and Serap Özdemir
ISBN: 979-8-89530-304-7

Introduction

Hyperbilirubinemia, defined as an elevation in the total serum bilirubin level above normal values, is observed in approximately 60% of term infants and approximately 80% of preterm infants (Kılıçarslan Törüner & Büyükgönenç, 2017). In newborns, the normal range of bilirubin in 100 ml of blood is 0.2-1.4 mg. When bilirubin levels in 100 ml of blood exceed 7 mg, it is termed hyperbilirubinemia (Sarıkaya Karabudak & Ergün, 2018). Any disturbance occurring at any stage of bilirubin metabolism leads to an elevation in blood bilirubin levels, resulting in hyperbilirubinemia (Kültürsay, 2014). Hyperbilirubinemia can arise from an increase in both direct (conjugated) and indirect (unconjugated) bilirubin levels, but in newborns, it primarily develops due to an increase in indirect (unconjugated) bilirubin levels (Karadaş Özdemir, 2023; Kültürsay, 2014; Özkan & Karakoç, 2021). Hyperbilirubinemia occurring in newborns can be either physiological or pathological (B. N. Doğan et al., 2019; Karadaş Özdemir, 2023; Kılıçarslan Törüner & Büyükgönenç, 2017; Kültürsay, 2014; Sarıkaya Karabudak & Ergün, 2018).

Physiological jaundice manifests within the first 24 hours after birth (or within 48 hours for preterm infants), peaks around the 3rd to 4th day, and begins to decline by the 5th to 7th day (B. N. Doğan et al., 2019; Kılıç & Bal Yılmaz, 2021; Kılıçarslan Törüner & Büyükgönenç, 2017). Physiological jaundice in newborns occurs because of inadequate erythrocyte breakdown and the liver's ability to excrete and conjugate bilirubin (B. N. Doğan et al., 2019; Üstün, 2019). In physiological jaundice, bilirubin levels begin to rise at a rate slower than 5 mg/dl per day. The bilirubin level typically peaks around the 2nd to 3rd day, reaching a maximum value of 5-6 mg/dl, and it is expected not to exceed 15-16 mg/dl. After the 5th to 7th days, a decline in bilirubin levels is anticipated (B. N. Doğan et al., 2019; Kılıç & Bal Yılmaz, 2021; Kılıçarslan Törüner & Büyükgönenç, 2017). Physiological jaundice may persist slightly longer in preterm newborns (B. N. Doğan et al., 2019).

Pathological jaundice is a condition that appears within the first 24 hours after birth, lasting more than 7 days in term newborns and 10-14 days in preterm newborns (B. N. Doğan et al., 2019; Kılıç & Bal Yılmaz, 2021; Kılıçarslan Törüner & Büyükgönenç, 2017; Üstün, 2019). In pathological jaundice, the daily rate of increase in serum bilirubin levels exceeds 5 mg/dl. Bilirubin levels can exceed 12 mg/dl in term infants and 15 mg/dl in preterm infants (Kılıçarslan Törüner & Büyükgönenç, 2017). Sometimes this value can reach 20 mg/dl, and very rarely, it can exceed 20 mg/dl (B. N. Doğan et al., 2019). When bilirubin levels exceed 20 mg/dl, it can lead to the development of a condition called kernicterus by crossing the blood-brain barrier (Çavuşoğlu, 2015; B. N. Doğan et al., 2019; Kılıç & Bal Yılmaz, 2021).

Factors contributing to the development of hyperbilirubinemia include infection, hematologic disorders, breastfeeding, inadequate nutrition, glucose-6-phosphate dehydrogenase (G6PD) enzyme deficiency, congenital hypothyroidism, polycythemia, hypothermia, asphyxia, hypoalbuminemia, and genetic predisposition (Karadaş Özdemir, 2023; Kılıçarslan Törüner & Büyükgönenç, 2017; Mei et al., 2022).

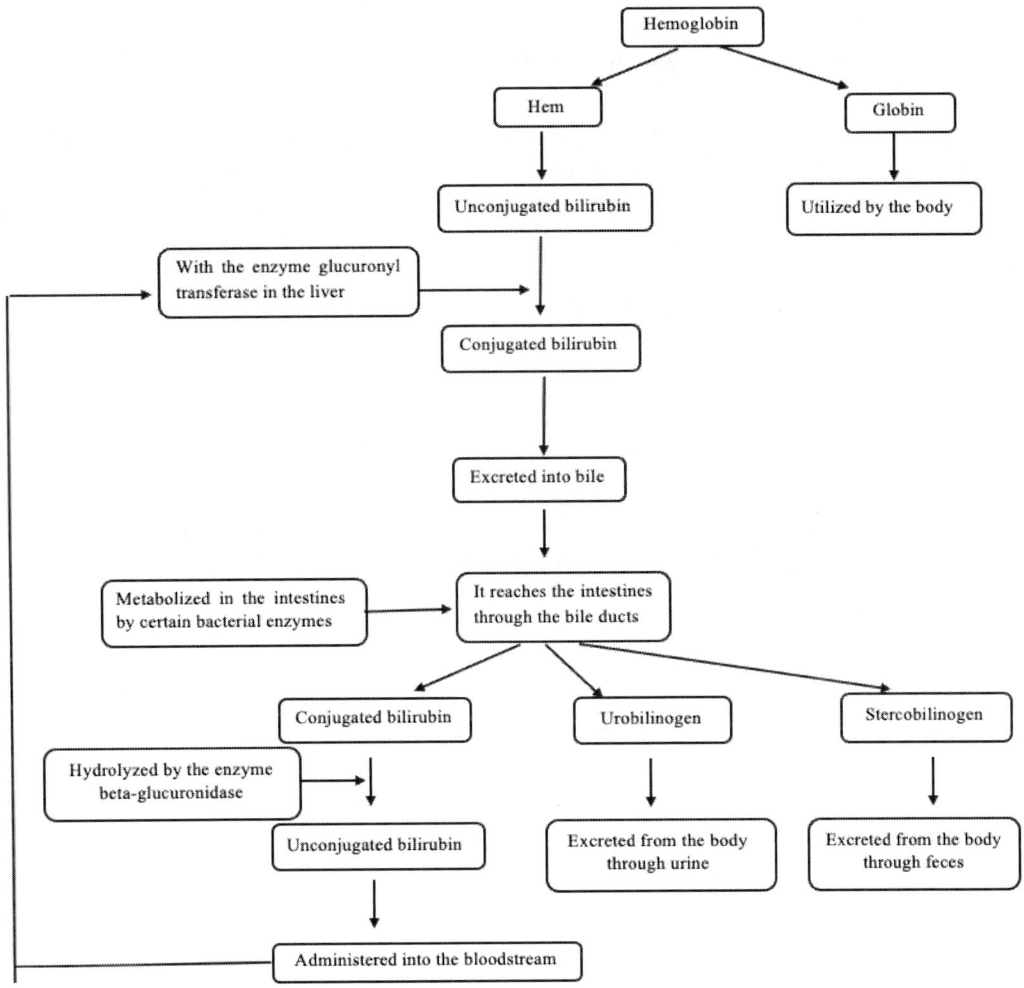

Figure 1. Bilirubin metabolism (Karadaş Özdemir, 2023; Kılıçarslan Törüner & Büyükgönenç, 2017; Lauer & Spector, 2011; Sarıkaya Karabudak & Ergün, 2018).

The Pathophysiology of Hyperbilirubinemia

The process of bilirubin metabolism is as follows: the breakdown of erythrocytes results in the formation of "heme" (Karadaş Özdemir, 2023; Kılıçarslan Törüner & Büyükgönenç, 2017; Sarıkaya Karabudak & Ergün, 2018) and "globin (protein)" (Kılıçarslan Törüner & Büyükgönenç, 2017). The protein "globin" is utilized by the body as needed (Kılıçarslan Törüner & Büyükgönenç, 2017). The breakdown of the "heme" portion of hemoglobin leads to the formation of unconjugated or indirect bilirubin, which is lipid-soluble (Karadaş Özdemir, 2023; Kılıçarslan Törüner & Büyükgönenç, 2017; Lauer & Spector, 2011; Sarıkaya Karabudak & Ergün, 2018). This unconjugated bilirubin then binds to albumin and is transported to the liver (Sarıkaya Karabudak & Ergün, 2018). "In the liver, bilirubin undergoes conjugation with glucuronic acid mediated by the enzyme glucuronyl transferase, resulting in the conversion of bilirubin into a water-soluble form termed direct or conjugated bilirubin (Karadaş Özdemir, 2023; Sarıkaya Karabudak & Ergün, 2018). Subsequently, the conjugated bilirubin, which is then excreted into bile, is discharged into the small intestine through the bile ducts (Karadaş Özdemir, 2023; Kılıçarslan Törüner & Büyükgönenç, 2017). Certain bacterial enzymes in the intestine facilitate the conversion of bilirubin into urobilinogen and stercobilinogen (Karadaş Özdemir, 2023). Urobilinogen is excreted in the urine, while stercobilinogen is eliminated from the body via the fecal route (Kılıçarslan Törüner & Büyükgönenç, 2017). Direct bilirubin, which cannot be excreted from the intestines, is converted back into indirect bilirubin by the enzyme beta-glucuronidase through hydrolysis in the intestinal lumen (Kılıçarslan Törüner & Büyükgönenç, 2017; Lauer & Spector, 2011). The resulting indirect bilirubin is reintroduced into the bloodstream (Lauer & Spector, 2011).

Bilirubin is a compound that arises from the breakdown of erythrocytes (Kılıçarslan Törüner & Büyükgönenç, 2017). Due to the shorter lifespan of fetal erythrocytes in newborns (60-70 days) compared to adult erythrocytes (120 days), there is an increase in production during the neonatal period (Karadaş Özdemir, 2023). For the formed bilirubin to be metabolized and eliminated from the body, it needs to bind to albumin and be transported to the liver, where it undergoes conjugation with glucuronic acid by the enzyme glucuronyl transferase. However, in newborns, due to the low levels of albumin (Kılıçarslan Törüner & Büyükgönenç, 2017; Lauer & Spector, 2011), immaturity of the liver, and inadequate glucuronyl transferase enzyme (Kılıçarslan Törüner & Büyükgönenç, 2017; Sarıkaya Karabudak & Ergün, 2018), bilirubin may not be sufficiently metabolized. Additionally, due to the incomplete development of newborns, the conversion of direct bilirubin to urobilinogen and stercobilinogen in the intestines, and its elimination from the body, may be challenging (Kılıçarslan Törüner & Büyükgönenç, 2017). These factors contribute to the development of hyperbilirubinemia in newborns.

Treatment of Hyperbilirubinemia

The purpose of hyperbilirubinemia treatment is to prevent bilirubin levels from reaching levels that surpass the blood-brain barrier or to reduce elevated bilirubin levels to normal values (Çoban et al., 2018; Kültürsay, 2014; Özdemir, 2020). Hyperbilirubinemia is commonly treated using phototherapy, exchange transfusion, or pharmacological agents such as phenobarbital, metalloporphyrins, and intravenous immunoglobulin (Çoban et al., 2018; Karadaş Özdemir, 2023; Kültürsay, 2014).

Phototherapy

Phototherapy is a method used for the treatment or prophylaxis of hyperbilirubinemia. During phototherapy, the light administered is absorbed by the skin, facilitating the conversion of bilirubin to a water-soluble form (lumirubin) (Karadaş Özdemir, 2023; Kılıçarslan Törüner & Büyükgönenç, 2017; Özkan & Karakoç, 2021; Sarıkaya Karabudak & Ergün, 2018). The water-soluble form of bilirubin can be excreted as bile and urine without conjugation by the liver (Özkan & Karakoç, 2021). The most effective method for the treatment of hyperbilirubinemia after exchange transfusion is phototherapy (B. N. Doğan et al., 2019). For phototherapy to be effective, it is necessary to expose as much of the newborn's body surface area to sufficient light as possible (Karadaş Özdemir, 2023; Sarıkaya Karabudak & Ergün, 2018). The best results are typically achieved with a treatment duration of approximately 24-48 hours (Sarıkaya Karabudak & Ergün, 2018).

It is recommended to initiate phototherapy when the bilirubin level exceeds 15 mg/dl for healthy term newborns within 24-48 hours after birth and exceeds 18 mg/dl for newborns aged 49-72 hours. For preterm newborns, phototherapy is recommended when the bilirubin level exceeds 10 mg/dl (Karadaş Özdemir, 2023; Kılıçarslan Törüner & Büyükgönenç, 2017).

As a result of increased bile secretion and intestinal peristaltic movements due to phototherapy, side effects such as frequent, watery, green-colored stools, light-induced skin rashes, elevated body temperature, fluid and electrolyte imbalance, dehydration, bronzing of the skin, increased metabolic rate, and lactose intolerance can occur (Kılıçarslan Törüner & Büyükgönenç, 2017; Sarıkaya Karabudak & Ergün, 2018).

Evidence-Based Nursing Practices Used in the Treatment of Hyperbilirubinemia

Evidence-based practices emerged with the aim of creating better conditions for patients facing unhealthy circumstances, and providing safe and adequate care. These practices evolved from the efforts of pioneers such as Florence Nightingale in the 1800s, to the medical profession in the 1970s, and towards the nursing profession in the late 1990s.

Evidence is defined as information obtained through scientific evaluations related to clinical practices (Şenyuva, 2016). Evidence-based practice is a problem-solving approach that involves collecting data, critically evaluating the results, and implementing the findings with the aim of improving clinical practice, patient care, and outcomes (Leal-Costa et al., 2024; Mackey & Bassendowski, 2017). The aim of evidence-based practices is to appropriately manage the acquired information, minimize costs in interventions, and enhance the quality of care provided to patients (Ceylan & Mete, 2023; Karataş Baran et al., 2020). Therefore, it is possible to say that the evidence-based practices used by nurses will improve the quality of care, leading to shorter hospital stays for patients and reducing the costs associated with care.

It is known that approximately 60% of term newborns and approximately 80% of preterm newborns can develop hyperbilirubinemia (Kılıçarslan Törüner & Büyükgönenç, 2017). Many of these newborns require hospital treatment. Long hospital stays during the critical newborn period, especially when the bond between the mother and baby is crucial, can hinder the development of a healthy mother-infant bond. Therefore, the use of evidence-based practices that can reduce the length of hospital stays for newborns is crucial. Reviewing the literature, studies examining the effectiveness of evidence-based practices related to hyperbilirubinemia include massage (E. Doğan et al., 2023; Eghbalian et al., 2017; Korkmaz & Işık Esenay, 2020; Suna Dağ & Yayan, 2019), home phototherapy (Chang & Waite, 2020), foot reflexology (Badr & Ibrahim, 2023; Basiri Moghadam et al., 2020; Jazayeri et al., 2021), probiotic use (Goodarzi et al., 2022), umbilical cord clamping time (Qian et al., 2020; Wilander et al., 2023), use of purgative mannans (Fakhri et al., 2019), regular position changes under phototherapy (Fei & Abdullah, 2015; Rashwan et al., 2023), tub baths, and sponge baths (Suna Dağ & Yayan, 2019).

Massage

When examining the literature, it is possible to see studies investigating the effectiveness of various practices supporting the treatment of hyperbilirubinemia. One of these is massage. Massage stimulates pressure receptors in the area, increasing vagal activity. Vagal activity, in turn, leads to increased peristaltic movements (Diego et al., 2005; Field et al., 2011). Therefore, we can state that massage has a positive effect on hyperbilirubinemia by increasing peristaltic movements. In a randomized controlled study examining the effect of massage therapy on total serum bilirubin levels in newborns undergoing phototherapy due to indirect hyperbilirubinemia in Turkey, the experimental group received massage therapy twice a day for 15 minutes each during phototherapy, while the control group received routine care. The total serum bilirubin levels of both groups were measured every 24 hours. After treatment, it was found that the total serum bilirubin level was significantly lower in the experimental group (Korkmaz & Işık Esenay, 2020). In another randomized controlled study conducted in our country with newborns with hyperbilirubinemia, the effect of massage on bilirubin levels was evaluated. In this study, the total bilirubin values of the newborns were measured using a non-invasive bilirubin device before the procedure and 6 hours and 12 hours after the procedure. It was found that there was a significant difference between the massage group and the control group in terms of bilirubin levels and duration of phototherapy (Suna Dağ & Yayan, 2019). In the randomized controlled study conducted by Doğan et al. (2023), phototherapy was applied twice a day to both the experimental and control groups. In the experimental group, newborns received a baby massage for 10 minutes immediately before phototherapy. Bilirubin levels were measured in both groups 2 hours after the end of phototherapy. At the end of the study, it was determined that the bilirubin levels of the newborns in the experimental group showed a significant decrease from the third day onward (E. Doğan et al., 2023). In a randomized controlled study conducted in Iran, the effect of massage on bilirubin levels was also investigated. The newborns in the massage group received a massage once a day for 15 minutes with circular movements applied to the limbs. No intervention was performed in the control group. The newborns' blood bilirubin levels were measured by obtaining intravenous blood samples. After the intervention, it was determined that there was a significant improvement in bilirubin levels in the massage group compared to the control group (Jazayeri et al., 2021). Eghbalian et al. (2017) conducted a randomized controlled study to examine the effect of massage on reducing bilirubin levels in newborns. In both the experimental and control groups, serum total bilirubin levels were measured and compared in the first four days of treatment. Significant differences in bilirubin levels between the two groups were found during the measurements obtained after the intervention (Eghbalian et al., 2017). Rashwan et al. (2023) investigated the effect of regular positional changes combined with gentle body massage during phototherapy on bilirubin levels. In the experimental group, in addition to routine care, gentle body massage was applied twice daily for three days, and positional changes from supine to lateral positions were made every two hours during phototherapy. It was found that the bilirubin levels of newborns in the experimental group were significantly lower compared to the control group (Rashwan et al., 2023). Therefore, it is possible to suggest that massage can be used as a supportive treatment in addition to phototherapy for newborns with hyperbilirubinemia.

Reflexology

Reflexology is a technique applied to reflex zones located in the ears, hands, and feet, corresponding to various endocrine glands, body parts, and organs, with the aim of aiding the normalization of the body (Cevik, 2013; H. D. Doğan, 2014; Stephenson & Dalton, 2003). In reflexology, applying pressure to reflex points stimulates both the peripheral and central nervous systems, facilitating the transmission of information to the brain, which then communicates with organs and endocrine glands, thereby facilitating the transmission of information (Cevik, 2013). Applications involving pressure, such as massage, can indeed stimulate the nerve endings of receptors that transmit information to the organs of the gastrointestinal system (Badr & Ibrahim, 2023). As a result, it is believed that by accelerating the passage of stool through the intestines, such interventions may have a positive effect on hyperbilirubinemia. Moghadam and colleagues (2016) examined the effect of foot reflexology on meconium passage in a randomized controlled study. At the end of the study, it was determined that the meconium passage times of the newborns in the experimental group were significantly faster, and their feeding intolerance was also lower (Basiri Moghadam et al., 2016). In a randomized controlled study, the effect of foot reflexology applied to newborns on bilirubin levels was investigated. At the end of the study, it was determined that the bilirubin levels of the newborns in the reflexology group decreased significantly compared to the control group (Jazayeri et al., 2021). Moghadam and colleagues (2020) investigated the impact of foot reflexology administered to newborns on bilirubin levels in a randomized controlled trial. Foot reflexology was administered in four sessions of 30 minutes each on the first day of life. Measurements of bilirubin levels and phototherapy requirements were conducted before the intervention, on the first-day post-intervention, and on the third and fifth days. Despite increasing bilirubin levels after birth in all three groups, it was found that bilirubin levels were significantly lower on the first and third days in the foot reflexology group compared to the other two groups. Additionally, a significant decrease in the need for phototherapy was observed among newborns in the foot reflexology group (Basiri Moghadam et al., 2020). In a randomized controlled study conducted by Badr and Ibrahim (2023), the effect of foot reflexology on the clinical outcomes of neonates with hyperbilirubinemia undergoing phototherapy was investigated. The neonates in the experimental group received foot reflexology (gastrointestinal zone point) once daily for five days. It was found that the total bilirubin levels of neonates receiving foot reflexology were lower than those in the control group on the fifth day, and the duration of phototherapy was also shorter (Badr & Ibrahim, 2023). In conclusion, it is possible to say that foot reflexology has a therapeutic effect on the bilirubin levels in neonates with hyperbilirubinemia and can be used to support phototherapy.

Probiotic-Prebiotic

Probiotics are beneficial microorganisms that have significant effects in preventing or treating certain pathological conditions (Goodarzi et al., 2022). Prebiotics are indigestible carbohydrates that not only enhance the activity of microorganisms in the gut but also increase the effects of probiotics (Taşdemir, 2017). Probiotics can improve the quality of intestinal contractions and shorten intestinal transit time (Goodarzi et al., 2022). It has been determined that probiotics administered to newborns along with a component that stimulates intestinal peristalsis reduce feeding intolerance, decrease hyperbilirubinemia, and its incidence (Zhang et al., 2017). In a study aimed at determining the effectiveness and safety of probiotic use in the treatment of neonatal hyperbilirubinemia, it was found that newborns receiving probiotics had only higher rates of early discharge from the hospital on the 3rd day of hospitalization, and their lengths of hospital stay were significantly shorter. However, no significant differences were observed on the 2nd, 4th, and 5th days of hospitalization. Therefore, it is stated that probiotics are not effective in shortening the duration of phototherapy in neonates with hyperbilirubinemia (Goodarzi et al., 2022). A systematic review published in the Cochrane examined whether prebiotic supplementation reduces the incidence of hyperbilirubinemia in term and preterm infants. At the conclusion of the study, it was determined that the available evidence from the existing studies did not provide reliable evidence regarding the effectiveness of prebiotics in hyperbilirubinemia (Armanian et al., 2019). The literature review has identified a limited number of studies examining the effect of probiotics and prebiotics on hyperbilirubinemia. It is recommended that comprehensive studies on this topic be conducted.

Position Change

Changing position can increase the body surface area exposed to phototherapy light, leading to a faster decrease in bilirubin levels. In their study, Rashwan et al. (2023) examined the effect of regular position changes combined with gentle body massage on bilirubin levels in newborns with hyperbilirubinemia undergoing phototherapy. In the experimental group, in addition to routine care, newborns received gentle body massage twice daily for 3 days, and position changes from supine to lateral were performed every 2 hours with phototherapy. At the end of the study, it was determined that newborns in the experimental group had significantly greater reductions in bilirubin levels, passed the stools more frequently, and had shorter hospital stays compared to the control group. It is stated that massage combined with position changes in newborns stimulates circulation and lymphatic flow, increasing bilirubin excretion, and reducing reabsorption (Rashwan et al., 2023). A systematic review has demonstrated that keeping newborns with hyperbilirubinemia in the supine position during phototherapy is as effective as periodic turning (Fei & Abdullah, 2015). A systematic review in Cochrane has indicated low-certainty evidence suggesting that there may be little to no difference between periodic position changes and not changing positions in newborns undergoing phototherapy in terms of the duration of phototherapy and the rate of bilirubin decrease within 24 hours after the start of phototherapy (Thukral et al., 2022). The available information in the literature may not be sufficient, indicating the need for further studies in this field.

Umbilical Cord Clamping Time

From the moment the newborn is born until the clamping of the umbilical cord, there is a transfer of blood from the placenta to the newborn. This phenomenon is referred to as "placental transfusion." (Karataş Baran et al., 2020). The duration of cord clamping is associated with the amount of blood transferred to the newborn. It is believed that the amount of blood transferred from the placenta to the newborn may affect the occurrence of hyperbilirubinemia in newborns. In a retrospective study conducted in China, the effect of delayed cord clamping compared to early cord clamping on hyperbilirubinemia was evaluated in term newborns. At the end of the study, it was determined that prolonging the cord clamping time from 90 seconds to 120 seconds led to a trend toward an increased risk of hyperbilirubinemia requiring phototherapy and polycythemia (Qian et al., 2020). Wilander et al. (2023) found no relationship between cord clamping time and bilirubin levels in their study (Wilander et al., 2023).

Other Studies

In a study conducted in our country, the effects of tub baths and sponge baths on the bilirubin levels of newborns were investigated. At the end of the study, both tub baths and sponge baths were found to significantly reduce bilirubin levels compared to the control group (Suna Dağ & Yayan, 2019).

Chang and Waite (2020) determined in their retrospective study that home phototherapy application successfully treated hyperbilirubinemia in the majority of newborns (Chang & Waite, 2020).

A randomized controlled trial conducted in Iran aimed to evaluate the efficacy of a herbal product used as a laxative and to expedite the passage of meconium (a plant-derived product specific to Iran and Asian countries called Purgative Manna) in preventing severe jaundice cases and reducing total bilirubin levels in newborns. Newborns were given 5 drops of the herbal product per kilogram of newborn weight for three days (divided into three doses per day). The treatment duration lasted for three days, and total serum bilirubin levels were measured every 24 hours (three times in total). At the end of the study, it was determined that the total bilirubin levels in the group treated with Purgative Manna were significantly lower compared to the placebo group. The risk of severe jaundice or requiring phototherapy in the Purgative Manna group was calculated to be 75% lower than in the placebo group (Fakhri et al., 2019).

A systematic review published in Cochrane evaluated the effectiveness of sunlight alone or in combination with filters and amplification devices in preventing and treating neonatal hyperbilirubinemia. At the end of the study, it was stated that sunlight could be an effective adjunct to phototherapy in low and middle-income countries, potentially facilitating the rotational use of limited phototherapy devices and providing more opportunities for mother-infant bonding (Horn et al., 2021).

Conclusion

In full-term newborns, approximately 60% experience hyperbilirubinemia, while in preterm newborns, the rate is around 80% (Kılıçarslan Törüner & Büyükgönenç, 2017). This condition is a significant concern. However, due to low albumin levels in newborns (Kılıçarslan Törüner & Büyükgönenç, 2017; Lauer & Spector, 2011), immaturity of the liver, and insufficient glucuronyl transferase enzyme (Kılıçarslan Törüner & Büyükgönenç, 2017; Sarıkaya Karabudak & Ergün, 2018), bilirubin may not be adequately metabolized. Additionally, in the sterile intestines of newborns, the conversion of bilirubin to urobilinogen and stercobilinogen, which facilitates its elimination from the body, may be impeded (Kılıçarslan Törüner & Büyükgönenç, 2017). These factors collectively increase the risk of developing hyperbilirubinemia in newborns.

Newborns with hyperbilirubinemia are often treated using phototherapy, exchange transfusion, or pharmacological agents such as phenobarbital, metalloporphyrins, and intravenous immunoglobulin (Çoban et al., 2018; Karadaş Özdemir, 2023; Kültürsay, 2014). In addition to these, there are studies indicating the beneficial effects of massage (E. Doğan et al., 2023; Eghbalian et al., 2017; Jazayeri et al., 2021; Korkmaz & Işık Esenay, 2020; Rashwan et al., 2023; Suna Dağ & Yayan, 2019) and reflexology (Badr & Ibrahim, 2023; Basiri Moghadam et al., 2016, 2020; Jazayeri et al., 2021) applications on reducing neonatal hyperbilirubinemia. Therefore, it can be stated that massage and reflexology can be used to support phototherapy. Besides massage and reflexology, there are limited studies reporting the beneficial effects of tub baths and sponge baths applied to newborns (Suna Dağ & Yayan, 2019), home phototherapy application (Chang & Waite, 2020), a herbal product used as a laxative and to expedite the passage of meconium called Purgative Manna (specific to Iran and Asian countries) (Fakhri et al., 2019), sunlight application in low and middle-income countries (Horn et al., 2021) on hyperbilirubinemia. When the literature is examined, there are limited studies on the effects of probiotics-prebiotics (Armanian et al., 2019; Goodarzi et al., 2022; Zhang et al., 2017), positional changes during phototherapy (Fei & Abdullah, 2015; Rashwan et al., 2023; Thukral et al., 2022), and umbilical cord clamping time (Qian et al., 2020; Wilander et al., 2023) on hyperbilirubinemia, yielding different results from each other. Therefore, it is recommended that more studies be conducted to investigate the effects of these practices on hyperbilirubinemia.

References

Armanian, A. M., Jahanfar, S., Feizi, A., Salehimehr, N., Molaeinezhad, M., & Sadeghi, E. (2019). Prebiotics for the prevention of hyperbilirubinaemia in neonates. *Cochrane Database of Systematic Reviews, 2019*(8). https://doi.org/10.1002/14651858.CD012731.pub2.

Badr, E. A., & Ibrahim, H. (2023). Effect of foot reflexology on neonates' clinical outcomes with hyperbilirubinemia undergoing phototherapy: A randomized controlled trial. *Journal of Neonatal Nursing, 29*(2), 361–367. https://doi.org/10.1016/j.jnn.2022.07.023.

Basiri Moghadam, M., Esmaeili, M., Khosravan, S., & Mojtabavi, S. J. (2020). Effects of foot reflexology on neonatal jaundice: A randomized sham-controlled trial. *European Journal of Integrative Medicine, 38*(November), 101173. https://doi.org/10.1016/j.eujim.2020.101173.

Basiri Moghadam, M., Khosravan, S., Mojtabavi, S. J., & Esmaeili, M. (2016). Effect of foot reflexology on meconium passage in healthy infants Basiri-Moghadam. *Complementary Medicine Journal, 6*(1522–1534).

Çavuşoğlu, H. (2015). Yüksek Riskli Yenidoğan ve Hemşirelik Bakımı. In H. Çavuşoğlu (Ed.), *Çocuk Sağlığı Hemşireliği* (pp. 57–110).

Cevik, K. (2013). Complementary and alternative therapy in nursing: Reflexology. *Journal of Ege University Nursing Faculty (JEUNF), 29*(2), 71–82.

Ceylan, B. K., & Mete, M. (2023). The concept of evidence-based nursing and evidence-generation situations. *Akşehir Meslek Yüksekokulu Sosyal Bilimler Dergisi, 15*, 121–132.

Chang, P. W., & Waite, W. M. (2020). Evaluation of home phototherapy for neonatal hyperbilirubinemia. *Journal of Pediatrics*, *220*, 80–85. https://doi.org/10.1016/j.jpeds.2020.01.004.

Çoban, A., Kaynak Türkmen, M., & Gürsoy, T. (2018). Turkish neonatal society guideline to the approach, follow-up, and treatment of neonatal jaundice. *Turkish Archives of Pediatrics*, *53*(1), 172–179. https://doi.org/10.5152/TurkPediatriArs.2018.01816.

Diego, M. A., Field, T., & Hernandez-Reif, M. (2005). Vagal activity, gastric motility, and weight gain in massaged preterm neonates. *Journal of Pediatrics*, *147*(1), 50–55. https://doi.org/10.1016/j.jpeds.2005.02.023.

Doğan, B. N., Aydin Ateş, N., & Ayar Kocatürk, A. (2019). The effect of hyperbilirubinemia on newborn and midwifery approach. *Journal of Cumhuriyet University Health Sciences Institute*, *4*(2), 06–11. http://www.cumhuriyet.edu.tr/sbe/index.php?cubid=1&Dil=TR&Id=1057.

Doğan, E., Kaya Dinç, H., & Günaydin, S. (2023). The effect of massage on the bilirubin level in term infants receiving phototherapy. *Explore*, *19*(2), 209–213. https://doi.org/10.1016/j.explore.2022.05.001.

Doğan, H. D. (2014). Healing art of hand: Reflexology. *European Journal of Basic Medical Sciences*, *4*(4), 89–94. https://doi.org/10.15197/sabad.2.4.16.

Eghbalian, F., Rafienezhad, H., & Farmal, J. (2017). The lowering of bilirubin levels in patients with neonatal jaundice using massage therapy: A randomized, double-blind clinical trial. *Infant Behavior and Development*, *49*(July), 31–36. https://doi.org/10.1016/j.infbeh.2017.05.002.

Fakhri, M., Farhadi, R., Mousavinasab, N., Hosseinimehr, S. J., Yousefi, S. S., Davoodi, A., & Azadbakht, M. (2019). Preventive effect of purgative manna on neonatal jaundice: A double blind randomized controlled clinical trial. *Journal of Ethnopharmacology*, *236*(June), 240–249. https://doi.org/10.1016/j.jep.2019.03.009.

Fei, S. L. W., & Abdullah, K. L. (2015). Effect of turning vs. supine position under phototherapy on neonates with hyperbilirubinemia: A systematic review. *Journal of Clinical Nursing*, *24*(5–6), 672–682. https://doi.org/10.1111/jocn.12712.

Field, T., Diego, M., & Hernandez-Reif, M. (2011). Potential underlying mechanisms for greater weight gain in massaged preterm infants. *Infant Behavior and Development*, *34*(3), 383–389. https://doi.org/10.1016/j.infbeh.2010.12.001.

Goodarzi, R., Saadat, S. H., Arshadzadeh, M., Khayam hengami, N., Darban, B., & Haghshenas, H. (2022). Efficacy and safety of probiotics in neonatal hyperbilirubinemia: Randomized controlled trial. *Journal of Neonatal Nursing*, *28*(4), 286–290. https://doi.org/10.1016/j.jnn.2021.10.003.

Horn, D., Ehret, D., Gautham, K. S., & Soll, R. (2021). Sunlight for the prevention and treatment of hyperbilirubinemia in term and late preterm neonates. *Cochrane Database of Systematic Reviews*, *7*, 1–40. https://doi.org/10.1002/14651858.CD013277.pub2.

Jazayeri, Z., Sajadi, M., Dalvand, H., & Zolfaghari, M. (2021). Comparison of the effect of foot reflexology and body massage on physiological indicators and bilirubin levels in neonates under phototherapy. *Complementary Therapies in Medicine*, *59*(September), 102684. https://doi.org/10.1016/j.ctim.2021.102684.

Karadaş Özdemir, F. (2023). Yenidoğan Sarılıkları. In S. Aktaş, Y. Aksoy Derya, & E. Toker (Eds.), *A'dan Z'ye Temel Ebelik* (pp. 285–293). İstanbul Tıp Kitapevi.

Karataş Baran, G., Atasoy, S., & Şahin, S. (2020). Evaluation of awareness and attitudes of nNurses towards evidence-based nursing practices. *Celal Bayar University Journal of Institute of Health Science*, *7*(3), 352–359. https://doi.org/10.34087/cbusbed.699410.

Kılıç, G., & Bal Yılmaz, H. (2021). The effect of massage on bilirubin level in new born infants. *Turkiye Klinikleri Journal of Pediatrics*, *30*(1), 84–87. https://doi.org/10.5336/pediatr.2020-79011.

Kılıçarslan Törüner, E., & Büyükgönenç, L. (2017). Yüksek Riskli Yenidoğan. In E. Kılıçarslan Törüner & L. Büyükgönenç (Eds.), *Çocuk Sağlığı: Temel Hemşirelik Yaklaşımları* (pp. 253–290). Nobel Tıp Kitapevleri.

Korkmaz, G., & Işık Esenay, F. (2020). Effects of massage therapy on indirect hyperbilirubinemia in newborns who receive phototherapy. *JOGNN - Journal of Obstetric, Gynecologic, and Neonatal Nursing*, *49*(1), 91–100. https://doi.org/10.1016/j.jogn.2019.11.004.

Kültürsay, N. (2014). Yenidoğan Sarılığı İnderkt Hiperbilirubinemi İzlem, Tanı, Tedavi. In S. Kansoy (Ed.), *Çocuk Sağlığı ve Hastalıkları* (pp. 49–55). Meta Basım Matbaacılık Hizmetleri.

Lauer, B. J., & Spector, N. D. (2011). Hyperbilirubinemia in the newborn. *Pediatrics in Review*, *32*(8), 341–349. https://doi.org/10.1542/pir.32-8-341.

Leal-Costa, C., Carrasco-Guirao, J. J., Adánez-Martínez, M. G., Ramos-Morcillo, A. J., Ruzafa-Martínez, M., Suárez-Cortés, M., Jiménez-Ruiz, I., Molina-Rodríguez, A., & Díaz-Agea, J. L. (2024). Does clinical simulation learning enhance evidence-based practice? A quasi-experimental study involving nursing students. *Clinical Simulation in Nursing*, *87*, 101494. https://doi.org/10.1016/j.ecns.2023.101494.

Mackey, A., & Bassendowski, S. (2017). The history of evidence-based practice in nursing education and practice. *Journal of Professional Nursing*, *33*(1), 51–55. https://doi.org/10.1016/j.profnurs.2016.05.009.

Mei, H., Dong, X., Wu, B., Wang, H., Lu, Y., Hu, L., Wang, J., Cao, Y., Zhang, R., Cheng, G., Wang, L., Li, Z., Yang, L., & Zhou, W. (2022). Clinical and genetic etiologies of neonatal unconjugated hyperbilirubinemia in the China Neonatal Genomes Project. *Journal of Pediatrics*, *243*(April), 53-60.e9. https://doi.org/10.1016/j.jpeds.2021.12.038.

Özdemir, Ö. M. A. (2020). Diagnosis and therapy of neonatal indirect hyper bilirubinemia. *Pamukkale Medical Journal*, *13*(2), 463–475. https://doi.org/10.31362/patd.663348.

Özkan, H., & Karakoç, H. (2021). Yenidoğan Sarılıkları. In R. Ekti Genç & H. Özkan (Eds.), *Ebeler için Yenidoğan Sağlığı ve Hastalıkları* (pp. 337–351). Anadolu Nobel Tıp Kitapevleri.

Qian, Y., Lu, Q., Shao, H., Ying, X., Huang, W., & Hua, Y. (2020). Timing of umbilical cord clamping and neonatal jaundice in singleton term pregnancy. *Early Human Development*, *142*(109), 104948. https://doi.org/10.1016/j.earlhumdev.2019.104948.

Rashwan, Z. I., Abohadida, R. M., Khonji, L. M., & Saleh, S. E.-S. (2023). Bundling gentle body massage along with regular position change under phototherapy among full-term neonates with hyperbilirubinemia: Is it effective? *Journal of Neonatal Nursing*, *29*(3), 464–470. https://doi.org/10.1016/j.jnn.2022.08.002.

Sarıkaya Karabudak, S., & Ergün, S. (2018). Yenidoğan Hastalıkları ve Hemşirelik Bakımı. In Z. Conk, Z. Başbakkal, H. Bal Yılmaz, & B. Bolışık (Eds.), *Pediatri Hemşireliği* (pp. 340–345). Akademisyen Kitapevi.

Şenyuva, E. (2016). Nursing education and evidence based pPractice. *Florence Nightingale Journal of Nursing*, *24*(1), 59–65. https://doi.org/10.17672/fnhd.88449.

Stephenson, N. L. N., & Dalton, J. A. (2003). Using reflexology for pain management. *Journal of Hoilistic Nursimg*, *21*(2), 179–191. https://doi.org/10.1177/0898010103252380.

Suna Dağ, Y., & Yayan, E. H. (2019). The effect on Bilirubin levels of massage, tub bath, and sponge bath in newborns with hyperbilirubinemia: A randomized controlled trial. *European Journal of Integrative Medicine*, *27*(March), 70–74. https://doi.org/10.1016/j.eujim.2019.03.003.

Taşdemir, A. (2017). Probiotics, prebıotics and synviotics. *Health Academy Kastamonu*, *2*(1), 71–88. https://doi.org/10.25279/sak.300045.

Thukral, A., Deorari, A., & Chawla, D. (2022). Periodic change of body position under phototherapy in term and preterm neonates with hyperbilirubinaemia. *Cochrane Database of Systematic Reviews*, *3*, 1–33. https://doi.org/10.1002/14651858.CD011997.pub2.

Üstün, N. (2019). Neonatal Jaundice. *Klinik Tıp Pediatri Dergisi*, *11*(4), 213–218.

Wilander, M., Sandblom, J., Thies-Lagergren, L., Andersson, O., & Svedenkrans, J. (2023). Bilirubin levels in neonates ≥35 weeks of gGestation receiving delayed cord clamping for an extended time—An observational study. *Journal of Pediatrics*, *257*, 113326. https://doi.org/10.1016/j.jpeds.2023.01.005.

Zhang, A. M., Sun, Z. Q., & Zhang, L. M. (2017). Mosapride combined with probiotics on gastrointestinal function and growth in premature infants. *Experimental and Therapeutic Medicine*, *13*(6), 2675–2680. https://doi.org/10.3892/etm.2017.4340.

Chapter 5

Evidence-Based Nursing Practices in Newborn Skin Care

Serap Özdemir*, PhD

Department of Pediatric Nursing, Gaziantep University Faculty of Health Science, Gaziantep, Türkiye

Abstract

Skin is a complex organ that serves as a protective barrier between the external environment and the organism and has many different functions covering the surface of the body. The skin structure and functions of term and preterm newborns are different from each other. The maturation of the skin structure and functions ensures the maintenance of neonatal fluid electrolytes, temperature, and metabolic balance. Skin care in the newborn is essential for healthy growth and development. All newborns receiving treatment and care in neonatal intensive care units are at risk for skin integrity. Various instruments, invasive interventions, phototherapy, and antiseptic use may disrupt skin integrity. Evaluation of the newborn's skin provides preliminary information about possible adverse events and is also effective in the decision of the care needed. It is necessary to use skin assessment tools developed for evidence-based practices appropriate for the gestational week of the newborn baby and to know and record the basic skin characteristics. Good care should be provided as a result of these evaluations. Skin care should include practices that protect skin integrity and prevent toxicity and sensitization that may arise from chemical exposure. Skin care includes bathing, skin-to-skin contact, cord care, perinea care, use of cleansing products and moisturizers. Evidence-based approaches to these care practices have been increasing in recent years. Knowing what these practices are guides neonatal nurses to protect the skin integrity of newborn babies. In this section, includes evidence-based nursing practices for newborn skin care.

Keywords: evidence-based practices, newborn, nursing, skin care

Introduction

The skin is a complex organ with many different functions covering the body surface and acting as a protective barrier between the external environment and the organism. The skin is

* Corresponding Author's Email: serapozdemir@gantep.edu.tr.

In: Evidence-Based Care Practices in Pediatric Nursing
Editors: Feyza Küçük and Serap Özdemir
ISBN: 979-8-89530-304-7

still functionally immature after birth. The adaptation of term newborn skin from the intrauterine period, which is an environment surrounded by amniotic fluid, to the extrauterine life, which is dry and cold, occurs approximately on the 14th day (Hoeger, 2019). Although it is said that term newborns are born with an anatomically good skin structure, it is known that the skin maturation of the newborn continues for up to one year (Johnson & Hunt 2019). The skin of newborns is structurally and functionally different from that of adults. The ratio of body surface area to body weight of newborns is 2-3 times higher than that of adults. Because of these characteristics, neonatal skin is thinner, more permeable, and more sensitive compared to adult skin. There are also differences in skin characteristics in term and preterm infants (Lund and Kuller 2013). The skin consists of three basic layers: epidermis, dermis, and hypodermis. Furthermore, the pH and vernix caseosa are important structures of newborn skin. The connection between the epidermis and dermis of newborns is weak, and the skin is less elastic and thinner. As birth weight decreases, the epidermis (stratum corneum) becomes thinner. This layer completes its maturation at 32-34 weeks of gestation (Owa et al., 2017; Visscher et al., 2015). The newborn is born with soft skin, covered with lanugo hair and vernix caseosa.

Skin Functions

Functions of newborn skin; maintaining fluid-electrolyte balance, preventing infection, maintaining a certain fluid content and providing humidity, protecting against allergens, reducing the absorption of substances that will harm physical and chemical microorganisms, protecting from the harmful effects of ultraviolet (UV) rays, making vitamin D, which provides absorption of calcium and phosphate, fat storage and immune system supportive functions (Johnson, 2016; Johnson & Hunt, 2019; Murakami et al., 2022; Rahma & Lane 2022). Additionally, massage, like kangaroo care, provides physiological, cognitive, and behavioral development to initiate and maintain a positive relationship with touch. Maintaining an effective skin barrier with ideal pH is very important in maintaining these functions (Kuller, 2016; Lund, 2016; Visscher et al., 2015).

Skin Structure

The term, preterm, and adult skin are structurally and functionally different. In newborn infants, the skin covers 2500 cm^2 of the body, while in adults this area is 18000 cm^2. In preterm infants, the skin constitutes 13% of body weight, whereas in adults it is 3%. The ratio of body surface area to body weight is five times higher in preterm infants and two-three times higher in term infants compared to adults. Considering these characteristics, it is known that neonatal skin is more sensitive, thinner, and more permeable than adult skin (Murakami et al., 2022; Rahma & Lane, 2022). The skin consists of three layers: hypodermis, dermis, and epidermis from the inside out. Furthermore, vernix caseosa and skin pH are components that significantly affect the structure of the skin. The newborn skin structure is shown in Figure 1 (Rahma & Lane, 2022; Visscher et al., 2021).

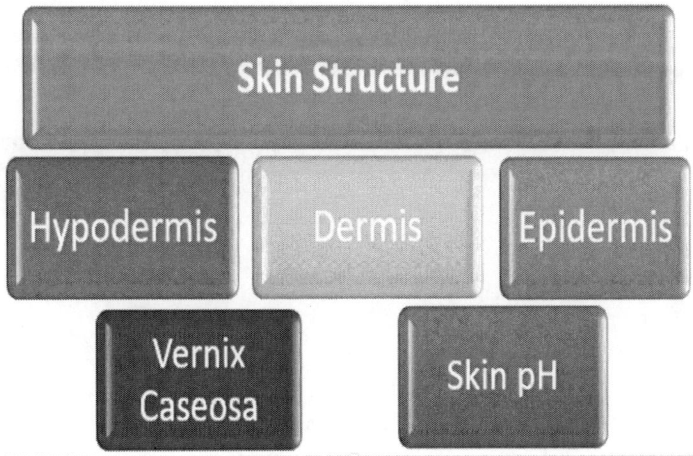

Figure 1. The structure of the newborn skin (Rahma & Lane, 2022; Visscher et al., 2021).

Epidermis

It is the outermost layer of the skin. It consists of flat cells and is 0.1 mm thick. This thickness can vary in different parts of the body. It has very few blood vessels and a thin structure. The epidermis begins to develop at 3 weeks of gestation and shows eight stages of epidermal differentiation between 5 and 26 weeks of gestation. This layer acts as a barrier, reducing fluid loss and preventing the absorption of harmful substances. Exposure to physical or chemical agents contributes to resistance against infections that may occur. Gestational age, epidermis thickness, and lipid content play an important role in protective functions (Menon, 2015; Sezer Efe & Bektaş, 2021). While the stratum corneum layer, which is the top layer of the epidermis that becomes mature in term newborns, is 2-3 layers at 30 weeks of gestation, it is absent in preterm babies born before 24 weeks of gestation. In these babies, the skin should be considered damaged and appropriate evaluation and care should be provided regularly (Johnson & Hunt, 2019; Visscher et al., 2015).

Dermis

It is the lowest part of the basal layer. It consists of two parts, reticular and papillary, and contains collagen and elastin fibers. These fibers provide strength and elasticity. This section contains blood, lymph vessels, sebaceous glands, nerves, and nerve roots, hair follicles extending to the hypodermis, and some of the sweat glands (Aredes et al., 2017; Menon, 2015; Owa et al., 2017). Dermis is involved in increasing endurance, temperature regulation, and sebum production. Sensations of touch, pain, and heat occur in this layer. Additionally, collagen and elastic fibers in the dermis layer prevent edema by preventing fluid accumulation (Aredes et al., 2017; Murakami et al., 2022). The frequent occurrence of edema in preterm infants is related to the scarcity of these structures. Ischemic injury and pressure ulcers occur with the slowing of blood flow with edema (Johnson, 2016; Visscher et al., 2021). In preterm infants, the connective tissue fibers between the dermis and epidermis are short and spaced, and the connection between these layers is very weak. Adhesive products, plasters, endotracheal tubes, electrodes, and umbilical catheters used in intensive care cause a faster deterioration of skin integrity (Kuller, 2016; Johnson, 2016). In Aredes et al., 2017, applications of pectin barrier and hydrophilic gel were used for the damage caused by the removal of adhesives on newborn skin. As a result, it was reported that pectin barrier applications protected skin integrity better.

Hypodermis

It is the innermost part of the skin. It connects the skin and muscle layer under the dermis. Connective tissue is largely rich in fat and contains blood vessels and nerves. It maintains body temperature, acts as a barrier against trauma, and stores energy (Kuller, 2016; Menon, 2015; Johnson, 2016). Insufficiency of the fat layer causes irregularities in temperature and blood glucose preterm infants (Lund & Kuller, 2013; Owa et al., 2017).

Skin pH

The pH value of the skin is alkaline at 6.4-7.5 in newborn babies. The skin structure gradually turns into an acid structure. The skin pH of a term newborn is 4.5-5.5. The acidic structure of the skin prevents the growth of pathogenic microorganisms. The neutral skin pH in preterm infants causes an increase in the number of bacteria and a change in the flora (Liversedge et al., 2018; Menon, 2015; Owa et al., 2017). Applications such as bathing, moisturizing lotion use, etc. can change the pH of newborn skin and damage the acid structure and bacterial flora (Johnson & Hunt 2019; Owa et al., 2017).

Vernix Caseosa

After birth, the skin of the newborn is covered with vernix caseosa, a sticky, thick, and cheesy structure. This structure is composed of sebum, cells from amniotic fluid, and shed lanugo hairs. This structure adapts to the external environment, prevents fluid loss, and acts as a barrier for the stratum corneum. The content of this structure consists of 80% water, 10% lipid and 10% protein, lysozyme, lactoferrin, fatty acids, lanugo, dead cells, sebum, vitamin E, and melanin (Kuller, 2016; Menon, 2015). It starts in the second trimester of pregnancy, begins to decrease in the last trimester, and dries up and disappears within 3-5 days after delivery (Visscher et al., 2021). Vernix caseosa has skin cleansing, moisturizing, maintaining heat balance, and reducing permeability (Murakami et al., 2022; Sezer Efe & Bektaş, 2021). Skin permeability is high because the dermis layer has not reached sufficient maturity. Skin permeability increases as the gestational age of a baby decreases. Skin permeability is also affected by the high ratio of body surface area to body weight (Stamatas et al., 2021). High skin permeability leads to easy absorption of low molecular substances through the skin. In this case, any substance that comes into contact with the skin (except medical treatment) is easily absorbed through the skin and can cause toxic effects (Murakami et al., 2022; Stamatas et al., 2021).

Assessment of Newborn Skin

The function of the skin barrier in newborn babies is completed 2-3 weeks after birth. The most basic element in meeting the care needs of neonatal skin is the evaluation of the skin and interventions aimed primarily at protecting and then caring for the skin of the newborn whose hospitalization is decided (Nist et al., 2016; Visscher et al., 2015). The main aim of skin care is to prevent possible traumas and support healthy skin development by protecting immature barrier functions and integrity (Lund, 2016; Visscher et al., 2015). During skin assessment in newborns, objective skin assessment tools appropriate for the neonatal period and developed based on scientific evidence should be used, and basic skin characteristics should be known and recorded. Furthermore, accurate and appropriate skin assessment provides information about the baby's gestational week, nutritional status, circulatory-respiratory functions, and systemic diseases (Sorte 2019; Visscher et al., 2015). In neonatal intensive care environments, skin integrity can be disrupted by physical and chemical causes. Physically; injury due to heat, abrasion, and friction can be seen during the removal of products such as adhesives that come into contact with the skin. Chemically; diaper dermatitis and various lotions can disrupt skin integrity. Proper skin assessment is important for early recognition, diagnosis, and adoption of the appropriate approach (Sezer Efe & Bektaş, 2021). The Association of Women's Health, Obstetric and Neonatal Nurse (AWHONN) first mentioned evidence-based skin care practices for newborn babies in 2001. Later, this guideline was regularly updated, and the latest 2018 guideline is still used all over the world (AWHONN, 2018). In line with this guideline, there is a wide range of care practices such as first baths for newborn babies, routine baths, diaper care, moisturizer, umbilical care, use of adhesives, and antiseptic use. Nurses have knowledge about care practices in line with this guide and apply them (Lund, 2016). While there are scales to evaluate the skin conditions of newborn babies, it has been reported that there are inadequacies related to standardization to protect the structure and functions of the skin (AWHONN, 2013).

The scales used in neonatal skin assessment are the Neonatal Skin Condition Scale (NSCS), the Neonatal Skin Risk Assessment Scale, the Neonatal / Pediatric Braden Q Scale, the Neonatal Tissue Viability Risk Assessment Tool (NTVRAT), the Northamphton Neonatal Skin Assessment Tool (NNSAT), Infant Skin Disorder Risk Assessment Tool (ISBRAT) (Sezer Efe & Bektaş 2021).

The general principles for newborn skin assessment are as follows:

- *Evaluating the skin every day or from top to bottom*; with this approach, nurses can diagnose skin problems and risks at an early stage and treatment can be started at an early stage (AWHONN, 2013).
- *Objective assessment of the skin with a valid and reliable measurement tool*; the use of these assessment tools will eliminate subjective assessment. Objective measurement tools should be standardized with validity and reliability appropriate for the gestational age of the baby (AWHONN, 2013).

- *Evaluation of risk factors that can cause disruption of skin integrity*; AWHONN has identified fifteen risk factors for this disruption. These include gestational age less than 32 years, edema, paralytic agents, CPAP and nasogastric/orogastric tubes, vasopressors, surgical wounds, electrodes, ostomies, monitors, probes, high-pressure ventilators and Extracorporeal Membrane Oxygenation (ECMO) (AWHONN, 2013).
- *Identification of treatment-related factors that can cause disruption in skin integrity*; These factors identified by AWHONN are heat injuries, removal of adhesives, abrasion or friction, pressure ulcers, infections, and diaper dermatitis (AWHONN, 2013).

Newborn Skin Problems

Skin integrity is the state in which there is no damage to the layers that make up the skin and the structure of the skin is considered normal (Lund, 2016). Although the necessary care and precautions are taken to maintain skin integrity in newborns, it may be impaired. While the skin protects the newborn from the harmful effects of the environment by acting as a protective barrier, impaired skin integrity can cause diseases and infections (Lund & Kuller 2013). The most common causes of neonatal skin problems are insufficient development of the stratum corneum layer, decreased connection between the epidermis and dermis, lack of dermal stability, and skin pH difference (Aredes et al., 2017). Disruption of skin integrity may be associated with congenital skin problems such as mechanical, chemical, thermal, or vascular problems. Appropriate care interventions should be taken immediately to prevent further damage to the skin damaged by any of these causes (Fox, 2011).

Newborn Skin Care

Skin care includes practices to maintain skin integrity and prevent toxicity and sensitization that may arise from chemical exposure. Skin care in the newborn is essential for healthy growth and development. Term and preterm infants differ in terms of skin structure and function. All newborns should be diagnosed, evaluated, and cared for considering these differences (AWHONN, 2018). Since it is known that the skin barrier is sensitive for the newborn, protection-oriented practices are recommended. Therefore, skin care, bathing, cleansing products, and moisturizing products should be selected appropriately, taking into account the skin structure and functions of the baby (Brogan & Rapkin 2017; Burdall et al., 2019). Treatment and care practices for damaged skin should be performed precisely with the necessary assessment and diagnosis (Sorte 2019; Visscher et al., 2015). Knowledge and implementation of evidence-based practices for neonatal skin care; skin-to-skin contact, bathing, use of cleansing products and moisturizers, cord care, and perineal care are very important for neonatal skin health. The newborn skin care practices are shown in Figure 2. (Burdall et al., 2019; Chalmers et al., 2020; Dessalegn et al., 2022; Lund et al., 2019).

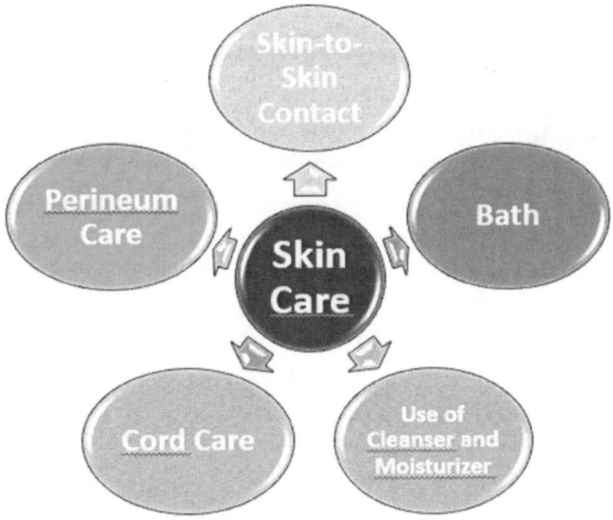

Figure 2. The newborn skin care practices (Burdall et al., 2019; Chalmers et al., 2020; Dessalegn et al., 2022; Lund et al., 2019).

Skin-to-Skin Contact

Skin-to-skin contact between mother and newborn in the first hour after birth without any complications is recommended by skin-to-skin care guidelines for neonatal care. This practice is also called kangaroo care. Skin-to-skin contact prevents hypothermia, stimulates breastfeeding, initiates mother-infant bonding, increases maternal satisfaction, and reduces neonatal stress. Furthermore, it ensures the colonization of newborn skin with beneficial maternal bacteria and supports the maturation/functioning of the immune system (Prescott et al., 2017).

Bath

Bathing is a nursing practice performed to prevent infections in newborn babies, to protect skin integrity, to maintain healthy development of the stratum corneum barrier and skin, and to maintain skin hydration and functions (AWHONN 2018; Burdall et al., 2019). This practice is cost-effective, protects the skin, increases family satisfaction, and provides comfort to the newborn (Brogan and Rapkin 2017; Taşdemir and Efe 2019).

Around the world, consensus decisions are needed on issues such as the frequency and duration of infant bathing, product use, and the temperature of the bath water and the environment (AWHONN, 2013). Bathing should be delayed until 24 hours after birth. If this is not possible for cultural reasons, bathing should be delayed for at least 6 hours. If the mother has a history of infectious disease, it should be done immediately. It is recommended that the baby is dressed according to the ambient temperature after bathing. This means one to two layers of clothing and hats compared to adults. It is recommended that the frequency of bathing in newborns should be 2-3 times a week routinely one week after birth and the duration of bathing should not be longer than 5-10 minutes. It is reported that the temperature of the bath water should be 38°C and the temperature of the room where bathing is performed should be 26-27°C (Kuller 2016). Additionally, the use of soap or shampoo-like products is not recommended for newborn bathing (AWHONN, 2018), and it is reported that the use of soap is particularly objectionable (AWHONN, 2013). The UK National Institute for Health and Clinical Excellence (NICE), in collaboration with the primary care center, opposes the addition of lotions or cleansers to bath water. Moist liquid cleansers are protective and help the acidity of the stratum corneum (pH 5.5-7.0) as they are formulated to be slightly acidic (NICE 2014).

Use of Cleansers and Moisturizers

One of the important approaches to establish neonatal skin integrity is to provide cleaning and moisturizing (Noor et al., 2016). It is being investigated how and with which product(s) the bathing and skin cleansing of newborn babies should be done. AWHONN (2018) does not recommend the use of cleansing products for newborn bathing. The effects of using only water or water and cleansing products during newborn bathing on skin barrier function are unknown. However, some studies have reported that the use of cleansing products with water or water with cleansing products had no effect on the skin pH of infants who received their first bath or more baths (Dizon et al., 2010; Garcia Bartels et al., 2010; Lavender et al., 2013; Lund et al., 2019). Lund et al. (2019) examined the pH, and TEWL stratum corneum hydration in the first bath of 100 term infants using only water or water and a cleansing product. As a result, it was determined that these parameters did not affect the skin barrier when water or a water cleansing product was used.

Due to the thin and sensitive skin structure of newborn babies, they are more prone to drying and cracking. These changes in the skin structure of infants can lead to disruption of skin integrity, changes in the skin barrier, and infections (Cleminson & Mcguire, 2021; Fernandes et al., 2011). Considering all these reasons, appropriate products should be used for infant skin care. The body surface area of newborn babies is larger than that of adults. The difference in the metabolic rate of newborn babies and the immaturity of their organ systems increases their sensitivity to chemical products. For this reason, the use of natural or synthetic products is very important for newborn skin whose skin development has not yet matured (Visscher et al., 2021). The use of products with inappropriate ingredients and properties can cause undesirable effects on neonatal skin integrity, moisture balance, pH, and imperceptible fluid losses (Noor et al., 2016; Summers et al., 2019).

Moisture is the definition of the amount of fluid in the skin at the cellular level. One of the most basic indicators of healthy skin is moisture. Water is needed for skin hydration. Water helps the skin to maintain its protective function, making it look supple and firm, and helps the rapid healing process when damage occurs.

When the skin of newborns begins to lose moisture after birth, changes occur in the skin. Within 90 days after birth, the function of the eccrine glands matures and the increase in moisture accelerates. This increase is evident in all parts of the newborn body and continues until one year of age, then reaches adult levels (Visscher et al., 2015). The use of moisturizing products in infants strengthens skin barrier functions by providing exogenous lipids that support epidermal lipid metabolism by trapping skin moisture (Nolan & Marmur 2012). By moisturizing the skin, the moisturizing product protects the integrity of the stratum corneum and the skin barrier, and at the same time treats dry skin (Johnson, 2016; Çağlar et al., 2020). The most important point in the use of these products is that whether the product content is natural or synthetic, it is necessary to choose components that will not cause allergic reactions that may occur. White petroleum jelly is an ideal and inexpensive product preferred for newborn babies with emollient properties that do not contain contact allergens (Johnson & Hunt 2019). Other ingredients such as white beeswax, sunflower oil, and phenoxyethanol are also used. These products are cosmetic agents that can penetrate the structure and function of the skin and produce visible changes (Noor et al., 2016). These agents are composed of multiple ingredients, including oil emulsions that can soften the skin, increase its elasticity, restore its homeostasis, prevent loss of transepidermal fluid and are applied topically (Noor et al., 2016). It has been reported that the effectiveness of the moisturizing product increases when applied to moist skin immediately after bathing (Fernandes et al., 2011). The characteristics of moisturizers to be applied to newborn babies are; perfume-free, dye and additive-free (Fernandes et al., 2011; Lavender et al., 2013). Considering cultural differences, it is known that each society uses different products. In the literature, it is reported that the most commonly used moisturizing products are mineral oils (almond, sunflower, soy, sesame, coconut, etc.), glycerin, and petrolatum (Cleminson & Mcguire 2021; Karagounis et al., 2019; Konar et al., 2020). It is important for families to have information about the ingredients used in the product, to reduce the use of some products with allergenic ingredients, and to reduce the side effects of the exposed product (Rengin et al., 2020). The use of moisturizers containing ceramide, cholesterol, palmitate, linoleate, or sunflower oil is recommended to eliminate neonatal skin dryness (Fernandes et al., 2011).

According to the results of a systematic review, the effects of using moisturizers on invasive infection in preterm infants are reported to be low. Since these products are cheap and easily accessible, their use in low- or middle-income countries and the conduct of randomized controlled trials were considered justified (Cleminson & Mcguire 2021). Karakoç & Ekici (2022) compared the effect of sunflower seed oil and liquid petroleum jelly on the protection of skin integrity in newborns. As a result, it was reported that these oils provide moisturization to the skin of the term baby and can be used safely in skin care. Çağlar et al. (2020) examined the effect of sunflower seed oil, almond oil, and a control group on skin condition scores and skin moisturization in the care of 90 preterm infants. As a result, it was determined that infants with oil application in terms of skin scores and moisturization were higher than the control group, but there was no difference between sunflower oil and almond oil. It was suggested that the use of these products in the skin moisturization of preterm infants is harmless and can be used safely. Summers et al. (2019) compared the effects of sunflower seed oil and mustard oil, which are natural vegetable oils, on the skin integrity of term and preterm infants. Consequently, it is reported that oils contribute to skin integrity when massaged regularly; additionally, sunflower seed oil protects the skin by giving faster results.

Cord Care

Cord care should be performed to ensure that the umbilical cord of the newborn baby dries quickly and to prevent infection. This care also protects the integrity of the skin in the abdominal region of the baby (Dessalegn et al., 2022; Kalufya et al., 2022; WHO, 2020). Cord care of newborns born in high mortality environments is recommended to apply chlorhexidine daily in the first week after birth. For newborns born in settings with low mortality rates, the basic approach is sufficient for newborns born in healthcare institutions and at home (WHO, 2020). The most basic approach to umbilical cord fall is to keep it dry and clean. The umbilical cord is expected to dry and fall off within 7-10 days in term babies and 2-3 weeks in preterm babies. Redness, swelling, and discharge are abnormal (Dessalegn et al., 2022). During cord care, antiseptic solutions should only be applied to the cord, and skin contact should be prevented because they are absorbed through the skin and may have systemic effects. When changing the diaper of the newborn, care should be taken to keep the cord outside to prevent contact with urine and stool (Sezer Efe et al., 2021).

When adequate hygiene cannot be provided, diluted chlorhexidine gluconate can be used as an antiseptic (Lyngdoh et al., 2018). Lyngdoh et al. (2018) randomly assigned 105 newborn babies to three groups to receive breast milk, 4% chlorhexidine, and dry cord care. In the end, they found that the chlorhexidine group was highly effective in reducing pathogenic bacterial colonization in the neonatal cord. Dry cord care was also reported to be more effective than breast milk in preventing infection. Gras-Le et al. (2017) followed the application of antiseptic umbilical care or dry umbilical care for 4 months in their study. As a result, it was reported that dry cord care was equivalent to an antiseptic solution in the prevention of omphalitis in developed countries. Based on this, it was suggested that dry cord care would be appropriate because antiseptic solutions are unnecessary, restrictive, and expensive. As a result of the systematic review conducted by Coffey & Brown (2017), it was reported that umbilical cord care practices in low and middle-income countries are not consistent, vary according to regions and cultures, the products used are very diverse, and the sources and costs of these products are unknown. It was pointed out that people living in these societies should adopt accepted practices and a behavior change approach should be established. Quattrin et al. (2016) compared 70% alcohol and dry cord care in the umbilical cord care of 200 newborn babies. While 70% alcohol was applied twice a day to the first group, the other group was provided with only air contact so that the cord remained outside the diaper. In conclusion, it was reported that dry cord care is an easy and reliable method for babies born in high-income hospital settings.

Perineum Care

Neonatal perineum care is one of the important practices in ensuring skin integrity. High-absorbency diapers should be used in newborn babies. Diapers should be changed frequently enough. Studies have reported that the frequency of diaper changes should be at least 5-6 per day (Baran & Çimen 2013; Ersoy-Evans et al., 2016). The most important perineal problem is atopic dermatitis. It occurs as a result of destruction in the perineum with deterioration of the skin barrier. It is known that soap and hard surfactants have an effect on this damage. Prolonged contact with urine and feces causes deterioration of skin integrity and irritation. In addition, the risk of dermatitis is high in babies with poorly cleaned diapers, diarrhea, antibiotic treatment, and prolonged skin exposure (Chittock et al., 2023).

Atopic dermatitis impairs the quality of life of the baby, family, and healthcare professionals and causes a burden of care (Perrett & Peters, 2020). The degree of dermatitis should be determined according to the redness and the area covered by the skin. Skin assessment scales should be used. Care should be provided with appropriate products (Sorte 2019; Visscher et al., 2015). It has been reported that water alone is ineffective because it cannot remove the fat-soluble substances from feces and its contents (Gelmetti, 2001). The first approach in the management of atopic dermatitis is the use of moisturizers. Regular use of moisturizers maintains skin moisture, repairs and strengthens the skin barrier, and prevents infection (Chalmers et al., 2020; Skjerven et al., 2020). Wipes containing alcohol should not be used in dermatitis care. During a diaper change, the area is cleaned with boiled, warmed water and soaked cotton wool without applying pressure and dried. The perineum area of the newborn is ventilated. After ensuring adequate dryness of the skin, a cream containing zinc oxide is applied. In cases of fungal infection, antifungal treatment should be used (Skjerven et al., 2020).

Hydrocolloid dressings are also used in the care of diaper rash. However, there are very limited studies on this subject. In the study by Qiao & Ge (2016), babies with diaper rash were divided into three groups, and hydrocolloid dressing, zinc oxide, and mupirocin were applied separately. As a result of the study, it was concluded that the hydrocolloid dressing had the least side effects and was more effective in the healing process. Techasatian & Kiatchoosakun (2022) compared appropriate moisturizer and skin care in their randomized controlled study on newborn babies for a 6-month period. Atopic dermatitis has been reported to show a significant reduction when using a moisturizer. In the study by Rehbinder et al. (2020), the relationship between prenatal maternal skin dryness and newborn babies' imperceptible fluid loss and atopic dermatitis was examined. As a result, it has been reported that dry skin in the early period is a marker for high imperceptible fluid loss and atopic dermatitis. In a systematic review of randomized controlled studies, the effects of moisturizer application on the prevention of atopic dermatitis in term and near-term healthy newborns were examined. As a result, it has been reported that topical moisturizer application may not prevent atopic dermatitis in term healthy newborns. Little data has also been reported on other neonatal skin and allergic outcomes (Priyadarshi et al., 2022).

It is known that moisturizing products such as olive oil, sunflower oil, and vaseline are also used for diaper rash care (Uysal et al., 2019). It has been reported that olive oil is useful in diaper rash care because it prevents the ammonia found in urine from contacting the skin (Özdemir, 2020; Pekyiğit et al., 2020). However, the scarcity of studies with a high level of evidence is remarkable, and it is reported that using olive oil and sunflower oil for a baby's dry skin can negatively affect the skin barrier (Taşdemir & Efe, 2019).

Conclusion

As a result, it is known that the skin of term and preterm newborns has structural and functional differences. The basic approach is to carry out appropriate evaluation and care practices by considering these differences. Skin, which is the largest organ of the body, is very important in protecting and improving newborn skin health. The most important approaches in newborn skin care are skin-to-skin contact, bathing, use of cleansing products, and moisturizers are evidence-based practices for cord care and perineal care. Testing these applications through scientific research guides newborn skin care.

Neonatal/neonatal intensive care nurses have a great responsibility to adopt evidence-based practices for newborn skin care and increase their practices. It should not be forgotten that during these applications, appropriate approaches should be determined, low-cost, reliable product(s) should be used, and the structural situations of underdeveloped, developed, and developing societies should be considered.

References

Aredes, N. D. A., Santos, R. & Fonseca, L. M. M. (2017). Skin care of premature newborns: Integrative review. *Revista Eletrônica de Enfermagem, 19*(a59): 1-23.

Association of Women's Health, Obstetric and Neonatal Nurses. (2018). Evidence-Based Clinical Practice Guideline: 4th ed. Washington, DC.

Association of Women's Health, Obstetric and Neonatal Nurses. (2013). Evidence-Based Clinical Practice Guideline: Neonatal Skin Care. 3rd ed. Washington, DC.

Baran, G., ve Çimen, S., (2013). The Effect of Protective Genital Care Protocol on Preventing Diaper Dermatit Development in 0–18-Month-Old Children Using Antibiotics. *Open Journal of Nursing*, 3(1), 153-161.

Brogan J, Rapkin G. (2017). Implementing evidence-based neonatal skin care with parent-performed, delayed immersion baths. Nurs Womens Health, 21(6):442-50.

Burdall O, Willgress L, Goad N. (2019). Neonatal skin care: Developments in care to maintain neonatal barrier function and prevention of diaper dermatitis. *Pediatric Dermatology*, 36(1), 31–35. https://doi.org/10.1111/pde.13714.

Chalmers, J. R., Haines, R. H., Bradshaw, L. E., Montgomery, A. A., Thomas, K. S., Brown, S. J., ... & Williams, H. C. (2020). Daily emollient during infancy for prevention of eczema: the BEEP randomised controlled trial. *The Lancet*, *395*(10228), 962-972.

Chittock, J., Kay, L., Brown, K., Cooke, A., Lavender, T., Cork, M. J., & Danby, S. G. (2023). Association between skin barrier development and early-onset atopic dermatitis: A longitudinal birth cohort study. *Journal of Allergy and Clinical Immunology*.

Cleminson, J. Ve Mcguire, W. (2021), Topical emollient for preventing infection in preterm infants. *Cochrane Database of Systematic Reviews,* (5).

Coffey, P. S., & Brown, S. C. (2017). Umbilical cord-care practices in low- and middle-income countries: a systematic review. BMC Pregnancy and Childbirth, 17(1), 68. https://doi.org/10.1186/s12884-017-1250-7.

Çağlar, S., Yıldız Kerimoğlu, G., Bakoğlu, İ., Salihoğlu, Ö. (2020), The effect of sunflower seed and almond oil on preterm ınfant skin: a randomized controlled trial. *Advances In Skın And Wound Care Journal*. 33(8), 1-6.

Dessalegn, N., Dagnaw, Y., Seid, K., & Wolde, A. (2022). Umbilical cord care practices and associated factor among mothers of neonates visiting mizan-tepi university teaching hospital southwest Ethiopia 2021. *Pediatric Health, Medicine and Therapeutics*, 227-234.

Dizon M, Galzote C, Estanislao R, Mathew N, Sarkar R. Tolerance of baby cleansers in infants: a randomized controlled trial. *Indian J Pediatr*. 2010; 47:959-963.

Ersoy-Evans, S., Akıncı, H., Doğan, S., ve Atakan, N., (2016). Diaper Dermatitis, A Review of 63 Children. *Pediatric Dermatology*, 33(3), 332-336.

Fernandes, J. D., Machado, M. C. R., Oliveria, Z. N. P. (2011), Children and newborn skin care and prevention. *Analis Brasileiros de Dermatolgia,* 86(1), 102-110.

Fox MD. Wound Care in the Neonatal Intensive Care Unit. *Neonatal Network* 2011; 30(5): 291-303.

Garcia Bartels N, Scheufele R, Prosch F, et al. Effect of standardized skin care regimens on neonatal skin barrier function in different body areas. *Pediatr Dermatol*. 2010; 27:1-8.

Gelmetti, C. (2001). Skin Cleansing in Children. *J Eur Acad Dermatol Venereol*. 15:12-5. 38.

Gras-Le Guen, C., Caille, A., Launay, E., Boscher, C., Godon, N., Savagner, C., Descombes, E., Gremmo-Feger, G., Pladys, P., Saillant, D., Legrand, A., Caillon, J., Barbarot, S., Christophe Roze, J., &

Giraudeau, B. (2017). Dry Care Versus Antiseptics for Umbilical Cord Care: A Cluster Randomized Trial. *Pediatrics,* 139(1), 1–8.

Hoeger, P. (2019). Physiology of neonatal skin. Hoeger P., Kinsler, V., Yani A., Harper, J., Oranje, A., Bodemer, C., Larralde, M., Luk, D., Vibhu, M. & Purvis, D. (Ed.), *Harper's textbook of pediatric dermatology*. New Jersey: Wiley-Blackwell. 56-62.

Johnson D. E. (2016). Extremely preterm infant skin care: A transformation of practice aimed to prevent harm. *Advances in Neonatal Care*. 16: S26–S32.

Johnson, E. & Hunt, R. (2019). Infant skin care: Updates and recommendations. *Current Opinion in Pediatrics, 31*(4): 476-481. doi:10.1097/MOP.0000000000000791.

Kalufya, N. A., Seif, S. A., & Masoi, T. J. (2022). Knowledge and practice of umbilical cord care among young mothers of neonates in Tabora region: Analytical cross-sectional study. *Medicine*, *101*(49).

Karagounis, T. K., Gittler, J. K., Rotemberg, V., Morel, K. D. (2019), Use of "natural" oils for moisturization: review of olive, coconut, and sunflower seed oil. *Pediatr Dermatology*, 36(1), 9–15.

Karakoç, I. B., Ekici, B. (2022), Maintaining skin ıntegrity in neonates with sunflower seed oil and liquid vaseline: a prospective randomized controlled study. *Adv Skin Wound Care*. 35(12),1-8.

Konar, M. C., İslam, K., Roy, A., Ghosh, T. (2020), Effect of virgin coconut oil application on the skin of preterm newborns: a randomized controlled trial. *Journal of Tropical Pediatrics*. 1-7.

Kuller J. M. (2016). Infant skin care products: What are the issues? *Advances in Neonatal Care*. 16: S3–S12.

Lavender T, Bedwell C, Roberts SA, et al. Randomized, con-trolled trial evaluating a baby wash product on skin barrier function in healthy, term neonates. *J Obstet Gynecol Neonatal Nurs*. 2013; 42:203-214.

Liversedge, H. L., Bader, D. L., Schoonhoven, L. & Worsley, P. R. (2018). Survey of neonatal nurses' practices and beliefs in relation to skin health. *Journal of Neonatal Nursing, 24*(2): 86-93.

Lund C. (2016). Issues in newborn skin care. *Advances in Neonatal Care*. 16: S1–S2.

Lund, C. H. & Kuller, J. (2013). Integumentary system. *Comprehensive neonatal nursing care, 5*: 299-333.

Lund, C., Kuller, J., Durand, D. J. (2019), Baby's first bath: changes in skin barrier function after bathing full term newborns with water vs liquid baby Cleanser. *Pediatr Dermatolgy*.1–5.

Lyngdoh, D., Kaur, S., Kumar, P., Gautam, V., & Ghai, S. (2018). Effect of topical application of human breast milk versus 4% chlorhexidine versus dry cord care on bacterial colonization and clinical outcomes of umbilical cord in preterm newborns. *Journal of Clinical Neonatology*, 7(1), 25. https://doi.org/10.4103/jcn.JCN_91_17.

Menon, G. (2015). Skin basics; structure and function. A. Pappas (Ed.) *Lipids and skin health*. Springer, Cham.

Merrill, L., (2015). Prevention, Ttreatment and Parent Education for Diaper Dermatitis. *Nursing for Women's Health*, 19(4), 324-337.

Murakami, M., Yonezawa, K., Shimizu, S., Haruna, M., Sasagawa, E., & Usui, Y. (2022). Newborn-oriented and environmental factors for newborns' skin barrier functions. *Japan Journal of Nursing Science*, *19*(2), e12457.

NICE (National Institute for Health and Clinical Excellence). (2014). Routine postnatal care of women and their babies. *NICE Clinical Guide* no 37.

Nist M. D., Rodgers E. A., Ruth B. M., Bertoni C. B., Bartman T., Keller L. A., Dail J. W., Gardikes-Gardikes R. & Shepherd E. G. (2016). Skin rounds: A quality improvement approach to enhance skin care in the neonatal intensive care unit. *Advances in Neonatal Care*. 16:S33–S41.

Nolan, K., & Marmur, E. (2012). Moisturizers: reality and the skin benefits. *Dermatologic therapy*, *25*(3), 229-233. doi:10.1111/ j.1529-8019.2012.01504.x.

Noor, N. M., Sarmidi, M. R., Khan, A. A., Talib, A., Aziz, A., Aziz, R., Hasham, R. (2016), Empty nano and micro-structured lipid carriers of virgin coconut oil for skin moisturisation. *IET Nanobiotechnology,* 10(4), 195–199.

Nourbakhsh, S. M., Rouhi-Boroujeni, H., Kheiri, M., Mobasheri, M., Shirani, M., Ahrani, S., ve Keivani, Z., (2016) Effect of Topical Application of the Cream Containing Magnesium 2% on Treatment of Diaper Dermatitis and Diaper Rash in Childen a Clinical Trial Study. *Journal of Clinical and Diagnostic Research*, 10(1), 4-6.

Owa, A., Oladokun, R. & Osinusi, K. (2017). Skin ph and transepidermal water loss values in children with diaper dermatitis in ibadan, nigeria. *Pediatric Dermatology, 34*(3): 303-307.

Özdemir, S. (2020). Bebek bakımında geleneksel uygulamalar. *Sağlık ve Toplum*, 30(3), 3-10.

Pekyiğit, A., Yıldız, D., Fidancı, B. E., Çalık, B. B., Dehmen, Ö., Koçak, T., Altıntaş, S. (2020). Annelerin bebek bakımında kullandıkları geleneksel uygulamaların kuşaklararası boyutu. *Turkish Journal of Family Medicine and Primary Care,* 14(4), 443-451. doi: 10.21763/tjfmpc.733696.

Priyadarshi, M., Balachander, B., Gupta, S., & Sankar, M. J. (2022). Topical emollient application in term healthy newborns: A systematic review. *Journal of global health*, *12*.

Qiao, X. P., ve Ge, Y. Z., (2016). Clinical Effect of Hydrocolloid Dressings in Prevention and Treatment of İnfant Diaper Rash. *Experimental and Therapeutic Medicine*, 12(6), 3665-3669.

Quattrin, R., Iacobucci, K., De Tina, A. L., Gallina, L., Pittini, C., & Brusaferro, S. (2016). 70% Alcohol Versus Dry Cord Care in the Umbilical Cord Care. Medicine, 95(14), e3207. https://doi.org/10.1097/ MD.0000000000003207.

Rahma, A., & Lane, M. E. (2022). Skin barrier function in infants: update and outlook. *Pharmaceutics*, *14*(2), 433.

Rehbinder, E. M., Endre, K. M. A., Carlsen, K. C. L., Asarnoj, A., Bains, K. E. S., Berents, T. L., ... & Winger, A. J. (2020). Predicting skin barrier dysfunction and atopic dermatitis in early infancy. *The Journal of Allergy and Clinical Immunology: In Practice*, *8*(2), 664-673.

Rengin, R., Kılıççıoğlu, E., & Sipahi, H. (2020). Bebek ve Çocuklara Yönelik Kozmetik Ürünlerin Güvenliliği. *Hacettepe University Journal of the Faculty of Pharmacy*, *41*(2), 117-132.

Sezer Efe, Y. & Bektaş, M. (2021). Yenidoğanda cilt bakımı ve kanıt temelli uygulamalar. *Türkiye Klinikleri Pediatric Nursing-Special Topics*, 58-62.

Sezer Efe, Y., Erdem, E., Tuncay, B., & Özbey, H. (2021). Annelerin Bebek Bakımında Kullandıkları Geleneksel Uygulamalar: Tanımlayıcı Bir Çalışma. *Journal of Traditional Medical Complementary Therapies*, *4*(3).

Skjerven, H. O., Rehbinder, E. M., Vettukattil, R., LeBlanc, M., Granum, B., Haugen, G., ... & Carlsen, K. C. L. (2020). Skin emollient and early complementary feeding to prevent infant atopic dermatitis (PreventADALL): a factorial, multicentre, cluster-randomised trial. *The Lancet*, *395*(10228), 951-961.

Sorte, D. (2019). Care of skin in neonate (neonatal skin care guidelines). *Nursing & Healthcare International Journal, 3*(1): 1-3.

Stamatas, G. N., Bensaci, J., Greugny, E., Kaur, S., Wang, H., Dizon, M. V., ... & Oddos, T. (2021). A predictive self-organizing multicellular computational model of infant skin permeability to topically applied substances. *Journal of Investigative Dermatology*, *141*(8), 2049-2055.

Summers, A., Visscher, M. O., Khatry, S. K., Sherchand, J. B., LeClerq, S. C., Katz, J., Tielsch, J. M., Mullany, L. C. (2019), Impact of sunflower seed oil versus mustard seed oil on skin barrier function in newborns: a community-based, cluster-randomized trial. *BMC Pediatrics*, 19(1).

Taşdemir, H. İ., & Efe, E. (2019). The effect of tub bathing and sponge bathing on neonatal comfort and physiological parameters in late preterm infants: A randomized controlled trial. *International journal of nursing studies*, *99*, 103377.

Taşdemir, H. İ., Efe, E. (2019). Skin care for infants: a systematic review of the evidence-based. *IJETHS*, 3(2), 50-65. doi: 10.18844/ijeths. v3i2.4562.

Techasatian, L., & Kiatchoosakun, P. (2022). Effects of an emollient application on newborn skin from birth for prevention of atopic dermatitis: a randomized controlled study in Thai neonates. *Journal of the European Academy of Dermatology and Venereology*, *36*(1), 76-83.

Uysal, G., Beydağ, K. D., Düzkaya, D. S. (2019). 0-12 aylık bebeği olan ebeveynlerin bebek bakımına ilişkin geleneksel uygulamaları. *Acıbadem Üniversitesi Sağlık Bilimleri Dergisi*, 10(2), 211-217.

Visscher, M. O., Adam R., Brink S. & Odio M. (2015). Newborn infant skin: physiology, development, and care. *Clin Dermatol, 33*(3): 271-280.

Visscher, M. O., Carr, A. N., & Narendran, V. (2021). Premature infant skin barrier maturation: Status at full-term corrected age. *Journal of Perinatology*, *41*(2), 232-239.

WHO, (2020). *Pregnancy, childbirth, postpartum and newborn care: a guide for essential practice.* Available at: https://apps.who.int/iris/handle/10665/249580 [accessed January 15, 2024].

Chapter 6

Evidence-Based Nursing Practices in Diaper Dermatitis

Esin Keskin[1,*], PhD
and Büşra Gül[2], MSc
[1]Department of Pediatric Hematology-Oncology, Behcet Uz Children's Hospital, Izmir, Türkiye
[2]Department of Pediatric Cardiology, Behcet Uz Children's Hospital, Izmir, Türkiye

Abstract

Newborns and babies have a different skin structure, composition, and function than adults. Researchers have found that although the epidermal barrier is intact at birth, it undergoes a rapid change due to external irritants in the subsequent neonatal period. The presence of skin damage is considered an indicator of quality of care in the acute care setting. Damaged skin is more permeable to irritants, susceptible to infections, and triggers the inflammatory process called dermatitis.

Baby diaper dermatitis, also known as diaper/napkin/nappy rash, is an acute and episodic inflammation, especially in the diaper area, manifested by the presence of erythema, papules, and pustules. Diaper dermatitis is a skin disease that is most common in infancy. Research shows that diaper dermatitis is the most common condition, accounting for 1 in 5 of pediatric dermatology admissions. One-third of babies may show clinical symptoms of diaper dermatitis at some period during infancy. Studies report that 7-35% of all babies have diaper rash between the ages of 9-12 months.

Although not a life-threatening condition, diaper dermatitis can become chronic if left untreated, causing babies to experience tenderness, pain, discomfort, and high levels of parental anxiety. Unpreventable diaper dermatitis occurs the risk of secondary infections and low life quality. Another risk is that the resistance of overhydrated skin cells to pressure and friction decreases, and as a result, pressure injuries develop.

Detection of the disease, diagnosis, and determination of its severity are the most important issues in the treatment of diaper dermatitis. International consensus on prevention and treatment in infants is limited. In this section, the evidence-based nursing practices for diaper dermatitis prepared in line with the current literature are included.

Keywords: diaper dermatitis, napkin rash, baby, nursing

---

* Corresponding Author's Email: esinkeskin21@gmail.com.

In: Evidence-Based Care Practices in Pediatric Nursing
Editors: Feyza Küçük and Serap Özdemir
ISBN: 979-8-89530-304-7

Introduction

What Is Diaper Dermatitis?

Skin integrity is of great importance in children because the skin is a protective barrier against physical, chemical, and biological threats. One of the skin problems, especially infection, that damages skin integrity is diaper dermatitis (Novitasari and Wanda, 2021). Diaper dermatitis (diaper rash, nappy rash, napkin dermatitis) is an acute inflammatory disorder occurring in the diaper area, which is common in infants and children (Adib-Hajbaghery et al., 2014; Mahayaty et al., 2021; Petek et al., 2022). DD is defined as a common cutaneous condition that occurs in the perineal and perianal region (Petek et al., 2022), where erythema, pustules, and papules may occur (Keskin & Didişen, 2023; Novitasari & Wanda, 2021) (Dastgheib et al., 2017; Gıynaş and Yardımcı, 2023). It is a non-immunological response to skin irritants that causes dehydration of skin cells (Mahayaty et al., 2021).

Although the epidermal barrier is intact in newborns, it undergoes rapid evolution depending on external factors exposed to it (Dunk et al., 2022). Therefore, diaper dermatitis is one of the most common skin complaints among babies (Keskin and Didişen, 2023; Price et al., 2021). All infants are at risk of DD to some degree (M. S. Esser et al., 2021). If left untreated, it can become chronic and cause pain, sensitivity, and stress in babies, while creating a troublesome situation for caregivers and causing anxiety (Blume-Peytavi et al., 2014; Gıynaş and Yardımcı, 2023; Keskin and Didişen, 2023; Özdemir, 2020).

Although it cannot be precisely determined because it is not generally seen as a disease by parents and most patients are treated at home (Stamatas and Tierney, 2014; Yilmaz & Yıldız, 2019), the prevalence of DD varies between 7% and 35% depending on the study population and age groups (Coughlin et al., 2014; Yildiz et al., 2023). A multinational study showed that while the prevalence of DD in children worldwide was 7%-43.8% in 2012, it increased significantly to 16%-65% in 2019 (Carr et al., 2020). Another study estimates that the prevalence of DD in children under 2 years of age is around 36%; this rate decreases significantly as age increases (Sukhneewat et al., 2019).

Diaper dermatitis accounts for one-fifth of pediatric dermatology visits (Lim & Carville, 2019). A large study in the United Kingdom reported a 25% incidence of diaper dermatitis in the first month of life (Chang and Nakrani, 2014). Little is known about the prevalence among infants monitored in the NICU (M. S. Esser and Johnson, 2022). A study conducted with a large sample in Hungary reported that the incidence of DD in the NICU was 25% (Csoma et al., 2016). Although the prevalence of DD in hospitalized infants is estimated to be between 5-67%, prevalence rates are not well documented (Cohen, 2017; Esser et al., 2021; Salsbury et al., 2023).

While diaper dermatitis can develop from the first postnatal week, its highest incidence occurs between 9 and 12 months of age (Mahayaty et al., 2021; Petek et al., 2022; Yilmaz and Yıldız, 2019). DD is considered to affect most infants at least once (Dunk et al., 2022).

Diaper Dermatitis Risk Factors

The etiology of diaper dermatitis is multifactorial. Obstruction of the barrier function due to the occlusive structure of the diaper is the most important underlying pathology (Atherton, 2016; Ersoy-Evans et al., 2016; Gıynaş and Yardımcı, 2023; Merrill, 2015). DD began to be seen in the 1960s with the development of disposable diapers (Bonifaz et al., 2013). Humidity, temperature, irritation, friction, exposure to urine and feces, and bacterial or fungal infections are the other main factors responsible for the formation of diaper rash (Ekim and Ocakçı, 2014; Keskin and Didişen, 2023; Stamatas and Tierney, 2014). It is also known that phototherapy treatment, antibiotics, high-protein diets or immunosuppressive agents have an effect on the development of DD (Alonso et al., 2013). All the etiological factors of diaper dermatitis are indicated in Figure 1 (Gıynaş and Yardımcı, 2023; Stamatas and Tierney, 2014).

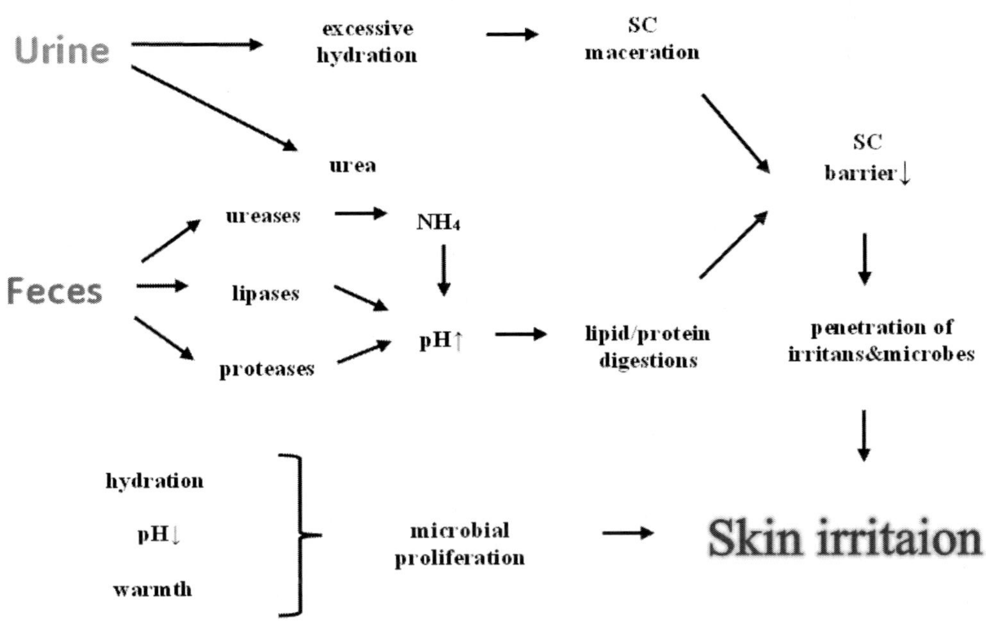

Figure 1. Physical and Biochemical Factors Affecting the Pathophysiology of Diaper Dermatitis (Gıynaş and Yardımcı, 2023; Stamatas and Tierney, 2014)

Increased Humidity

The most important predisposing factor in the etiology of DD is excessive hydration of the stratum corneum. There is a correlation between skin wetness and the severity of DD (Atherton and David Atherton, 2016; Stamatas and Tierney, 2014). The stratum corneum is almost entirely responsible for the barrier function of the epidermis (Atherton, 2016). An excessively humid environment increases the sensitivity of the stratum corneum to friction, disrupts the functions of the epidermal barrier, increases its permeability, thus increasing its reaction to chemical and enzymatic irritants and accelerating the passage of microorganisms into the skin (Alonso et al., 2013; Gıynaş and Yardımcı, 2023; Keskin and Didişen, 2023; Yilmaz and Yıldız, 2019). Prolonged contact of skin damage caused by increased humidity with urine, feces, wound drainage, and sweat results in inflammation and erosion and increases susceptibility to fungal infection (Tammel et al., 2019). Sometimes even long-term contact with water or sweat can be sufficient for the development of erythema and dermatitis (Yilmaz and Yıldız, 2019).

Friction

In most cases, friction between the skin and the fabric of the diaper appears to be an important factor (Atherton, 2016). Friction alone at the contact points between skin-skin and skin-diaper is not a sufficient factor for the development of diaper dermatitis (Gıynaş and Yardımcı, 2023). Friction damages epidermal integrity, especially when combined with increased humidity (Yilmaz and Yıldız, 2019). Overly wet skin and friction with the diaper diaper can cause further damage or maceration of the SC. As a result, skin permeability increases and compounds can penetrate the living epidermis, causing irritation (Rahma and Lane, 2022). This is a very important predisposing factor for diaper dermatitis. This is evidenced by the fact that the lower abdominal region, inguinal, genital, and gluteal areas, where the skin contacts the diaper the most, are the places where diaper dermatitis develops most often (Yilmaz and Yıldız, 2019).

Urine and Feces

Urine and feces are the primary contaminants of the diaper area, and both contribute to irritant diaper dermatitis. Multifactors contribute to the irritating potential of urine and feces. Urine can have acidic or basic pHs (4.6-8) and feces typically have a basic pH (6.5-7.5). Skin pH can vary between body regions, but is generally between 4.5-6.0 (Coughlin et al., 2014). Contact with urine and feces changes skin pH, increases hydration, increases skin barrier sensitivity, and, at the same time, increased activation of fecal enzymes paves the way for diaper rash (Ekim and Ocakçı, 2014; Gıynaş and Yardımcı, 2023).

Urea in urine is broken down by bacteria, causing ammonia to appear. Although ammonia is not the primary cause of the development of diaper dermatitis, it may contribute to the development of diaper dermatitis by disrupting epidermal integrity and increasing permeability (Gıynaş and Yardımcı, 2023; Klunk et al., 2014). Additionally, the higher the pH of the urine, the higher the risk of developing DD (Atherton, 2016). Increased activation of fecal enzymes also paves the way for diaper rash (Ekim & Ocakçı, 2014; Steele, 2017). Proteolytic enzymes in feces become more active at high pH (Coughlin et al., 2014). The rate of protease and lipase enzymes in the baby stool is high, and these enzymes have irritating effects (Gıynaş and Yardımcı, 2023; Mahayaty et al., 2021; Merrill, 2015).

When stool and urine mix, bacteria with urease activity in the stool break down the urea in the urine and convert it into ammonia. The release of ammonia increases the skin pH, the increased pH stimulates the activity of the digestive enzymes protease and lipase found in the stool, which can easily cause irritation to the skin (Akpinar and Göçmen, 2014; Dunk et al., 2022; Yilmaz and Yıldız, 2019). Proteins and lipids tend to break down in the stratum corneum. The skin barrier is disrupted (Akpinar and Göçmen, 2014; Atherton & David Atherton, 2016; Coughlin et al., 2014). Proteolytic enzymes increase permeability to bile salts and other potential irritants. Bile salts potentiate the irritating activity of fecal enzymes (Stamatas and Tierney, 2014). Poor barrier function makes the skin susceptible to irritants and microbial invasion, leading to localized skin inflammation (Blume-Peytavi et al., 2014). In cases where appropriate care is not provided and long-term contact with urine and feces continues, secondary infection may occur with increased bacterial and fungal colonization (Ekim and Ocakçı, 2014).

The correlation between the number of bowel movements and the frequency of DD supports the harmful role of feces on the skin. Diarrhea increases the risk of DD, which may be due to higher concentrations of residual digestive enzymes associated with shorter transit times (Stamatas and Tierney, 2014). Additionally, there is an increased in the action of fecal enzymes such as lipase and protease during periods of diarrhea (Owa et al., 2016). When severe diarrhea develops, the moisture content in the closed gland area increases further, and, at the same time, since intestinal transit is rapid, the number of digestive enzymes in the stool also increases. This causes the skin's barrier function to further deteriorate. On the other hand, bile salts increase the activity of protease. Therefore, persistent diaper dermatitis may occur in children with short bowel syndrome and conjugated hyperbilirubinemia (Yilmaz and Yıldız, 2019).

Improper Skin Care

Another factor that may affect the incidence of diaper dermatitis is diaper use (Mahayaty et al., 2021; Petek et al., 2022). In a prospective study examining factors related to the recovery time of diaper dermatitis in infants, the frequency of changing diapers ≤10 times a day was found to be a risk factor for recovery time (Yokoyama et al., 2022). In addition to the use of diapers, not using skin barriers is another factor that may cause the incidence of dermatitis (Mahayaty et al., 2021).

Chemical Agents

Chemical substances used for detergent, soap, and antiseptic purposes have high irritation and allergenicity potential. This condition plays an important role in the development of diaper dermatitis and the exacerbation of diaper dermatitis symptoms. Another factor that increases the severity of diaper dermatitis is laundry that is not rinsed well (Gıynaş and Yardımcı, 2023).

Nutrition

Feeding with solid foods and consumption of cow's milk are factors that affect the risk of DD in babies (Keskin and Didişen, 2023). Diaper rash is more common in formula-fed babies than in breast-fed babies (Ak and Dolgun, 2021; Ersoy-Evans et al., 2016). Because the feces of formula-fed babies have a higher pH, higher protease and lipase activity, and higher urease content, the potential for skin irritation in the diaper area is higher (Blume-Peytavi et al., 2014; Merrill, 2015; Stamatas and Tierney, 2014). While the gram-positive bacterial flora is higher in breast-fed babies, there is a mixed bacterial flora in cow's milk-fed babies (Shin, 2005).

Additionally, biotin and zinc deficiency are other causes of diaper rash (Keskin & Didişen, 2023). The highest prevalence of diaper dermatitis occurs in infants between 9 and 12 months of age; This may be due to the introduction of solid foods during this period, which causes a high frequency of bowel movements and urination in some babies (Mahayaty et al., 2021).

Antibiotic Use

The use of broad-spectrum antibiotics for various reasons increases the risk of developing diaper dermatitis (Atherton, 2016; Yilmaz and Yıldız, 2019). Antibiotics disrupt the normal intestinal and skin flora, causing changes in stool and skin pH. As a result, colonization with Candida species is triggered and can cause diarrhea (Cohen, 2017; Owa et al., 2016).

Microorganisms

Since the diaper area is wet and closed, it is an area prone to maceration and the settlement of microorganisms such as candida, staphylococci, and streptococci (Akpinar and Göçmen, 2014). Microorganisms alone are not an effective factor in the development of diaper dermatitis. However, factors such as humidity, temperature, airlessness of the diaper area, organic compounds in the stool, and diarrhea, which cause diaper dermatitis in the closed area, create a suitable environment and facilitate the entry of microorganisms into the epidermis from the fragile stratum corneum layer (Gıynaş and Yardımcı, 2023; Stamatas and Tierney, 2014; Yilmaz and Yıldız, 2019).

Hospitalization

In the context of hospitalization, hospitalized children, especially infants, are at higher risk for this health problem. DD is associated with some additional risk factors from the hospital environment, making babies more at risk for developing this health problem. The risk of DD also increases in children diagnosed with an infectious disease and hospitalized for eight days or more (Novitasari and Wanda, 2021).

Diaper Dermatitis Symptoms

The diagnosis of diaper dermatitis is made clinically, and the first clinical symptom may be dry skin. In the initial period, asymptomatic mild erythema, mild maceration, and edema are observed on a limited surface area (Dunk et al., 2022; Yilmaz and Yıldız, 2019). The areas most affected by DD are the hips, genitals, abdomen, perianal region, lower abdomen, intertriginous folds, and thighs, but the entire area under the diaper can be affected (Blume-Peytavi et al., 2014; Petek et al., 2022; Stamatas and Tierney, 2014). As we progress from the mild to moderate phase, erythema becomes more prominent with maceration affecting a larger surface area and can be accompanied by superficial erosions and discomfort (Blume-Peytavi et al., 2014; Dunk et al., 2022; Yildiz et al., 2023). This is often accompanied by discomfort or pain. Severe DD exhibits skin erosion with papules, pustules, and open sores (Cohen, 2017; Lim and Carville, 2019; Salsbury et al., 2023; Stamatas and Tierney, 2014).

The anatomical location and affected surface area are also key factors in defining the severity of DD, with these changes and lesions often occurring in similar areas associated with distressing conditions. The common understanding is that DD should only be present where the diaper surrounds the skin surface (Dunk et al., 2022). As the condition progresses, it can be characterized by moderate erythema with maceration affecting a larger surface area and the potential for skin breakdown leading to exudative or ulcerated lesions or secondary infections (Dunk et al., 2022).

Diagnosis

A good history and physical examination are very important for the diagnosis of diaper dermatitis. While evaluating, the time of onset, the nature of the lesions, the changes in their structure, the location of the lesions, the accompanying itching, previous diseases, the use of antibiotics, diarrhea, the frequency of changing the diaper, the structure of the diaper, how the diaper care is done, which protective or cleaning products are used in the diaper care. It is necessary to pay attention to the issues. The appearance of the lesions and the culture result are important in making the diagnosis (Yilmaz and Yıldız, 2019). The degree of diaper dermatitis can be determined clinically with the help of a visual like Figure 2 (Buckley et al., 2016; Keskin and Didişen, 2023).

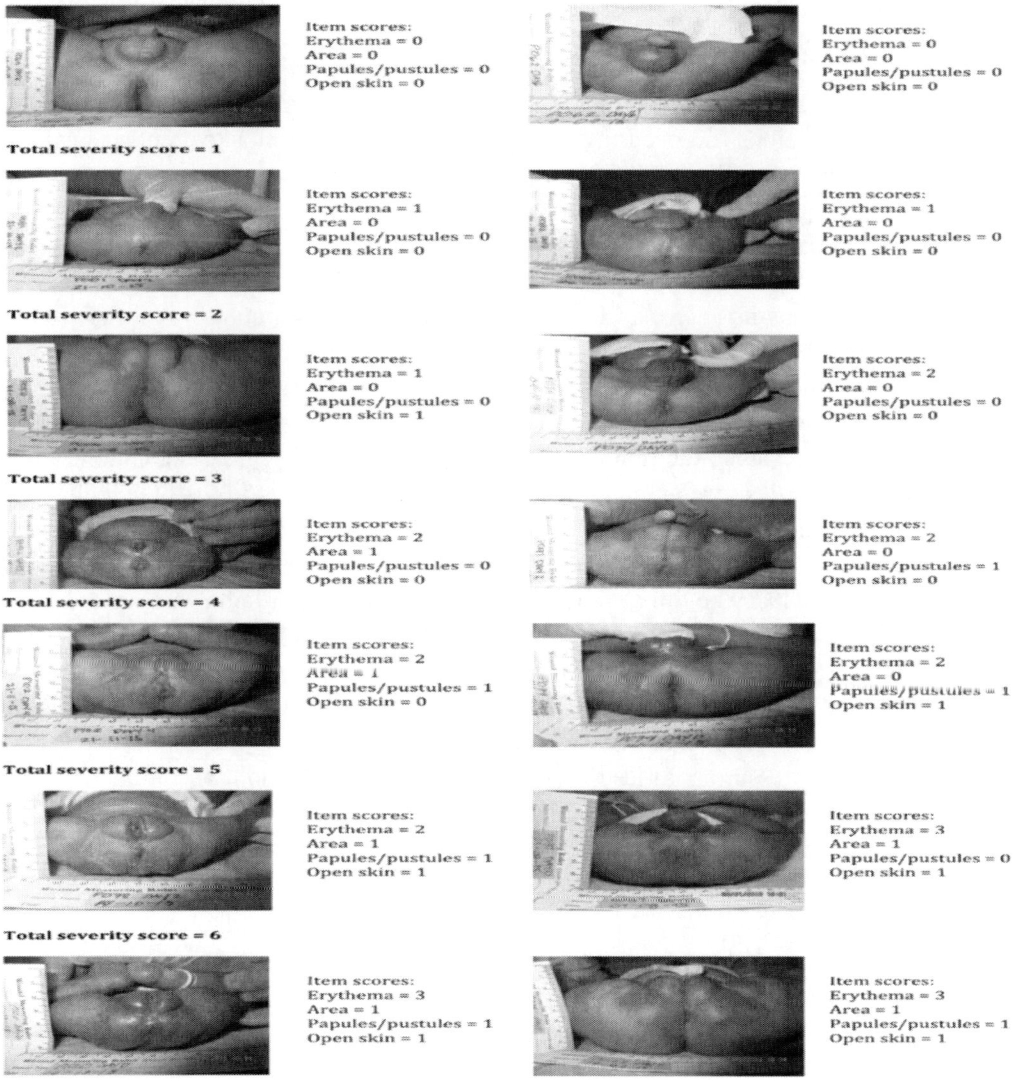

Figure 2. Visuals are helpful in detecting DD severity (Buckley et al., 2016; Keskin & Didişen, 2023).

Diaper Dermatitis Complications

Complications of DD are rare, as it can be easily treated with good skin care practices, barrier creams, and the treatment of underlying infections. In rare cases, or when diaper dermatitis is left untreated, complications such as severe pain, severe skin rashes, and bacterial and fungal infections can occur (Merrill, 2015; Shin, 2014). Long-term ongoing diaper dermatitis may further increase the risk of atopic dermatitis or infection (Yokoyama et al., 2022).

The risk of developing secondary infections in DD is potentially dangerous for immunocompromised patients (Lim & Carville, 2019). Secondary infections further exacerbate the prognosis (Shin, 2005). These infections prolong the hospital stay of babies monitored in the hospital (Esser and Schierholz, 2016; Yilmaz and Yıldız, 2019). All these complications affect health-related quality of life and also cause treatment to be costly and difficult (Black et al., 2011; Lim and Carville, 2019).

The most common types of microorganisms observed in infected diaper dermatitis areas are Candida albicans and Staphylococcus aureus (Gıynaş and Yardımcı, 2023; Vila et al., 2020). Bacterial infections can occur in many different forms, the most common of which are impetigo and bacterial folliculitis (Shin, 2014). In bacterial diaper dermatitis, infections caused by streptococci and staphylococci are most frequently encountered (Merrill, 2015). The diagnosis of bacterial infections in the gland area is usually made by gram staining and culture (Shin, 2014; Yilmaz and Yıldız, 2019).

Candidal infections usually manifest as erythematous, well-circumscribed red lesions in the inguinal folds, buttocks, thighs, genitals, and abdominal areas. It is the most common complication of diaper dermatitis, where pustules and vesicles can also be found at the edges of the lesions (Önder et al., 2007; Shin, 2014). C. albicans colonization is usually seen in diaper dermatitis that lasts longer than 72 hours (Keskin and Didişen, 2023). Colonization by different Candida species, predominantly Candida albicans, occurs in 70–80% of DDs, and therefore diaper rash can be considered as diaper dermatitis cannidiasis (DDC), also called Candida (Bonifaz et al., 2013). Candidal gland dermatitis is diagnosed by smear and culture (Yilmaz & Yıldız, 2019). The development of oral candidiasis in infants with candidal diaper dermatitis is also noteworthy (Merrill, 2015). A significant relationship was found between the rate or severity of diaper dermatitis according to the presence of candida albicans in the mouth (thrush) and in the diaper areas of children (Vila et al., 2020).

Overhydrated skin cells have reduced resistance to pressure and friction, increasing the risk of developing pressure injuries (Black et al., 2011; Lim and Carville, 2019). If left untreated, diaper dermatitis can result in severe ulcerations or erosions that are borderline serious (Merrill, 2015). Additionally, infants who have experienced DD also face the risk of recurrent DD (Lim and Carville, 2019).

Evaluation of Diaper Dermatitis

Early recognition of DD clinical symptoms and determination of their severity are very important for early treatment (Yildiz et al., 2023). Diaper dermatitis is diagnosed by seeing the rash and ruling out other potential causes. In addition to the physical examination, a comprehensive history should be taken, including information such as the duration of the rash, pain, and itching, type of diaper used, hygiene practices and cleaning routine, exposure to potential irritants, antibiotic use, nutrition, frequency of urination and defecation, and skin trauma (Table 1) (Merrill, 2015; Shin, 2014).

Table 1. Factors to consider in diaper dermatitis evaluation (Merrill, 2015)

Duration of rash
Symptoms (pain and itching)
Hygiene practices and cleaning routine (frequency of diaper changes, type of cleanser, wipes or wipes, exposure to irritants such as perfumes and dyes)
Type of diaper used (cloth or disposable)
Skin trauma (friction of the cloth; strong cleaning)
Recent use of antibiotics or other medications
Urination and defecation frequency
Products applied to the skin (barrier creams, powder, home remedies)
Diet (formula/milk, breastfeeding, new foods)
Recent gastrointestinal diseases

Diaper Dermatitis Management, Prevention and Evidence-Based Care

The need for consistency in the management of diaper dermatitis is crucial to providing quality care. Adherence to consistent, evidence-based treatment regimens has the potential to reduce the incidence and severity of diaper dermatitis in infants (Esser and Schierholz, 2016). The best approach to DD management lies in prevention (Akın and Celasin, 2023; Stamatas and Tierney, 2014). In general, approaches that improve DD are considered effective prevention measures (Blume-Peytavi et al., 2014). Prevention comes from evidence-based standards of care that use tools and algorithms that support optimal skin care and positive patient outcomes (Sharp, 2022).

After DD develops, the general goal should be to heal tissue damage, reduce infection, and prevent the recurrence of DD in the ongoing process (Ekim and Ocakçı, 2014; Merrill, 2015; Shin, 2014). The management of DD can be pharmacological and non-pharmacological. The "ABCDE" approach (Air, Barrier, Cleaner, Diaper, and Education), a nonpharmacological intervention, plays an important role in both the prevention and treatment of DD (Klunk et al., 2014; Mahayaty et al., 2021; Merrill, 2015; Novitasari and Wanda, 2021; Shin, 2014). Keys to effectiveness here are preventing or reducing inflammation, repairing skin damage, and preventing recurrence (Merrill, 2015; Novitasari and Wanda, 2021).

Air

Ventilation is an easy, safe, and effective way to prevent and manage DD in infants (Merrill, 2015). Baby skin care best practices recommend frequent diaper changes to keep the perineal skin clean and dry (Salsbury et al., 2023). Exposing the skin to air for as long as possible reduces the time and friction of the skin in direct contact with the wet surface (Merrill, 2015; Stamatas and Tierney, 2014). The baby with DD should be allowed to ventilate by not tying the diaper intermittently throughout the day. Additionally, for hot application during ventilation periods, the lamp should be used for 30 minutes at 3-4 hour intervals can be used (Ak and Dolgun, 2021).

Oxygen has attracted attention as a preferred treatment method in wound care in recent years. The decrease in oxygen in the inflammation area is a factor that delays wound healing. Because regional metabolism accelerates during the healing process of tissues. Meeting the increasing energy need is related to the presence of oxygen. Oxygen accelerates wound healing by ensuring collagen accumulation on the wound surface and tissue regeneration (Bennardop et al., 2018; Kaufman et al., 2018; Yip, 2015). It is known that oxygen therapy applied by inhaling high-pressure oxygen in diabetic foot, crush syndrome, and chronic wounds increases fibroblastic activity and collagen synthesis (Özer, 2021; Öztaş, 2021). Humidified oxygen is continuously applied to the wound surface through a thin tube from the oxygen distributor system. An attempt is made to obtain a high benefit from oxygen by covering the wound with a dressing (Hayes et al., 2017; Kaufman et al., 2018). It is predicted that oxygen, which plays an active role in every stage of wound healing, will also be beneficial in the treatment of diaper dermatitis. In a recent study, it was determined that oxygen at room air density accelerated healing in newborns with diaper dermatitis (Doğan and Kaya, 2024). There is not enough research in the literature for evidence-based practices regarding the use of oxygen in the treatment of diaper dermatitis.

Barrier Usage

Barriers used on the skin have a protective effect on the skin from long-term exposure to moisture (Ekim and Ocakçı, 2014). Studies have shown that patients may benefit from using moisturizers to maintain or increase skin barrier function (Bender et al., 2017; Tammel et al., 2019). Overall, the evidence seems to suggest that common and essential ingredients in skin care products are beneficial for protection and/or hydration and that regular application may be more important than certain specific ingredients (Fastner et al., 2023). The application of protective creams or ointments at each diaper change is recommended as an additional protective or preventive measure and for the treatment of mild to moderate DD. They form a lipid film on the skin surface and protect it from contact with moisture and irritants (Stamatas and Tierney, 2014).

The main components of skin protective products are petrolatum (vaseline), zinc oxide, dimethicone, and acrylate thermopolymer (Avşar and Karadağ, 2018; Stamatas and Tierney, 2014). The most recommended products are those based on zinc oxide (ZnO) and/or petroleum jelly (e.g. Vaseline). However, there are limited data to support the effectiveness of zinc oxide ointment in preventing diaper dermatitis (Rahma and Lane, 2022). Additionally, some studies indicate that zinc oxide is more difficult to clean, increasing the risk of skin being damaged by the cleansing process (Alonso et al., 2013). Many formulations contain zinc oxide, which exhibits mild anti-inflammatory effects (Aitken and Williams, 2014). The positive effects of 20% zinc oxide or vaseline-based creams in increasing the activation of barriers have been shown in studies (Ekim and Ocakçı, 2014).

Vaseline can be applied over other creams and ointments to prevent the diaper from sticking. The barrier can be placed over topical antifungals and topical steroids when necessary (Klunk et al., 2014). Vaseline has also been proven to be a good moisturizer that can penetrate the upper layers of the corneal sublayer. Specifically, it reduces water loss through the epidermis, which is associated with dermatitis and contributes to the healing of damaged tissues and maintenance of skin moisture. Additionally, it is easy to apply and remove, inexpensive, and widely available (Alonso et al., 2013). However, a study on global differences in skin care practices reports that infants using petroleum jelly-based products in NICUs are more likely to develop DD, while those using oil-based emollients have lower rates (Jani et al., 2023).

Emerging evidence supports the use of 5% dexpanthenol to relieve the symptoms of diaper dermatitis. A number of studies have shown that dexpanthenol improves skin barrier function due to reduced fluid loss (Gehring and Gloor, 2011; Wananukul et al., 2006). Dexpanthenol is rapidly absorbed and metabolized from the skin surface. It increases the synthesis of components in the fatty tissue of the skin. It supports healing and provides moisture to the skin. For this reason, it is recommended to prefer creams containing dexpanthenol in skin care (Hebert, 2021; Peltier et al., 2023). In a study conducted with caregivers, it was stated that the application of a cream containing dexpanthenol before sleeping reduced nighttime sleep disturbance in newborns with diaper dermatitis. It has been reported that the symptoms regressed the day after the application and disappeared completely in 2-3 days (Peltier et al., 2023). However, the literature on dexpanthenol is not sufficient (Rahma and Lane, 2022).

Taurine, another dermatitis care product, stimulates lipid synthesis on the epidermis surface and protects against oxidative stress. It prevents the skin from drying out by providing moisture. The combination of barrier creams consisting of taurine, zinc salts, and dexpanthenol is also thought to be useful in the treatment of diaper dermatitis (Hebert, 2021). The combined treatment applied twice a day for 30 days was found to be more effective than applying topical antifungal, corticosteroid, or zinc oxide alone (Dall'Oglio et al., 2021).

Coconut oil (CO) may be a suitable alternative to petroleum-based products. Unrefined organic CO from Cocos nucifera contains saturated fatty acids (medium chain triglycerides) and is mostly lauric acid (Karagounis et al., 2019; Pupala et al., 2019). A randomized trial of CO in preterm infants reported improved scores for neonatal skin conditions compared with routine care (Strunk et al., 2018). Topically applied CO has a low reported risk of allergy or side effects (Pupala et al., 2019; Salam et al., 2015; Strunk et al., 2018). In a study evaluating the effectiveness and safety of organic coconut oil for the prevention of DD among 150 infants admitted to a Level II NICU, organic coconut oil applied to the perineal area at each diaper change and the standard of care control reduced diaper dermatitis in 150 infants admitted to the NICU. It has not been found to significantly prevent it (Salsbury et al., 2023).

In a study, it was determined that the anti-inflammatory and cell regeneration stimulating effects of aloe vera accelerated the healing of diaper rash, and the study stated that aloe vera was also suitable for long-term use (Yagi et al., 2002). It is accepted that applying olive oil to the area helps eliminate diaper rash by preventing the ammonia found in urine from contacting the skin (Akın and Celasin, 2023; Özdemir, 2020). However, as a result of research, there are also findings that the use of olive oil or sunflower oil for the baby's dry skin may negatively affect the skin barrier (Tasdemir and Efe, 2019). Other ingredients used include cod liver oil, aloe barbadensis, and dimethicone (Stamatas and Tierney, 2014).

Although the mechanism of action in inflammatory diseases is not clearly known, the use of menthol is also common. Menthol is thought to play a protective role against inflammation (Cheng and An, 2022). In a study conducted with newborns with diaper dermatitis, it was found that the use of menthol drops in the treatment of diaper rash was more effective than topical clotrimazole. The treatment period was shorter in the menthol group and no side effects were observed. Topical menthol application may be an effective method in candida infection due to diaper dermatitis (Sabzghabaee et al., 2011).

In a study comparing the healing rates of henna, a traditional method, with hydrocortisone cream in diaper dermatitis care after 5 days of application, an improvement was observed in almost all of the children in the henna group. Henna diaper has been evaluated as a suitable traditional method in dermatitis care because it has a significantly higher recovery rate than the hydrocortisone group and no side effects are observed (Keshavarz et al., 2016).

It is important that the creams used for diaper rash are colorless, odorless, and do not contain antiseptic properties (Ekim and Ocakçı, 2014). Products that are close to physiological pH values should be preferred. Convince parents not to over-clean the area and irritate the skin. Cleaning should be done only for feces and not urine (Klunk et al., 2014). During diaper changes, it is not necessary to completely remove the barrier cream or ointment to prevent additional damage to the skin; the skin in the diaper area should be gently patted, not rubbed. A beneficial effect after the application of a barrier cream may also be related to decreased skin hydration (Stamatas and Tierney, 2014).

The powder should not be used on babies (Ak and Dolgun, 2021). Applying powder under the baby, which continues to be used today, will not benefit the baby and may also negatively affect the baby's health (Akın and Celasin, 2023). Powder accumulates between the skin folds and is suitable for the colonization of microorganisms. It also poses a risk of aspiration because it obstructs the respiratory tract of babies (Akın and Celasin, 2023; Akpinar and Göçmen, 2014; Coughlin et al., 2014; Gözen et al., 2011; Özdemir, 2020).

If conventional measures fail in moderate to severe cases, topical corticosteroids and topical antifungal medications can be prescribed for treatment and applied under barrier cream (Ersoy-Evans et al., 2016; Stamatas and Tierney, 2014). Topical steroids are often used to reduce inflammation caused by various forms of irritant dermatitis. Although evidence in adults is sparse, hydrocortisone 1% cream or desonide 0.05% for diaper dermatitis have been recommended for use in infants with diaper dermatitis (Tammel et al., 2019). It is necessary to avoid long-term use of corticosteroids. It is rapidly absorbed and enters the systemic circulation in a short time. Although it is very effective in treatment, the risk of toxic effects is high. Cases of Cushing's syndrome due to overdose topical steroid use with a diagnosis of diaper dermatitis have been reported in the literature (Arı et al., 2009; Tekin et al., 2013; Türkmen et al., 2014). The absorption of topical agents increases, especially due to the high permeability of the skin structure of newborns. Covering the skin surface with products such as baby diapers also contributes to increased dermal absorption. For this reason, it is recommended to be careful against the risk of toxicity and not to use topical corticosteroids more than twice a day (Yilmaz and Yıldız, 2019).

In a study comparing the effect of breast milk and topical 1% hydrocortisone cream in the treatment of diaper dermatitis, no difference was seen in rash scores at the end of 1 week. It has been stated that breast milk alone is as effective as hydrocortisone in the treatment of diaper dermatitis (Farahani et al., 2013). It is recommended to teach mothers about the positive effects of breast milk on the healing of diaper rash (Ak and Dolgun, 2021). For safety reasons, it is beneficial to keep the use of hydrocortisone among the last options.

Cleaning

Providing skin care has a significant impact on the prevention and treatment of a number of skin conditions (Fastner et al., 2023). The main purpose of cleaning the diaper area is to remove contaminants from the skin without disrupting the skin barrier. Cleansing the skin surface is to cleanse the area without irritating the skin or causing dermatitis (Coughlin et al., 2014; Rahma and Lane, 2022). Proper cleaning of the perianal area is essential in case of diaper rash. Washing the perianal area is important in preventing the development of bacterial colonization (Ekim and Ocakçı, 2014). Wiping should be done from front to back (Akpinar and Göçmen, 2014).

Cleaning agents range from water to soap to synthetic detergents to impregnated disposable wipes (Coughlin et al., 2014). Cleansing of the perianal area is done by considering skin physiology such as normal flora, bacteria, and skin pH. Water and a soft cloth can be used to clean the perianal area without rubbing the skin harshly (Mahayaty et al., 2021). Using water to clean the perianal area is an effective intervention that does not require large costs and does not cause irritation. (Mahayaty et al., 2021). The aim of diaper rash treatment is to clean urine and feces and keep them dry and clean. If possible, wet wipes should not be used, and if they are used, wet wipes that do not contain alcohol should be preferred (Ak and Dolgun, 2021).

It has been stated in the literature that Candida infection is significantly more common in patients using wet wipes for diaper cleaning (Ersoy-Evans et al., 2016). However, a study showed that water alone was not sufficient to remove fecal material from the diaper area (Lavender et al., 2012). To solve this problem, baby cleansing wipes were developed and quickly replaced traditional cleaning practices (Rahma and Lane, 2022). Most baby wipe formulations should contain a large percentage of water, preservatives, surfactants, and emollients. The rationale for each component is listed in Table 2 (Rahma and Lane, 2022).

Wipes that are free of alcohol, perfume, essential oils, and harsh detergents can be used to cleanse the skin and are a suitable solution in some cases. Wipes have been shown to be equivalent in terms of skin softness when compared to cleansing with water and cotton, and are therefore recommended as a good alternative (Bender et al., 2017; Lavender et al., 2012).

However, wipes can cause complications, especially due to the presence of preservatives such as methylisothiazolinone. Using wet wipes (baby wipes) to clean the perianal area is as mild as using water with no change in skin condition. However, wet wipes contain preservatives and fragrances that have the potential to be topically sensitizing, so the use of wet wipes is not recommended if damage to skin integrity has occurred (Li et al., 2012; Mahayaty et al., 2021). Additionally, the use of alcohols such as isopropanol in baby wipes is strictly not recommended due to the irritating and drying properties of these solvents (Rahma and Lane, 2022).

It is very important to use water and appropriate cleaners when cleaning the diaper rash area. Soap is defined as alkaline salts of fatty acids, and due to its high pH rate, it changes the skin pH level in an alkaline direction. At the same time, another side effect of soap is that the calcium and magnesium salts contained in soap create residues on the skin, and these residues increase skin irritation (Ekim and Ocakçı, 2014). The skin should be gently cleansed, avoiding excessive use of soap. In the case of stool, cotton oils or petroleum jelly can be used in addition to water (Alonso et al., 2013).

Table 2. Recommended Requirements for Ingredients in Baby Wipe Formulations (Rahma & Lane, 2022)

Component	Reason	Suggestion
Water	As a vehicle for cleaning ingredients	Highly purified
Protectors	To prevent microbial growth on products	It should not alter the normal cutaneous microbiome; use only regulatory-approved materials
Surfactants	Water alone is ineffective in removing water-insoluble skin impurities; for optimum cleaning	It should effectively remove feces and urine; and should not contain harsh surfactants, especially sodium lauryl sulfate
Softeners	To minimize friction and replenish SC lipids	Must have a positive effect on skin barrier function
pH buffering compounds	To maintain a healthy skin pH	The skin pH should be maintained at ±5.5

Diaper

It is important to change newborns' diapers every 2 hours and babies' diapers every 3 to 4 hours. It is reported in the literature that diaper rash decreases by increasing the frequency of changing diapers (Ersoy et al., 2016; Ak and Dolgun, 2021). The diaper should also be changed every time the baby soils his/her diaper. Cloths produced with new technology increase the possibility of the skin remaining dry due to their intense absorbent properties. (Akpinar and Göçmen, 2014). The use of disposable diapers is recommended because they contain absorbent ingredients such as hydrocellulose gel, which are very good at preventing moist conditions on the skin. Disposable diapers with super absorbent gel, an outer porous fabric layer, and an absorbent outer layer have been shown to reduce the incidence of diaper dermatitis. (Mahayaty et al., 2021).

Education

Family education aimed at reducing the incidence of diaper dermatitis in infants is also important (Li et al., 2022). For effective prevention, parents and caregivers need proven information for guidance and assistance (Blume-Peytavi et al., 2014). Diaper hygiene is an important part of education for parents and caregivers of newborns. Diaper dermatitis is a preventable condition, and all parents should be educated on common methods to reduce the likelihood of this condition by adhering to proper diaper hygiene and meticulous skin care practices. Measures taken to restore healthy skin and prevent recurrent events can be safely provided in the home environment by parents and other caregivers (Merrill, 2015). As care management for children prioritizes treatment of the main problem related to medical diagnosis, DD has become less of a concern and family-centered care is required. Family-centered care emphasizes the important role that the family plays in every childcare intervention and decision (Novitasari and Wanda, 2021).

Conclusion

Diaper dermatitis, one of the most common dermatological problems in newborns and infants, has a complex and multifactorial etiology. The prevention and management of diaper dermatitis is possible with a comprehensive understanding of its etiology and elimination of risk factors. The fundamental responsibility of nurses is to possess an understanding of the predisposing factors associated with diaper dermatitis, the implementation of strategies to prevent its occurrence and the provision of educational guidance to parents. Secondarily, in the event of nappy dermatitis developing, it is to provide appropriate care in accordance with the available evidence base. Evidence-based practices shorten the duration of the patient's hospital stay, reduce costs, increase the quality of care and satisfaction. In order to maintain professional standards of conduct and practice, nurses should adhere to the most current guidelines for their respective fields of practice. This is a requisite aspect of professional practice, as it enables nurses to deliver optimal care based on the most current evidence-based practices.

Disclamier

None.

References

Adib-Hajbaghery, M., Mahmoudi, M., & Mashaiekhi, Mahdi. (2014). Shampoo-Clay Heals Diaper Rash Faster Than Calendula Officinalis. *Nurs Midwifery Stud*, *3*(2), 14180.

Aitken, J., & Williams, F. L. R. (2014). A systematic review of thyroid dysfunction in preterm neonates exposed to topical iodine. *Archives of Disease in Childhood - Fetal and Neonatal Edition*, *99*(1), F21–F28. https://doi.org/10.1136/archdischild-2013-303799.

Ak, Ö. B., & Dolgun, G. (2021). Doğum Sonu Dönemde Yenidoğanda Yapılan Kanıta Dayalı Uygulamalar ve Ebelik. *Samsun Sağlık Bilimleri Dergisi*, *6*(1), 18–27. https://doi.org/10.47115/jshs.742123.

Akın, H. Y. S., & Celasin, N. Ş. (2023). Dünyada ve Türkiye'de Annelerin Geleneksel Bebek Bakımı Uygulamaları Farklı mıdır? *Göbeklitepe Sağlık Bilimleri Dergisi*, *6*(12), 1–11. https://doi.org/10.55433/gsbd/189.

Akpinar, F., & Göçmen, İ. (2014). Yenidoğanlarda Deri Bakımı. *Maltepe Medical Journal*, *6*(2). http://www.who.int/reproductive-health/publi-.

Alonso, C., Larburu, I., Bon, E., González, M. M., Iglesias, M. T., Urreta, I., & Emparanza, J. I. (2013). Efficacy of petrolatum jelly for the prevention of diaper rash: A randomized clinical trial. *Journal for Specialists in Pediatric Nursing*, *18*(2), 123–132. https://doi.org/10.1111/jspn.12022.

Arı, M. E., Çetinkaya, S., TÜFEKÇİ, B. S., Takçi, Ş., & Nazlier, K. (2009). Türkiye Çocuk Hastalıkları Dergisi / Turkish Journal of Pediatric Disease. *Turkhis J Pediatr Dis*, *3*(2), 48–52.

Atherton, D. J. (2016). Understanding irritant napkin dermatitis. *International Journal of Dermatology*, 7–9.

Avşar, P., & Karadağ, A. (2018). İnkontinansa Bağlı Dermatit: Değerlendirme, Önleme ve Tedavi. *Journal of Hacettepe University Faculty of Nursing*, *5*(1), 69–77. https://orcid.org/0000-0001-6436-1647.

Bender, J. K., Faergemann, J., & Sköld, M. (2017). Skin Health Connected to the Use of Absorbent Hygiene Products: A Review. *Dermatology and Therapy*, *7*(3), 319–330. https://doi.org/10.1007/s13555-017-0189-y.

Bennardop, L., Del Duca, E., Dastoli, S., Schipani, G., Scali, E., Silvestri, M., & Nisticò, S. (2018). Potential applications of topical oxygen therapy in dermatology. *Dermatology Practical & Conceptual*, 272–276. https://doi.org/10.5826/dpc.0804a04.

Black, J. M., Gray, M., Bliss, D. Z., Kennedy-Evans, K. L., Logan, S., Baharestani, M. M., Colwell, J. C., Goldberg, M., & Ratliff, C. R. (2011). MASD Part 2. *Journal of Wound, Ostomy & Continence Nursing*, *38*(4), 359–370. https://doi.org/10.1097/WON.0b013e31822272d9.

Blume-Peytavi, U., Hauser, M., Lünnemann, L., Stamatas, G. N., Kottner, J., & Garcia Bartels, N. (2014). Prevention of diaper dermatitis in infants - A literature review. *Pediatric Dermatology*, *31*(4), 413–429. https://doi.org/10.1111/pde.12348.

Bonifaz, A., Tirado-Sánchez, A., Graniel, M. J., Mena, C., Valencia, A., & Ponce-Olivera, R. M. (2013). The Efficacy and Safety of Sertaconazole Cream (2 %) in Diaper Dermatitis Candidiasis. *Mycopathologia*, *175*(3–4), 249–254. https://doi.org/10.1007/s11046-013-9642-3.

Buckley, B. S., Mantaring, J. B., Dofitas, R. B., Lapitan, M. C., & Monteagudo, A. (2016). A New Scale for Assessing the Severity of Uncomplicated Diaper Dermatitis in Infants: Development and Validation. *Pediatric Dermatology*, *33*(6), 632–639. https://doi.org/10.1111/pde.12988.

Carr, A. N., DeWitt, T., Cork, M. J., Eichenfield, L. F., Fölster-Holst, R., Hohl, D., Lane, A. T., Paller, A., Pickering, L., Taieb, A., Cui, T. Y., Xu, Z. G., Wang, X., Brink, S., Niu, Y., Ogle, J., Odio, M., & Gibb, R. D. (2020). Diaper dermatitis prevalence and severity: Global perspective on the impact of caregiver behavior. *Pediatric Dermatology*, *37*(1), 130–136. https://doi.org/10.1111/pde.14047.

Chang, M. W., & Nakrani, R. (2014). Six Children With Allergic Contact Dermatitis to Methylisothiazolinone in Wet Wipes (Baby Wipes). *Pediatrics*, *133*(2), e434–e438. https://doi.org/10.1542/peds.2013-1453.

Cheng, H., & An, X. (2022). Cold stimuli, hot topic: An updated review on the biological activity of menthol in relation to inflammation. *Frontiers in Immunology*, *13*. https://doi.org/10.3389/fimmu.2022.1023746.

Cohen, B. (2017). Differential Diagnosis of Diaper Dermatitis. *Clinical Pediatrics*, *56*(5_suppl), 16S-22S. https://doi.org/10.1177/0009922817706982.

Coughlin, C. C., Frieden, I. J., & Eichenfield, L. F. (2014). Clinical approaches to skin cleansing of the diaper area: Practice and challenges. *Pediatric Dermatology*, *31*(s1), 1–4. https://doi.org/10.1111/pde.12461.

Csoma, Z. R., Meszes, A., Ábrahám, R., Kemény, L., Tálosi, G., & Doró, P. (2016). Iatrogenic Skin Disorders and Related Factors in Newborn Infants. *Pediatric Dermatology*, *33*(5), 543–548. https://doi.org/10.1111/
pde.12960.

Dall'Oglio, F., Musumeci, M. L., Puglisi, D. F., & Micali, G. (2021). A novel treatment of diaper dermatitis in children and adults. *Journal of Cosmetic Dermatology*, *20*(S1), 1–4. https://doi.org/10.1111/jocd.14091.

Dastgheib, L., Pishva, N., Saki, N., Khabnadideh, S., Kardeh, B., Torabi, F., Arabnia, S., & Heiran, A. (2017). Efficacy of topical Coriandrum sativum extract on treatment of infants with diaper dermatitis: A single blinded non-randomised controlled trial. *Malaysian Journal of Medical Sciences*, *24*(4), 97–101. https://doi.org/10.21315/mjms2017.24.4.11.

Doğan, E., & Kaya, H. D. (2024). The effect of oxygen on diaper dermatitis in infants: A randomized controlled trial. *Journal of Neonatal Nursing*. https://doi.org/10.1016/j.jnn.2024.01.009.

Dunk, A. M., Broom, M., Fourie, A., & Beeckman, D. (2022). Clinical signs and symptoms of diaper dermatitis in newborns, infants, and young children: A scoping review. *Journal of Tissue Viability*, *31*(3), 404–415. https://doi.org/10.1016/j.jtv.2022.03.003.

Ekim, A., & Ocakçı, A. F. (2014). Yenidoğan Cilt Bakımında Güncel Yaklaşımlar. *Cumhuriyet Nursing Journal*, *3*(2), 30–37.

Ersoy-Evans, S., Akinci, H., Doğan, S., & Atakan, N. (2016). Diaper Dermatitis: A Review of 63 Children. *Pediatric Dermatology*, *33*(3), 332–336. https://doi.org/10.1111/pde.12860.

Esser, M. S., & Johnson, T. S. (2020). An Integrative Review of Clinical Characteristics of Infants with Diaper Dermatitis. *Advances in Neonatal Care*, *20*(4), 276–285. https://doi.org/10.1097/ANC.00000
00000000682.

Esser, M. S., & Johnson, T. S. (2022). An Adaptation of the Skin Safety Model to Guide Diaper Dermatitis Research in the NICU. *Neonatal Network*, *41*(1), 38–44. https://doi.org/10.1891/11-T-747.

Esser, M. S., Ngui, E. M., & Johnson, T. S. (2021). Contributing factors to diaper dermatitis and NICU length of stay. *Journal of Neonatal Nursing*, *27*(5), 358–364. https://doi.org/10.1016/j.jnn.2021.03.006.

Esser, M., & Schierholz, E. (2016). Diaper Dermatitis: What Do We Do Next? *Advances in Neonatal Care*, *16*, S21–S25. https://doi.org/10.1097/ANC.0000000000000316.

Farahani, L. A., Ghobadzadeh, M., & Yousefi, P. (2013). Comparison of the Effect of Human Milk and Topical Hydrocortisone 1% on Diaper Dermatitis. *Pediatric Dermatology*, *30*(6), 725–729. https://doi.org/10.1111/pde.12118.

Fastner, A., Hauss, A., & Kottner, J. (2023). Skin assessments and interventions for maintaining skin integrity in nursing practice: An umbrella review. *International Journal of Nursing Studies*, *143*, 104495. https://doi.org/10.1016/j.ijnurstu.2023.104495.

Gehring, W., & Gloor, M. (2011). Effect of Topically Applied Dexpanthenol on Epidermal Barrier Function and Stratum Corneum Hydration. *Arzneimittelforschung*, *50*(07), 659–663. https://doi.org/10.1055/s-0031-1300268.

Gıynaş, T., & Yardımcı, F. (2023). Yeni doğanlarda deri bakımı: Bez dermatiti ve yönetimi. *Health Care Academician Journal*, *10*(2), 302–314. https://doi.org/10.52880/sagakaderg.1195064.

Gözen, D., Çağlar, S., & Doğan, Z. (2011). 0-24 Ay Arası Bebeği Olan Annelerin Pişiği Önleme ve Bakımına Yönelik Uygulamaları*. *Cilt 19-Sayı*, *1*, 17–22.

Hayes, P. D., Alzuhir, N., Curran, G., & Loftus, I. M. (2017). Topical oxygen therapy promotes the healing of chronic diabetic foot ulcers: a pilot study. *Journal of Wound Care*, *26*(11), 652–660. https://doi.org/10.12968/jowc.2017.26.11.652.

Hebert, A. A. (2021). A new therapeutic horizon in diaper dermatitis: Novel agents with novel action. *International Journal of Women's Dermatology*, *7*(4), 466–470. https://doi.org/10.1016/j.ijwd.2021.02.003.

Jani, P., Mishra, U., Buchmayer, J., Maheshwari, R., D'Çruz, D., Walker, K., Gözen, D., Lowe, K., Wright, A., Marceau, J., Culcer, M., Priyadarshi, A., Kirby, A., Moore, J. E., Oei, J. L., Shah, V., Vaidya, U., Khashana, A., Godambe, S., … Satardien, M. (2023). Global variation in skin injures and skincare practices in extremely preterm infants. *World Journal of Pediatrics*, *19*(2), 139–157. https://doi.org/10.1007/s12519-022-00625-2.

Karagounis, T. K., Gittler, J. K., Rotemberg, V., & Morel, K. D. (2019). Use of "natural" oils for moisturization: Review of olive, coconut, and sunflower seed oil. *Pediatric Dermatology*, *36*(1), 9–15. https://doi.org/10.1111/pde.13621.

Kaufman, H., Gurevich, M., Tamir, E., Keren, E., Alexander, L., & Hayes, P. (2018). Topical oxygen therapy stimulates healing in difficult, chronic wounds: a tertiary centre experience. *Journal of Wound Care*, *27*(7), 426–433. https://doi.org/10.12968/jowc.2018.27.7.426.

Keshavarz, A., Zeinaloo, A. A., Mahram, M., Mohammadi, N., Sadeghpour, O., & Maleki, M. R. (2016). Efficacy of Traditional Medicine Product Henna and Hydrocortisone on Diaper Dermatitis in Infants. *Iranian Red Crescent Medical Journal*, *18*(5). https://doi.org/10.5812/ircmj.24809.

Keskin, E., & Didişen, N. A. (2023). The Validity and Reliability Study of the Turkish Version of the Scale for Assessing the Severity of Uncomplicated Diaper Dermatitis in Infants. *Journal of Basic and Clinical Health Sciences*, *7*(3), 21–29. https://doi.org/10.30621/jbachs.1101510.

Klunk, C., Domingues, E., & Wiss, K. (2014). An update on diaper dermatitis. *Clinics in Dermatology*, *32*(4), 477–487. https://doi.org/10.1016/j.clindermatol.2014.02.003.

Lavender, T., Furber, C., Campbell, M., Victor, S., Roberts, I., Bedwell, C., & Cork, M. J. (2012). Effect on skin hydration of using baby wipes to clean the napkin area of newborn babies: assessor-blinded randomised controlled equivalence trial. *BMC Pediatrics*, *12*(1), 59. https://doi.org/10.1186/1471-2431-12-59.

Li, C., Zhu, Z., & Dai, Y. (2012). Diaper Dermatitis: A Survey of Risk Factors for Children Aged 1 - 24 Months in China. *Journal of International Medical Research*, *40*(5), 1752–1760. https://doi.org/10.1177/030006051204000514.

Li, Y., Jiang, Y., Kang, Q., & Lu, Q. (2022). Summary of the best evidence summary on prevention strategies for diaper dermatitis in infants. *Journal of Shanghai Jiaotong University (Medical Science)*, *42*(3), 357–363. https://doi.org/10.3969/j.issn.1674-8115.2022.03.014.

Lim, Y. S. L., & Carville, K. (2019). Prevention and Management of Incontinence-Associated Dermatitis in the Pediatric Population: An Integrative Review. *Journal of Wound, Ostomy and Continence Nursing*, *46*(1), 30–37. https://doi.org/10.1097/WON.0000000000000490.

Mahayaty, L., Nurhaeni, N., Wanda, D., & Fitriah. (2021). Perianal Care Proven to Reduce the Incidence of Diaper Dermatitis. *Indian Journal of Forensic Medicine & Toxicology*, *15*(1), 1212–1217. https://doi.org/10.37506/ijfmt.v15i1.13582.

Merrill, L. (2015). Prevention, Treatment and Parent Education for Diaper Dermatitis. *Nursing for Women's Health*, *19*(4), 324–337. https://doi.org/10.1111/1751-486X.12218.

Novitasari, P. D., & Wanda, D. (2021). Evidence-based nursing intervention to reduce skin integrity impairment in children with diaper dermatitis: A systematic review. *Pediatria Medica e Chirurgica*, *43*(s1). https://doi.org/10.4081/pmc.2021.265.

Önder, M., Adışen, E., & Velagiç, Z. (2007). Diaper dermatit. *Çocuk Sağlığı ve Hastalıkları Dergisi*, *50*, 129–135.

Owa, A. B., Oladokun, R. E., & Osinusi, K. (2016). Diaper dermatitis among children in Ibadan, Nigeria: frequency and predisposing factors. *Eur. J. Pediat. Dermatol*, *26*, 135–141.

Özdemir, S. (2020). Bebek Bakımında Geleneksel Uygulamalar. *Sağlık ve Toplum*, *20*(3), 3–10.

Özer, E. E. (2021). Hiperbarik Oksijen Tedavisi Uygulanan Diyabetik Ayak Yaralarında İyileşme ve Ampütasyon Sonuçlarını Etkileyen Faktörler. *Muğla Sıtkı Koçman Üniversitesi Tıp Dergisi*, *8*(1), 23–28. https://doi.org/10.47572/muskutd.732398.

Öztaş, P. (2021). Yara İyileşmesi, Bakımı ve Tedavisi. *Ankara Eğitim ve Araştırma Hastanesi Tıp Dergisi*, *54*(2), 341–351. https://doi.org/10.20492/aeahtd.931499.

Peltier, E., de Salvo, R., Ehret, A., Trapp, S., Lakomsky, D., & El Shazly, M. A. (2023). Evaluation of a 5% dexpanthenol-containing ointment for the treatment of infant irritant diaper dermatitis through the lens of the caregiver—A real-world data observational study. *Health Science Reports*, *6*(1). https://doi.org/10.1002/hsr2.1033.

Petek, T. H., Petek, M., Petek, T., & Varda, N. M. (2022). *Emerging Links between Microbiome Composition and Skin Immunology in Diaper Dermatitis: A Narrative Review*. https://doi.org/10.3390/children.

Price, A. D., Lythgoe, J., Ackers-Johnson, J., Cook, P. A., Clarke-Cornwell, A. M., & MacVane Phipps, F. (2021). The BaSICS (Baby Skin Integrity Comparison Survey) study: A prospective experimental study using maternal observations to report the effect of baby wipes on the incidence of irritant diaper dermatitis in infants, from birth to eight weeks of age. *Pediatrics and Neonatology*, *62*(2), 138–145. https://doi.org/
10.1016/j.pedneo.2020.10.003.

Pupala, S. S., Rao, S., Strunk, T., & Patole, S. (2019). Topical application of coconut oil to the skin of preterm infants: a systematic review. *European Journal of Pediatrics*, *178*(9), 1317–1324. https://doi.org/10.1007/
s00431-019-03407-7.

Rahma, A., & Lane, M. E. (2022). Skin Barrier Function in Infants: Update and Outlook. *Pharmaceutics*, *14*(2), 433. https://doi.org/10.3390/pharmaceutics14020433.

Sabzghabaee, A. M., Nili, F., Ghannadi, A., Eizadi-Mood, N., & Anvari, M. (2011). Role of menthol in treatment of candidial napkin dermatitis. *World Journal of Pediatrics*, *7*(2), 167–170. https://doi.org/10.1007/s12519-011-0253-0.

Salam, R. A., Darmstadt, G. L., & Bhutta, Z. A. (2015). Effect of emollient therapy on clinical outcomes in preterm neonates in Pakistan: a randomised controlled trial. *Archives of Disease in Childhood - Fetal and Neonatal Edition*, *100*(3), F210–F215. https://doi.org/10.1136/archdischild-2014-307157.

Salsbury, S. A., Arikat, S. O., Martin, M. D., Haack, S., Castro, S., Frazier, M., Weakley, D., & Lemke, J. H. (2023). Coconut oil versus standard of care for the prevention of diaper dermatitis in the neonatal intensive care unit: A randomized clinical trial. *Journal of Neonatal Nursing*. https://doi.org/10.1016/j.jnn.
2023.10.014.

Sharp, M. (2022). Diaper Dermatitis Algorithm Quality Improvement Initiative To Decrease Incidence of and Severity of Diaper Dermatitis Using A Reliable and Valid Scoring Tool in the Neonatal Intensive Care Unit (NICU). *World Council of Enterostomal Therapists Journal*, *42*(3).

Shin, H. T. (2005). Diaper dermatitis that does not quit. *Dermatologic Therapy*, *18*(2), 124–135. https://doi.org/10.1111/j.1529-8019.2005.05013.x.

Shin, H. T. (2014). Diagnosis and Management of Diaper Dermatitis. *Pediatric Clinics of North America*, *61*(2), 367–382. https://doi.org/10.1016/j.pcl.2013.11.009.

Stamatas, G. N., & Tierney, N. K. (2014). Diaper dermatitis: Etiology, manifestations, prevention, and management. *Pediatric Dermatology*, *31*(1), 1–7. https://doi.org/10.1111/pde.12245.

Steele, R. W. (2017). Diaper Dermatitis: Facts and Misinformation. *Clinical Pediatrics*, *56*(5), 6S-7S. https://doi.org/10.1177/0009922817704929.

Strunk, T., Pupala, S., Hibbert, J., Doherty, D., & Patole, S. (2018). Topical Coconut Oil in Very Preterm Infants: An Open-Label Randomised Controlled Trial. *Neonatology*, *113*(2), 146–151. https://doi.org/10.1159/000480538.

Sukhneewat, C., Chaiyarit, J., & Techasatian, L. (2019). Diaper dermatitis: a survey of risk factors in Thai children aged under 24 months. *BMC Dermatology*, *19*(1), 7. https://doi.org/10.1186/s12895-019-0089-1

Tammel, K., Benike, D., & Sievers, B. (2019). A Novel Approach to Treating Moderate to Severe Incontinence-Associated Dermatitis and Intertriginous Dermatitis: A Case Series. *Journal of Wound, Ostomy and Continence Nursing*, *46*(5), 446–452. https://doi.org/10.1097/WON.0000000000000564

Tasdemir, H. I., & Efe, E. (2019). Skin care for infants: A systematic review of the evidence-based. *International Journal of Emerging Trends in Health Sciences*, *3*(2), 50–65. https://doi.org/10.18844/ijeths.v3i2.4562.

Tekin, M., Topaloğlu, N., Yıldırım, Ş., Fatih Binnetoğlu, K., Kaymaz, N., Aylanç, H., Battal, F., & Aşık, Z. (2013). Topikal Steroid Kullanımına Bağlı İyatrojenik Adrenokortikal Yetmezlik. *International Journal of Clinical Research*, *1*(2), 74–75.

Türkmen, A. V., Atilla Nursoy, M., Türkmen, S., & Yazıcı, M. (2014). İktiyozisli bir bebekte topikal kortikosteroid kullanımına bağlı iatrojenik Cushing sendromu: Bir vaka takdimi. *Çocuk Sağlığı ve Hastalıkları Dergisi*, *57*, 2730.

Vila, T., Sultan, A. S., Montelongo-Jauregui, D., & Jabra-Rizk, M. A. (2020). Oral Candidiasis: A Disease of Opportunity. *Journal of Fungi*, *6*(1), 15. https://doi.org/10.3390/jof6010015.

Wananukul, S., Limpongsanuruk, W., Singalavanija, S., & Wisuthsarewong, W. (2006). Comparison of Dexpanthenol and Zinc Oxide Ointment with Ointment Base in the Treatment of Irritant Diaper Dermatitis from Diarrhea: A Multicenter Study. *J Med Assoc Thai*, *89*(10), 1654–1662.

Yagi, A., Kabash, A., Okamura, N., Haraguchi, H., Moustafa, S. M., & Khalifa, T. I. (2002). Antioxidant, Free Radical Scavenging and Anti-Inflammatory Effects of Aloesin Derivatives in *Aloe vera*. *Planta Medica*, *68*(11), 957–960. https://doi.org/10.1055/s-2002-35666.

Yildiz, I., Kizilca, O., Haksayar, A., & Demirkale, Z. H. (2023). Pediatricians' Knowledge, Attitudes, and Therapeutic Approaches Regarding Diaper Dermatitis: A Common Condition with Many Different Practices. *Clinical, Cosmetic and Investigational Dermatology*, *16*, 901–910. https://doi.org/10.2147/CCID.S405414.

Yilmaz, G., & Yıldız, S. (2019). Bez Dermatiti ve Hemşirelik Bakımı. *Journal of Nursing Science*, *2*(2), 31–37. http://dergipark.gov.tr/hbd.

Yip, W. L. (2015). Evaluation of the clinimetrics of transcutaneous oxygen measurement and its application in wound care. *International Wound Journal*, *12*(6), 625–629. https://doi.org/10.1111/iwj.12356.

Yokoyama, M., Yonezawa, K., Matsubara, M., Hikita, N., Sasagawa, E., & Haruna, M. (2022). The factors related to recovery time of diaper dermatitis in infants: A prospective observational study. *Japan Journal of Nursing Science*, *19*(4). https://doi.org/10.1111/jjns.12492.

Chapter 7

Evidence-Based Nursing Practices in Umbilical Cord Care

Esra Cumur Baskır[1,*], MSc
and Zeynem Yildirim Balkan[2], PhD
[1]Department of Child Health and Disease Nursing, Florence Nightingale Faculty of Nursing, Istanbul, Türkiye
[2]University Cerrahpaşa, Turkey Department of Nursing, Faculty of Health Sciences, Tekirdag Namık Kemal University, Tekirdag, Türkiye

Abstract

Approximately 2.5 million neonatal deaths occur every year in the world, most of them in low- and middle-income countries (Rosa Mangeret et al., 2022). Umbilical cord infections are among the main causes of these deaths. The umbilical cord, which is cut after the birth of a newborn, is an entry point for bacteria. Bacteria can rapidly colonize the moist cord and reach the bloodstream, causing sepsis and death (Aku et al., 2023; Şener Taplak and Bayat, 2016). The umbilical cord care applied to newborns prevents bacterial colonization and accelerates the natural separation time of the cord. The umbilical cord care applied to newborns aims to prevent bacterial colonization and accelerate the natural cord separation time (Shen et al., 2023). Neonatal deaths can be significantly reduced with the prevention of sepsis by providing appropriate, effective, and safe umbilical care. Against this, the best umbilical care in the postpartum period is still controversial (Quattrin et al., 2016; Abbaszadeh et al., 2016). The World Health Organization (WHO) recommends dry umbilical cord care in countries where obstetric care is adequate and neonatal mortality rates are low. However, in cases where infection rates are high and poor hygienic conditions exist, they recommend the use of topical antiseptics (World Health Organization, 2013; World Health Organization, 2017). Despite these recommendations, umbilical cord care practices are still affected by unreliable traditional practices and inequalities in healthcare. The effectiveness and safety of umbilical care should be investigated to ensure the best results during this period, which is critical for babies' lives (Reis et al., 2020). Evidence-based umbilical cord care practices such as topical human milk application, and application of antiseptic solutions such as chlorhexidine, 70% alcohol, triple dye, povidone iodide, and arnica montana extracts are of great importance in reducing morbidity and mortality due to sepsis.

* Corresponding Author's Email: esracumur25@gmail.com.

In: Evidence-Based Care Practices in Pediatric Nursing
Editors: Feyza Küçük and Serap Özdemir
ISBN: 979-8-89530-304-7

In this section, evidence-based interventions in umbilical cord care for newborns will be discussed in light of literature information.

Keywords: umbilical cord, care of the umbilicus, omphalitis, newborn, nursing care

Introduction

The umbilical cord forms a physical and psychological link between the mother and baby throughout pregnancy. Through this connection; the nutrients and oxygen in the maternal blood are transferred to the fetal blood, and wastes in the fetal blood are eliminated (Israel et al., 2023). With the cutting of the cord after birth, mother and baby are physically and symbolically separated. Within 5-15 days after birth, the cord stump dries, falls off, and the wound heals (Quattrin et al., 2016). The newly cut umbilical cord is susceptible to infections. The main reason for these infections is that in the neonatal period when the resistance to infection is very low, the umbilical cord creates an entry to an open source of infection in the skin (Aku et al., 2023; Şener Taplak and Bayat, 2016). The umbilical cord stump can be colonized by some gram-positive and negative bacteria, including S. Epidermidis, Escherichia coli and Klebsiella pneumonia, group A and B Streptococci, more specifically Staphylococcus aureus (Al-Shehri, 2019). Since the umbilical cord is an important bacterial colonization site in this respect, it can lead to omphalitis (Quattrin et al., 2016; Abbaszadeh et al., 2016). Omphalitis is an infection around the navel. Foul odor, redness, yellowish-green discharge, and tenderness around the navel are signs of infection (Bindler et al., 2014). Among the reasons that increase the risk of omphalitis; these include infection in the mother, birth under non-sterile conditions, long labor, home birth, umbilical catheterization, low birth weight, and inadequate cord care (Al-Shehri, 2019). As a result, omphalitis can cause neonatal sepsis and mortality. Therefore, omphalitis is a medical emergency that requires appropriate treatment to avoid negative sequelae (Al-Shehri, 2019; Abbaszadeh et al, 2016). Worldwide, 2.5 million infant deaths occur each year, the majority of which are caused by infections, accounting for 47% of all under-five deaths (Rosa Mangeret et al., 2022). The majority of deaths occur in countries with low socioeconomic status, with 75% of total neonatal deaths occurring in South Asia and Africa (Ans et al., 2023). Umbilical cord infection is responsible for more than 15% of neonatal sepsis and neonatal deaths and is the third leading cause of neonatal death worldwide (Aku et al., 2023; Kinanu et al., 2016). Due to the resulting risk of infection, umbilical cord care practice trends have changed frequently over many years (Kanisek et al., 2015). The main aim of umbilical care in newborns is to accelerate the natural detachment of the umbilical cord and shorten the detachment time, while preventing bacterial invasion and reducing the risk of umbilical infection (Shen et al., 2023).

Although there are different practices in the literature regarding umbilical cord care, each practice has advantages and disadvantages. In this section, evidence-based practices used in umbilical cord care will be discussed and reliable practices that can be used in umbilical cord care will be identified.

Research

'Umbilical cord care' describes procedures used to facilitate cord detachment and prevent bacteria from settling in the umbilical stump of the newborn (Israel et al., 2023). Although there is consensus that cutting the cord with a sterile cutting instrument (knife or scissors) and clean hands are important to prevent infection, it is not clear what is the best care for umbilical cord care (Quattrin et al., 2016; Abbaszadeh et al., 2016). The World Health Organization recommends that in areas with high neonatal mortality (30 or more neonatal deaths per 1000 live births), umbilical care of newborns born at home should be performed with a daily solution of chlorhexidine (4% chlorhexidine digluconate aqueous solution or gel, giving 4% chlorhexidine). In newborns born at home in environments with low risk of infection and in health facilities, it is recommended to keep the navel clean and dry as umbilical care (World Health Organization, 2013; World Health Organization, 2017). The basic principle in the care of the umbilical cord of the newborn is to keep the umbilicus and its surroundings clean and dry. After bathing the newborn, the umbilical cord must be kept dry. The umbilical cord should be checked for bleeding (Siroosbakht et al., 2021). Furthermore, the baby's diaper should be placed under the umbilical cord so that the umbilical cord remains outside, preventing the cord from coming into contact with the baby's diaper (Toksöz, 2023).

In routine umbilical care, dry care can be recommended in terms of low cost and ease of implementation (World Health Organization, 2013). Dry care, also called natural drying, is leaving the umbilical cord exposed to air without the use of routine topical agents (Toksöz, 2023; Çaksak et al., 2019). However, to leave the cord for natural drying, there are rules to be considered such as keeping the cord area clean and dry, following an aseptic technique, washing hands before touching the umbilical cord, cleaning the area with sterile water if the umbilical cord is contaminated, and drying with clean and dry gauze after cleaning (Toksöz, 2023; Conk et al., 2013). In a study conducted in Italy, dry umbilical cord care was reported to be an easy, simple, and reliable method in healthy newborns born in a high-income hospital (Quattrin et al., 2016). In a Slovenian study, the umbilical cord was classified according to its clinical status as healthy umbilical cord, umbilical cord at risk, and unhealthy umbilical cord. Dry umbilical cord care has been recommended for a healthy umbilicus and care with antiseptic solutions for at-risk or unhealthy umbilicus (Nosan and Paro Panjan, 2017). In regions with a low incidence of omphalitis, such as Spain, dry cord care remains the most appropriate approach (Castellanos, 2019). A French study compared the use of dry care and antiseptics in umbilical cord care. This study found that in high-income countries, the use of antiseptics is unnecessary, restrictive, and expensive and could be replaced by dry care (Guen et al., 2017). In a study examining the duration of umbilical cord separation, it was found that dry umbilical cord care is a safe practice that allows umbilical cord separation in a short time (López Medina et al., 2020). Although dry care is recommended in umbilical care, antiseptic agents are used, especially in environments where the risk of infection is high. There are many antiseptic solutions used. The main ones are chlorhexidine, 70% alcohol, triple dye, breast milk, povidone iodide, and arnica montana extracts (Toksöz, 2023; Çaksak et al., 2019; Coscia et al., 2021). With the use of topical antiseptics, the risk of infection in the newborn is reduced by preventing or reducing bacterial colonization on the skin or umbilical cord (Toksöz, 2023; Sankar et al., 2016).

Among the different antiseptics available, chlorhexidine (4% chlorhexidine, 7.1% chlorhexidine digluconate solution or gel) is the most studied agent in newborn babies (Shariff et al., 2016). Studies show a significant reduction in bacterial colonization rates in the umbilical cord after chlorhexidine treatment (Nosan and Paro Panjan, 2017; Sankar et al., 2016). Chlorhexidine is a broad-spectrum bisbiguanide that is effective against gram-negative and gram-positive microorganisms and has antibacterial properties. It is harmless to the sensitive skin of newborns (Israel et al., 2023). In a study, the use of chlorhexidine in umbilical cord care was found to reduce the risk of sepsis that may occur in the neonatal intensive care unit (Gathwala et al., 2013). In a study comparing the effect of breast milk, 4% chlorhexidine and the topical effects of dry care application on the clinical outcomes of bacterial colonization in preterm newborns, it was concluded that 4% chlorhexidine was highly effective in reducing pathogenic bacterial colonization of the cord (Lyngdoh et al., 2018). Even one use of chlorhexidine significantly reduces the risk of infection. High-quality evidence shows that umbilical cord care with chlorhexidine reduces the risk of omphalitis by 50% and neonatal deaths by 12% (Nosan ve Paro Panjan, 2017). Routine use of chlorhexidine is indicated in regions or settings with high incidences of omphalitis and associated neonatal mortality (Castellanos et al., 2019; López Medina, 2019). Since chlorhexidine is an evidence-based practice, its use will lead to the best outcomes in neonatal health (Owusu, 2023).

70% alcohol has been recommended in umbilical care for a long time, but recently it has been observed that it is less effective than other antiseptics in drying the navel and preventing infections (Çaksak et al., 2019). In a systematic review, topical alcohol application was found to be effective in reducing Enterococcus coli colonization (Imdad et al., 2013). In another Argentine study, leaving dry after body bathing with neutral soap and alcoholic care was compared in terms of colonization and duration of navel fall. While the fall time was shorter in dry care, colonization was found to be less in alcoholic care (Covas Mdel; 2011). In a meta-analysis study examining alcohol use versus dry care for the umbilical cord in newborns, it was shown that alcohol application prolonged the cord separation time, while there was no significant difference in terms of omphalitis risk (Al-Shehri, 2019). A different study compared the occurrence of adverse events and time to cord separation between neonates treated with dry cord care and neonates treated with 70% alcohol. It was reported that umbilical cord separation time was prolonged in newborns treated with 70% alcohol, but no significant adverse effects occurred in either group (Quattrin et al., 2016).

Triple dye (Brillant Green, Crystal Violet, and Proflavinehemisulfate) is an effective antiseptic against gram-positive bacteria (Çaksak et al., 2019). In a UK study comparing triple dye with alcohol, the umbilical cord was dropped 3 days earlier in babies who received alcohol umbilical care. Infection control was achieved in both applications (Golombek et al., 2002). In a systematic review, topical triple dye application was compared with both dry cord care and alcohol application. It was reported to significantly reduce Staphylococcus aureus bacterial colonization (Imdad et al., 2013).

Human milk is known to have antibacterial and antiviral effects. Human milk includes large amounts of IgA antibodies, and these appear to have an inhibitory effect on skin infections. In addition to provide excellent immune support, human milk promotes musculoskeletal repair and growth (Allam et al., 2015). Lactoferrin, found in human milk, helps babies resist Escherichia Coli. It also reduces the risk of infectious diseases in babies, which are usually caused by microorganisms such as viruses. Some studies report that infusion of colostrum into the oral cavity has a positive effect on gastrointestinal functions and can prevent ventilator-associated pneumonia (Ji and Zhang, 2016; Frank et al., 2019). Human milk can also effectively prevent otitis media, respiratory diseases, diarrhea, and gastrointestinal diseases (Shen et al, 2023). Administration of human milk to the cord root is one of the cultural cord care practices used in Turkey. According to the World Health Organization, the large number of immunological and anti-infective agents found in human milk may also be beneficial in terms of antibacterial factors. Colostrum contains significant amounts of components that act as natural antimicrobial agents and protective factors that provide passive immunity (Allam et al., 2015; Abbaszadeh et al., 2016). The effect of topical application of human milk in umbilical cord care was examined on the incidence of omphalitis and the duration of umbilical cord separation. The cord care model with topical breast milk was found to reduce the risk of omphalitis and accelerate cord separation time compared to dry open treatment (Kasiati et al., 2013). As a result of a study, it was found that topical application of human milk to the remaining part of the cord decreased the cord separation time and can be used as an easy, inexpensive, and noninvasive method in cord care (Allam et al., 2015). Another study compared the effect of topical use of human milk and chlorhexidine solution on cord separation time in umbilical cord care of the newborn. It has been shown that topical application of breast milk in umbilical cord care shortens the cord separation time and can be used as an easy, inexpensive, and harmless method in umbilical cord care (Abbaszadeh et al., 2016). In another study comparing human milk, chlorhexidine, and dry cord care methods, all three methods were found to be effective in controlling bacterial colonization in the umbilical cord (Yaghoobi et al., 2019).

Povidone iodide is an effective method in umbilical care due to its broad-spectrum antibiotic properties. However, there are opinions that its use in newborns is contraindicated due to its thyroid toxicity effect (Çaksak et al., 2019).

In a study evaluating the effect of arnica montana on cord separation, the umbilical cord of infants was treated with a natural dermo-protective powder containing arnica montana. The use of a natural skin protectant powder containing Arnica montana has been found to shorten the cord separation time and reduce the risk of complications (Coscia et al., 2021).

Conclusion

Infections are an important cause of morbidity and mortality for the newborn. The umbilical cord is an important source of infection. It is possible to reduce the risk of morbidity and mortality by providing appropriate umbilical cord care. Therefore, evidence-based umbilical cord care practices gain importance. The use of topical antiseptics is an intervention that can reduce cases of infection in newborns by preventing or reducing bacterial colonization of the skin or umbilical cord. Although the antiseptics used have advantages and disadvantages, it is a clinical fact that they reduce the risk of omphalitis. The most commonly used solutions for umbilical cord care are chlorhexidine and 70% alcohol. The World Health Organization recommends dry care for umbilical care in developed countries and especially chlorhexidine as a topical agent in developing countries where infectious diseases are common. More interventional studies are needed to clarify the effectiveness of the antiseptics used.

Disclaimer

The authors declare that they have no competing interests.

References

Abbaszadeh, F., Hajizadeh, Z., & Jahangiri, M. (2016). Comparing the impact of topical application of human milk and chlorhexidine on cord separation time in newborns. *Pakistan journal of medical sciences*, 32(1), 239.

Abbaszadeh, F., Hajizadeh, Z., & Jahangiri, M. (2016). Comparing the impact of topical application of human milk and chlorhexidine on cord separation time in newborns. *Pakistan journal of medical sciences*, 32(1), 239.

Aku, N. O., Amakulor, G., & Onuorah, C. (2023). Prevalent cord-stump care practices among mothers of infants: Against the backdrop of chlorhexidine digluconate gel scale-up. *Journal of Neonatal Nursing*, 29(2), 350-355.

Aku, N. O., Amakulor, G., & Onuorah, C. (2023). Prevalent cord-stump care practices among mothers of infants: Against the backdrop of chlorhexidine digluconate gel scale-up. *Journal of Neonatal Nursing*, 29(2), 350-355.

Allam, N. A., Wafa, A., & Talat, A. M. (2015). The effect of topical application of mother milk on separation of umbilical cord for newborn babies. *American Journal of Nursing Science*, 4(5), 288-296.

Al-Shehri, H. (2019). The use of alcohol versus dry care for the umbilical cord in newborns: A systematic review and meta-analysis of randomized and non-randomized studies. *Cureus*, 11(7).

Al-Shehri, H. (2019). The Use of Alcohol versus Dry Care for the Umbilical Cord in Newborns: A Systematic Review and Meta-analysis of Randomized and Non-randomized Studies. *Cureus*, 11 (7), e5103.

Ans, M., Hussain, M., Ahmed, F., Khan, K. J., Abbas, S., & Sultan, M. (2023). Umbilical Cord Care Practices and Cord Care Education of Mothers Attending Health Care (Pakistan Prospect). *Health*, 15(1), 20-32.

Bindler RCM, Ball JW, London LM, Davidson MR, (2014). Anne ve Çocuk Hemşireliği Klinik Uygulama Becerileri Kitabı. 50-51. NC Şahiner, A Açıkgöz, MD Bal (Çev Ed), Nobel Akademik Yayıncılık, Ankara.

Castellanos, J. L. L., Muñuzuri, A. P., Campillo, C. W. R., López, E. S., Fernández, I. B., Redondo, M. D. S., ... & Luna, M. S. (2019). Recommendations for the care of the umbilical cord in the newborn. *Anales de Pediatría* (English Edition), 90(6), 401-e1.

Chen, Y. C., Song, Y., & Song, B. P. (2017). Study on the timing of umbilical cord ligation in neonates. *Laboratory Medicine and Clinical*, 14(1), 106–108.

Conk, Z., Başbakkal, Z., Yılmaz, H. B., & Bolışık, B. (2013). *Pediatri hemşireliği.* Akademisyen Tıp Kitapevleri.

Coscia, A., Boscarino, G., Di Chiara, M., Faccioli, F., Pedicino, R., Onestà, E., ... & Terrin, G. (2021). Umbilical cord medication in healthy full-term newborns: a before-after uncontrolled quality improvement study. *European Journal of Pediatrics*, 180, 505-511.

Covas Mdel C, Alda E, Medina MS, Ventura S, Pezutti O, Paris De Baeza A, et al, (2011). Alcohol versus bath and natural drying for term newborns umbilical cord care: a prospective randomized clinical trial. *Arch Argent Pediatr*. 109 (4), 305-13.

Çaksak, A., Yıldız, D., Eren Fidancı, B., & Çalık B. (2019). Evidence Based Practices in Umbilical Cord Care. *Eurasian JHS*;2(1):20-26.

Frank, N. M., Lynch, K. F., Uusitalo, U., Yang, J., Lönnrot, M., Virtanen, S. M., Hyöty, H., & Norris, J. M. (2019). The relationship between breastfeeding and reported respiratory and gastrointestinal infection rates in young children. *BMC Pediatrics*, 19(1), 339. Published 2019 Sep 18. https://doi.org/10.1186/s12887-019-1693-2.

Gathwala, G., Sharma, D., & Bhakhri, B. K. (2013). Effect of topical application of chlorhexidine for umbilical cord care in comparison with conventional dry cord care on the risk of neonatal sepsis: a randomized controlled trial. *Journal of tropical pediatrics*, 59(3), 209-213.

Golombek SG, Brill PE, Salice AL, (2002). Randomized trial of alcohol versus triple dye for umbilical cord care. *Clin Pediatr* (Phila). 41 (6), 419-23.

Guen, G. L., Caille, A., Launay, E., Boscher, C., Godon, N., Savagner, C., ... & Giraudeau, B. (2017). Dry care versus antiseptics for umbilical cord care: a cluster randomized trial. *Pediatrics,* 139(1).

Imdad, A., Bautista, R. M. M., Senen, K. A. A., Uy, M. E. V., Mantaring III, J. B., & Bhutta, Z. A. (2013). Umbilical cord antiseptics for preventing sepsis and death among newborns. *Cochrane Database of Systematic Reviews*, (5).

Israel, C. E., Attama, K. O., Opara, H. C., Ihudiebube-Splendor, C. N., & Omotola, N. J. (2023). Knowledge and use of chorhexidine gel in umbilical cord care among postpartum women at Poly General Hospital, Enugu, Southeast Nigeria: a cross-sectional study. *International Health,* ihad061.

Israel, C. E., Attama, K. O., Opara, H. C., Ihudiebube-Splendor, C. N., & Omotola, N. J. (2023). Knowledge and use of chorhexidine gel in umbilical cord care among postpartum women at Poly General Hospital, Enugu, Southeast Nigeria: a cross-sectional study. *International Health*, ihad061.

Ji, F. T., & Zhang, Y. X. (2016). A study on the safety and feasibility of colostrum oral application to very low birth weight infants. *Nursing Research*, 30(11), 3882–3885.

Kanisek, S., Prlić, N., Barać, I., & Nemet, L. D. (2015). Differences in newborn umbilical cord care. *Medicinski Glasnik,* 12(2).

Kasiati, K., Santoso, B., Yunitasari, E., & Nursalam, N. (2013). Topical Breastmilk: Nursing Care of Newborn Umbilical Cord Model. *Jurnal Ners*, 8(1), 9-16.

Kinanu, L., Odhiambo, E., Mwaura, J., & Habtu, M. (2016). Cord care practices and omphalitis among neonates aged 3-28 days at Pumwani Maternity Hospital, Kenya. *Journal of Biosciences and Medicines*, 4(01), 27.

López-Medina, M. D., Linares-Abad, M., López-Araque, A. B., & López-Medina, I. M. (2019). Dry care versus chlorhexidine cord care for prevention of omphalitis. Systematic review with meta-analysis. *Revista latino-americana de enfermagem*, 27, e3106.

López-Medina, M. D., López-Araque, A. B., Linares-Abad, M., & López-Medina, I. M. (2020). Umbilical cord separation time, predictors and healing complications in newborns with dry care. *PLoS One*, 15(1), e0227209.

Lyngdoh, D., Kaur, S., Kumar, P., Gautam, V., & Ghai, S. (2018). Effect of topical application of human breast milk versus 4% chlorhexidine versus dry cord care on bacterial colonization and clinical outcomes of umbilical cord in preterm newborns. *Journal of Clinical Neonatology*, 7(1), 25. https://doi.org/
10.4103/JCN.JCN 91 17.

Nosan, G., & Paro-Panjan, D. (2017). Umbilical cord care: national survey, literature review and recommendations. *The Journal of Maternal-Fetal & Neonatal Medicine*, 30(14), 1655-1658.

Owusu, L. B., Zakaria, A. F. S., Agyapong, S., Akokre, R., & Adebanji, A. O. (2023). Care of the newborn's umbilical cord: The perspectives of mothers in a developing country. *Journal of Neonatal Nursing*, 29(6), 832-838.

Quattrin, R., Iacobucci, K., De Tina, A. L., Gallina, L., Pittini, C., & Brusaferro, S. (2016). 70% alcohol versus dry cord care in the umbilical cord care: a case–control study in Italy. *Medicine,* 95(14), e3207.

Reis, M. R., de Sousa, M. C., de Souza Silva, L., Conceição, L. R. R., de Andrade Silvestre, M., Sudário, C. D. P. S., ... & Salge, A. K. M. (2020). Factors associated with umbilical cord stump healing practices: literature review. *Open Journal of Obstetrics and Gynecology*, 10(8), 1067-1078.

Rosa-Mangeret, F., Benski, A. C., Golaz, A., Zala, P. Z., Kyokan, M., Wagner, N., ... & Pfister, R. E. (2022). 2.5 million annual deaths—are neonates in low-and middle-income countries too small to be seen? A bottom-up overview on neonatal morbi-mortality. *Tropical medicine and infectious disease*, 7(5), 64.

Sankar, M. J., Chandrasekaran, A., Ravindranath, A., Agarwal, R., & Paul, V. K. (2016). Umbilical cord cleansing with chlorhexidine in neonates: a systematic review. Journal of Perinatology, 36(1), S12-S20.

Shariff, J. A., Lee, K. C., Leyton, A., & Abdalal, S. (2016). Neonatal mortality and topical application of chlorhexidine on umbilical cord stump: a meta-analysis of randomized control trials. *Public Health*, 139, 27-35.

Shen, J., Shen, M., & Jin, A. (2023). Application of breast milk smears in umbilical care of full-term newborn. *Biotechnology and Genetic Engineering Reviews*, 1-11.

Shen, J., Shen, M., & Jin, A. (2023). Application of breast milk smears in umbilical care of full-term newborn. *Biotechnology and Genetic Engineering Reviews*, 1-11.

Siroosbakht, S., Aarabi, N., & Rezakhaniha, B. (2021). Bathing or not bathing: which is better for Umbilical Cord Separation Time and bacterial colonization in neonates? *Archives of Pediatric Infectious Diseases*, 9(2).

Şener Taplak, A., & Bayat, M. (2016). Yenidoğanlarda Göbek Bakımında Kanıta Dayalı Uygulamalar. *Florence Nightingale Hemşirelik Dergisi*, 23(3), 252. https://doi.org/10.17672/fnhd.64484.

Toksöz, F. (2023). Sağlıklı Yenidoğanın Doğum Sonrası Temel Hijyenik Bakım Gereksinimleri. *Hitit Medical Journal,* 5(2), 117-121.

World Health Organization. (2013). Recommendations on Postnatal Care of the Mother and Newborn. https://www.who.int/publications/i/item/9789241506649.

World Health Organization. (2017). WHO Recommendations on newborn health: guidelines approved by the WHO guidelines review com- mittee. 2017. Available from https://apps.who.int/iris/handle/10665/259269 [accessed October 6, 2024].

Yaghoobi, M., Bolandi, B., Namaei, M., & Faal, G. (2019). Comparing the effect of topical application of breast milk, chlorhexidine and dry cord care methods on bacterial colonization in umbilical cord of preterm neonates in NICU: a randomized clinical trial. *Electronic Physician*, 11(2).

Chapter 8

Evidence-Based Nursing Practices in Relieving Colic Infants

Aylin Kurt*, PhD

Department of Nursing, Faculty of Health Science, Bartın University, Bartın, Türkiye

Abstract

Infantile colic is defined as restlessness and crying spells that have been present for more than three weeks, at least three days a week, exceeding three hours a day, and cannot be explained for any other reason. It is a common reason for infants to be brought to the physician. Despite numerous suggested risk factors, its exact etiology remains unknown. There is no definitive method for treating infantile colic that can be considered both effective and safe. This condition causes anxiety for families and pediatricians alike, as the crying and restlessness in infants can suggest a range of potential underlying issues, including infections, gastrointestinal problems, trauma, nutritional issues, drug reactions, neurological causes, and cardiovascular diseases. Continuous crying in a baby can cause parents to feel frustrated, and inadequate, lose concentration and patience, fear harming the baby, and stop breastfeeding early.

In this section, we discuss methods used to reduce the symptoms of infantile colic, such as massage, manipulative therapies (such as chiropractic, osteopathy, cranial osteopathy, craniosacral therapy, and cranial manipulation), dietary changes, and the use of probiotics and prebiotics (synbiotics). Additionally, parent education programs offer a range of techniques to help parents care for their infants. These techniques include calming strategies for crying infants, understanding infants' needs, general care recommendations such as sleep and feeding advice, stress reduction, and empathic counseling for parents. Understanding infants' needs is crucial for providing appropriate care.

Keywords: infants, colic, pediatric nursing

* Corresponding Author's Email: akurt@bartin.edu.tr.

In: Evidence-Based Care Practices in Pediatric Nursing
Editors: Feyza Küçük and Serap Özdemir
ISBN: 979-8-89530-304-7

Introduction

Infantile colic is a syndrome that is most common in infancy, has no known cause, occurs in attacks, and is characterized by clenched fists, abdominal rigidity, flatulence, pulling of the legs toward the abdomen, and excessive crying that is very difficult to stop (Zeevenhooven et al., 2018). Infantile colic is defined as unexplained and uncontrollable crying spells that last for more than three hours a day, occurring more than three days a week and continuing for at least three weeks. These crying spells usually occur in the afternoon and/or evening hours (Wessel et al., 1954). The incidence of infantile colic varies depending on the population studied and ranges from 3% to 40% (Ellwood et al., 2020; Hjern et al., 2020; Wolke et al., 2019). Infantile colic can be a challenging situation for infants, families, and healthcare professionals to manage (Gordon et al., 2019). Frequent and prolonged crying spells can cause significant behavioral problems in the baby's sleep, rest, and feeding (Uysal et al., 2017).

Infantile colic is a condition that is more prevalent in boys during early childhood (Alagöz & Ertekin, 2013; Gelfand, 2016; Hannula et al., 2020; Mutlu et al., 2020; Vaziri et al., 2018). Maternal smoking during pregnancy and after childbirth, as well as nicotine replacement therapy, can trigger infantile colic and increase the risk (Johnson et al., 2015; Sarasu et al., 2018; Zeevenhooven et al., 2018). Furthermore, research has shown that smoking inside the household can increase the likelihood of infantile colic in babies (Alagöz & Ertekin, 2013). In their study examining the factors affecting infants with colic, Uysal et al. (2017) found that 59.3% of the infants were male, 46.4% were fed with a combination of breast milk and formula in a bottle, and infantile colic was more common in younger infants. Additionally, advanced maternal age was identified as a risk factor. (Johnson et al., 2015; Sarasu et al., 2018; Zeevenhooven et al., 2018).

Nurses who work with families and children often encounter cases of infantile colic. Parents of infants with colic can experience a range of emotions, including anger, frustration, fatigue, guilt, and depression (Sung, 2018). The mental state of the mother is particularly impacted (Twomey et al., 2012; Zeevenhooven et al., 2018). To calm a baby with infantile colic, it can be helpful to use soothing methods such as patting the back and rhythmic rocking in a quiet environment before resorting to analgesics. However, it is important to note that these methods may only provide temporary relief and should not be relied upon as the sole solution. It is also important to consider consulting a healthcare professional for further guidance (Akçay Didişen et al., 2020). It is important for parents that their baby remains calm (Sarasu et al., 2018). It should not be forgotten that family counseling is the most effective solution in dealing with infantile colic, and plans should be made accordingly (Lam et al., 2019).

Nurses should adopt a family-centered approach to caring for colicky infants. During this period, the family is at the center of the baby's life. Nurses should assist the family in identifying practices that soothe and calm the baby (Lam et al., 2019). It has been observed that infants are less likely to cry and are more relaxed and peaceful when they are with their parents (Gordon et al., 2019; Salisbury et al., 2012). In their study of infants with colic and their parents, Salisbury et al. (2012) found that infants in the group receiving family-centered care cried less, were fed more quickly, and had longer sleep durations compared to the group receiving standard pediatric care. Therefore, strengthening parental self-efficacy in the care of colicky infants is an important aspect of nursing care (Lam et al., 2019; Zeevenhooven et al., 2018).

Evidence-Based Nursing Practices in Relieving Colic Infants

The uncertain cause of infantile colic, the lack of effective treatment, and the ambiguity of whether it is a part of normal development or a disease, as well as the absence of a standard protocol, make treatment difficult (Sung, 2018). It is believed that treatment is necessary due to the potential to cause unrest within the family and harm the parent-child relationship (Benninga et al., 2016; Zeevenhooven et al., 2017, 2018). Firstly, it is important to inform parents that infantile colic will naturally decrease after 3-4 months and is not a chronic illness. It should also be emphasized that the baby's development will continue during this time, and parents should be gentle and calm with their baby (Lam et al., 2019). It is recommended to provide parents with advice on nutrition, diet, and baby care (Akçam & Aslan, 2019).

The interventions applied in the treatment of infantile colic are dietary therapy and behavioral therapy. Behavioral therapy is the most widely accepted method (Bagci et al., 2020; Çelik, 2016; Ellwood et al., 2020; Johnson et al., 2015; Salisbury et al., 2012; Savino et al., 2015).

Dietary Practices

Dietary approaches to infantile colic can be considered as approaches for both mother and baby (Çelik, 2016). Food consumed by the mother can cause sensitivity in the baby through breast milk. It is recommended that the mother's diet exclude allergenic foods such as citrus fruits, eggs, cola, cow's milk, chocolate, legumes, nuts, and dairy products (Iacovou et al., 2012). Herbal teas may be beneficial in improving the symptoms of infantile colic (Alagöz & Ertekin, 2013).

To determine the effectiveness of a diet application, it should be continued and monitored for at least two weeks. If it is effective, it is recommended to continue (Savino et al., 2015). Additionally, if the mother indicates that crying is due to the food she eats, and crying resumes when she starts consuming the food again, the mother should avoid consuming these foods for a few months (Reinthal et al., 2011).

Infantile colicky babies who are fed with breast milk should continue to receive breast milk and should not receive formula (Hall et al., 2012). Breastfeeding at night can help the baby sleep and reduce infantile colic due to the presence of melatonin in breast milk (Savino et al. 2014). For formula-fed babies, the first approach is to recommend prebiotic hydrolyzed formulas and support a low-allergen maternal diet (Savino et al., 2015).

Mothers may use herbal products such as fennel, cumin, dill, lemon balm, yarrow, chamomile, ginger, licorice root, and mint for the treatment of infantile colic, based on the advice of healthcare professionals or their social circles (Alves et al., 2012; Çetinkaya, 2021; Evans & Lorentz, 2022). These herbs have been reported to have antispasmodic effects and are effective in reducing infantile colic pain and durations of crying (Alagöz & Ertekin, 2013; Ertekin, 2013). Plant teas have the property of causing diarrhea and reducing iron absorption

(Johnson et al., 2015). Furthermore, studies with a higher level of evidence are needed to demonstrate that these plants can be used safely in children before recommending them (Johnson et al., 2015; Perry et al., 2019).

Another approach is that when babies receive sufficient amounts of probiotics, the microbial balance in their intestines is regulated, resulting in positive effects on the baby's health (Foster et al., 2022). Probiotics are used as an effective method for relief from infantile colic pain (Perry et al., 2019; Simonson et al., 2021). In a study conducted by Savino and Tarasco (2010), the symptoms of colic were found to be more effectively treated with probiotics than in the control group. In their 2015 study, Mi et al. found that probiotics significantly reduced crying time in infants with colic and were effective in treating colic. According to the systematic review in Cochrane, there is no conclusive evidence that probiotics are more effective in preventing infantile colic, but a decrease in daily crying time has been observed (Ong et al., 2019; Perry et al., 2019).

Many studies have been conducted on the use of probiotics in the treatment of infantile colic (Perry et al., 2019; Simonson et al., 2021). There are differences between the results of these studies and data on the efficacy of probiotics are controversial. In a study by Chau et al. in 2015, regression in colic symptoms was found when Lactobacillus Reuteri preparation was given to breastfed colicky infants. In their systematic review study, Anabrees et al. concluded that the use of probiotics in breastfed infants may bring positive results, but their efficacy in formula-fed infants is controversial (Simonson et al., 2021).

In general, it has been observed that the effects of nutritional approaches are difficult to demonstrate with certainty and may be dangerous to apply (Ong et al., 2019; Perry et al., 2019). Therefore, it is not recommended to try any type of formula in breastfed infants with infantile colic and hypoallergenic formulas in formula-fed infants with low suspicion of food allergy (Zamanillo-Campos et al., 2022). It is very important to ensure the continuation of breastfeeding, especially in breastfed infants (Verduci et al., 2021).

Another method used to relieve colicky babies is herbal teas. Many herbal teas such as fennel, chamomile, lemon oil, cinnamon, and ginger have been used by the public for years (Harputluoğlu et al., 2022). There are reservations about the use of these teas as a treatment, such as the lack of a certain standard of dosage and ingredients, damage to the breastfeeding process, and possible side effects due to the toxins they contain (Harputluoğlu et al., 2022). In addition to the negative aspects, scientific studies have not provided conclusive evidence that these methods reduce colic symptoms (Gavish et al., 2023).

Behavioral Methods

Factors such as the limited effectiveness of the drugs used for Kolik, their side effects, and the difficulty of long-term use (Cabanillas-Barea et al., 2023; Kesavelu, 2023); the insufficient effectiveness of dietary therapy (Zeevenhooven et al., 2018), and the severity of symptoms causing significant anxiety (Zeevenhooven et al., 2017) have led nurses and parents to seek behavioral options.

The initial approach for infants without any health risks is non-invasive and non-pharmacological treatments (Savino et al., 2015). The methods included in the '5S technique' for the treatment of infantile colic are recommended to be used before medication. The 5S technique consists of Swaddling, Side or Stomach positioning, Shhh sound, Swinging, and Sucking (Botha et al., 2020; Reinthal et al., 2011).

Behavioral treatment methods include massage, rocking, car rides, carrying, pacifier use, swaddling, warm application to the abdomen, hair dryer sound, swinging in a hammock, vacuum cleaner sound, laying on the mother's chest, white noise, acupuncture, chiropractic treatment, reflexology, and other similar practices (Azeez et al., 2023; Ellwood et al., 2020; Sarasu et al., 2018; Zeevenhooven et al., 2018). However, studies on the effectiveness of these methods for infantile colic in babies are limited, and there is insufficient evidence to support their use (Biagioli et al., 2016; Hall et al., 2012; Johnson et al., 2015).

The following are some of the behavioral therapy methods.

White Noise

The sound is a mixture of various frequencies from the environment and is a constant, droning, noisy, and monotonous sound that covers all disturbing sounds from the external environment. It also includes intrauterine sounds; therefore, when it is heard, it is similar to the sounds of the uterus and has been found to be effective in calming infants with colic (Sezici & Yiğit, 2018). In the literature, it has been found that playing white noise to infants with colic reduces their crying time, increases their duration of sleep, and is effective in reducing colic pain levels (Çelik, 2016; Sezici & Yiğit, 2018).

Massage

It is reported that massage, which is a systematic touch, reduces the stress level of infants, stimulates the neuro-endocrine system, and increases nutrient absorption. Massage is widely used in infants with infantile colic (Sheidaei et al., 2016; Zeevenhooven et al., 2018). Massage applied to the abdomen for fifteen minutes helps outflow of gas and stool and can alleviate contraction and pain in the intestines. In the literature, the application of massage in infantile colic has been proven to be effective in sleep, emptying, crying, and colic attacks (Sheidaei et al., 2016). It also reduces the stress level of the baby and increases mother-baby bonding (Mansouri et al., 2018).

Acupuncture

Acupuncture, which has a wide variety of approaches, is an ancient Asian medical practice. According to Western medicine, it is defined as 'sensory stimulation of the nervous system'. Since it affects the central nervous system, it has been proven to be effective in reducing the symptoms of infantile colic (Landgren & Hallström, 2017). In studies on the symptoms of infantile colic with acupuncture, it was found that there was a decrease in anxiety and stress, flatulence, and crying (Lee et al., 2018; Reinthal et al., 2011). However, they concluded that acupuncture should not be recommended regularly in infants because it is a needle intervention (Perry et al., 2019; Skjeie et al., 2018). On the other hand, some studies have found no benefit (Perry et al., 2019). They concluded that studies with a larger population are needed to determine the use, effectiveness, and safety of acupuncture and are not recommended (Dobson et al., 2014; Hjern et al., 2020).

Manual Therapy

The applications of manual therapy are very diverse. They include osteopathy, spinal manipulation, visceral osteopathy, and craniosacral therapy (Miller et al., 2012). Although most studies on manual therapy and infantile colic have shown positive data supporting its use as a moderately safe approach, no consensus has yet been reached on the best manual therapy approach for infantile colic. Chiropractic is a manual massage method applied to the chroniosacral region along the individual's spinal cord (Castejón-Castejón et al., 2019). In randomized controlled trials, it was found that chiropractic application is an effective method that reduces crying time and increases sleep duration in infants with infantile colic (Castejón-Castejón et al., 2019; Miller et al., 2012). In another study against these studies, chiropractic application was found to be an ineffective method in infants with infantile colic (Miller et al., 2012). The use of chiropractic application in the treatment of infants with colic is still controversial (Dobson et al., 2014).

Reflexology

It is a technique in which light pressure is applied to reflex points on the hands, ears, and feet to activate the human body's own healing and bring the body into a state of deep relaxation. In other words, each organ actually has a point where it is reflected in the feet and hands, and each organ is in a relationship with this reflection area (Hannula et al., 2020). Studies evaluating the application of reflexology in infantile colic are limited. According to a study conducted by Hannula et al. (2020) in infants with infantile colic, it was shown that there was a significant decrease in colic symptoms in the group in which reflexology was applied compared to the control group. Icke and Genc (2018) examined the effectiveness of reflexology application in infants with infantile colic and found that reflexology reduced the infantile colic scale score.

Conclusion

Infantile colic is a difficult condition to deal with for the infant, family, and healthcare professionals. Frequent and prolonged crying bouts may cause significant behavioral problems in the baby's sleep, rest, and feeding. On the other hand, caring for a baby with colic can be challenging for the whole family. There are some studies using pharmacologic, nonpharmacologic, and nutritional approaches to reduce symptoms in infants with infantile colic. Although these studies show that various pharmacological, nutritional, and behavioral interventions are effective in the treatment of infantile colic, there is no easy and definitive solution to the problem. However, dietary practices, and behavioral methods (white noise, massage, acupuncture, manual therapy, and reflexology) may be effective in increasing the sleep duration of infants and decreasing colic severity and crying duration.

References

Akçam, M., & Aslan, N. (2019). Colicum infantum. *Journal of Clinical Medicine Pediatrics*, *11*(1), 29–33.

Akçay Didişen, N., Yavuz, B., Özalp Gerçeker, G., Albayrak, T., Atak, M., & Başbakkal, D. Z. (2020). Infantile colic in infants aged one-six months and the practices of mothers for colic. *The Journal of Pediatric Research*, *7*(3), 223–229. https://doi.org/10.4274/jpr.galenos.2019.72687.

Alagöz, H., & Ertekin, V. (2013). Incidence, risk factors and different treatment options of infantile colic in eastern of turkey. *Journal of Contemporary Medicine*, *3*(1), 1–6. https://doi.org/10.5455/ctd.2013-90.

Alves, J. G. B., De Brito, R. D. C. C. M., & Cavalcanti, T. S. (2012). Effectiveness of mentha piperita in the treatment of infantile colic: A crossover study. *Evidence-Based Complementary and Alternative Medicine*, *2012*. https://doi.org/10.1155/2012/981352.

Azeez, G. K., Al-Rabati, A., & Hasan, S. S. (2023). The effectiveness of massaging, swaddling, and reflexology intervention in mothers' practices regarding infantile colic. *Journal of Medicinal and Chemical Sciences*, *6*(10), 2273–2281. https://doi.org/10.26655/JMCHEMSCI.2023.10.2.

Bagci, H., Cinar Yucel, S., & Bagcı, H. (2020). A systematic review of the studies about therapeutic rouch after the year of 2000. *International Journal of Caring Sciences*, *13*(1), 231–240. www.international journalofcaringsciences.org.

Benninga, M. A., Nurko, S., Faure, C., Hyman, P. E., St James Roberts, I., & Schechter, N. L. (2016). Childhood functional gastrointestinal disorders: Neonate/toddler. *Gastroenterology*, *150*(6), 1443-1455.e2. https://doi.org/10.1053/j.gastro.2016.02.016.

Biagioli, E., Tarasco, V., Lingua, C., Moja, L., & Savino, F. (2016). Pain-relieving agents for infantile colic. *Cochrane Database of Systematic Reviews*, *2016*(9), 1–86. https://doi.org/10.1002/14651858.CD009999.pub2.

Botha, E., Helminen, M., Kaunonen, M., Lubbe, W., & Joronen, K. (2020). The effects of an infant calming intervention on mothers' parenting self-efficacy and satisfaction during the postpartum period: A randomized controlled trial. *Journal of Perinatal and Neonatal Nursing*, *34*(4), 300–310. https://doi.org/10.1097/JPN.0000000000000510.

Cabanillas-Barea, S., Jiménez-del-Barrio, S., Carrasco-Uribarren, A., Ortega-Martínez, A., Pérez-Guillén, S., & Ceballos-Laita, L. (2023). Systematic review and meta-analysis showed that complementary and alternative medicines were not effective for infantile colic. *Acta Paediatrica, International Journal of Paediatrics*, *112*(7), 1378–1388. https://doi.org/10.1111/apa.16807.

Castejón-Castejón, M., Murcia-González, Gil, J. L. M., Todri, J., Rancel, M. S., Lena, O., & Chillón-Martínez, R. (2019). Effectiveness of craniosacral therapy in the treatment of infantile colic. A randomized controlled trial. *Complementary Therapies in Medicine*, *47*, 102164. https://doi.org/10.1016/j.ctim.
2019.07.023.

Çelik, M. Y. (2016). Infantile colic and nursing approaches: review. *Turkiye Klinikleri Journal of Nursing*, *8*(4), 335–342. https://doi.org/10.5336/nurses.2015-47999.

Çetinkaya, B. (2021). Complementary and alternative therapies for infantile colic: A systematic review of the literature. *Alternative Therapies in Health and Medicine*, *27*(2), 42–47.

Chau, K., Lau, E., Greenberg, S., Jacobson, S., Yazdani-Brojeni, P., Verma, N., & Koren, G. (2015). Probiotics for infantile colic: A randomized, double-blind, placebo-controlled trial investigating lactobacillus reuteri DSM 17938. *The Journal of Pediatrics*, *166*(1), 74–78. https://doi.org/10.46299/isg.2021.mono.med.ii-254-266.

Dobson, D., Lucassen, P., Miller, J., Vlieger, A., Prescott, P., & Lewith, G. (2014). Manipulative therapies for infantile colic. *Cochrane Database of Systematic Reviews*, *20*(5), A114–A114. https://doi.org/10.1089/acm.2014.5303.abstract.

Ellwood, J., Draper-Rodi, J., & Carnes, D. (2020). Comparison of common interventions for the treatment of infantile colic: A systematic review of reviews and guidelines. *BMJ Open*, *10*(2), e035405. https://doi.org/10.1136/bmjopen-2019-035405.

Evans, C., & Lorentz, W. P. (2022). Efficacy and safety of a colic relief remedy in infantile colic. *Global Pediatric Health*, *9*, 1–7. https://doi.org/10.1177/2333794X221100810.

Foster, J. P., Dahlen, H. G., Fijan, S., Badawi, N., Schmied, V., Thornton, C., Smith, C., & Psaila, K. (2022). Probiotics for preventing and treating infant regurgitation: A systematic review and meta-analysis. *Maternal and Child Nutrition*, *18*(1), 1–15. https://doi.org/10.1111/mcn.13290.

Gavish, L., Korchia, G., Cohen, S., & Maor, Y. (2023). A real-world evaluation of an herbal treatment for infantile colic reported by 1218 parents in Israel. *Journal of Pediatric Nursing*, *69*, e39–e44. https://doi.org/10.1016/j.pedn.2022.12.002.

Gelfand, A. A. (2016). Infant colic. *Seminars in Pediatric Neurology*, *23*(1), 79–82. https://doi.org/10.1016/j.spen.2015.08.003.Infant.

Gordon, M., Gohil, J., & Banks, S. S. C. (2019). Parent training programmes for managing infantile colic. *Cochrane Database of Systematic Reviews*, *2019*(12), 1–53. https://doi.org/10.1002/14651858.CD012459.pub2.

Hall, B., Chesters, J., & Robinson, A. (2012). Infantile colic: A systematic review of medical and conventional therapies. *Journal of Paediatrics and Child Health*, *48*(2), 128–137. https://doi.org/10.1111/j.1440-1754.2011.02061.x.

Hannula, L., Puukka, P., Asunmaa, M., & Mäkijärvi, M. (2020). A pilot study of parents' experiences of reflexology treatment for infants with colic in Finland. *Scandinavian Journal of Caring Sciences*, *34*(4), 861–870. https://doi.org/10.1111/scs.12790.

Harputluoğlu, N., Bağ, Ö., Tuncel, T., & Bekem Soylu, Ö. (2022). The frequency of use of complementary and alternative medicine in infantile colic and factors affecting method Selection. *Meandros Medical and Dental Journal*, *23*(3), 349–354. https://doi.org/10.4274/meandros.galenos.2022.82712.

Hjern, A., Lindblom, K., Reuter, A., & Silfverdal, S. A. (2020). A systematic review of prevention and treatment of infantile colic. *Acta Paediatrica, International Journal of Paediatrics*, *109*(9), 1733–1744. https://doi.org/10.1111/apa.15247.

Iacovou, M., Ralston, R. A., Muir, J., Walker, K. Z., & Truby, H. (2012). Dietary management of infantile colic: A systematic review. *Maternal and Child Health Journal*, *16*(6), 1319–1331. https://doi.org/10.1007/s10995-011-0842-5.

Icke, S., & Genc, R. (2018). Effect of reflexology on infantile colic. *Journal of Alternative and Complementary Medicine*, *24*(6), 584–588. https://doi.org/10.1089/acm.2017.0315.

Johnson, J. D., Cocker, K., Chang, E., & Army, T. (2015). Infantile colic: recognition and treatment. *American Family Physician*, *92*(7), 577–582.

Kesavelu, D. (2023). Alleviating gasto-intestinal discomfort in infants: quest for effective interventions. *Medical Research Archives*, *11*(9), 1–14. https://doi.org/10.18103/mra.v11i9.4459.

Lam, T. M. L., Chan, P. C., & Goh, L. H. (2019). Approach to infantile colic in primary care. *Singapore Medical Journal*, *60*(1), 12–16. https://doi.org/10.11622/smedj.2019004.

Landgren, K., & Hallström, I. (2017). Effect of minimal acupuncture for infantile colic: A multicentre, three-armed, single-blind, randomised controlled trial (ACU-COL). *Acupuncture in Medicine*, *35*(3), 171–179. https://doi.org/10.1136/acupmed-2016-011208.

Lee, D., Lee, H., Kim, J., Kim, T., Sung, S., Leem, J., & Kim, T. H. (2018). Acupuncture for infantile colic: A systematic review of randomised controlled trials. *Evidence-Based Complementary and Alternative Medicine*, 7526234. https://doi.org/10.1155/2018/7526234.

Mansouri, S., Kazemi, I., Baghestani, A. R., Zayeri, F., Nahidi, F., & Gazerani, N. (2018). A placebo-controlled clinical trial to evaluate the effectiveness of massaging on infantile colic using a random-effects joint model. *Pediatric Health, Medicine and Therapeutics*, *Volume 9*, 157–163. https://doi.org/10.2147/phmt.s185214.

Mi, G. L., Zhao, L., Qiao, D. D., Kang, W. Q., Tang, M. Q., & Xu, J. K. (2015). Effectiveness of Lactobacillus reuteri in infantile colic and colicky induced maternal depression: a prospective single blind randomized trial. *Antonie van Leeuwenhoek, International Journal of General and Molecular Microbiology*, *107*(6), 1547–1553. https://doi.org/10.1007/s10482-015-0448-9.

Miller, J. E., Newell, D., & Bolton, J. E. (2012). Efficacy of chiropractic manual therapy on infant colic: A pragmatic single-blind, randomized controlled trial. *Journal of Manipulative and Physiological Therapeutics*, *35*(8), 600–607. https://doi.org/10.1016/j.jmpt.2012.09.010.

Mutlu, B., Erkut, Z., Avcı, Ş., Girgin, S. S., & Gönen, İ. (2020). The practices used by mothers to infantile colic and their perceptions on the benefits of the practices. *Online Turkish Journal of Health Sciences*, *5*(1), 8–16. https://doi.org/10.26453/otjhs.583087.

Ong, T. G., Gordon, M., Banks, S. S. C., Thomas, M. R., & Akobeng, A. K. (2019). Probiotics to prevent infantile colic. *Cochrane Database of Systematic Reviews*, *2019*(3), 1–50. https://doi.org/10.1002/14651858.CD012473.pub2.

Perry, R., Leach, V., Penfold, C., & Davies, P. (2019). An overview of systematic reviews of complementary and alternative therapies for infantile colic. *Systematic Reviews*, *8*(1), 1–16. https://doi.org/10.1186/s13643-019-1191-5.

Reinthal, M., Lund, I., Ullman, D., & Lundeberg, T. (2011). Gastrointestinal symptoms of infantile colic and their change after light needling of acupuncture: A case series study of 913 infants. *Chinese Medicine*, *6*(1), 28. https://doi.org/10.1186/1749-8546-6-28.

Salisbury, A. L., High, P., Twomey, J. E., Dickstein, S., Chapman, H., Liu, J., & Lester, B. (2012). A randomized control trial of integrated care for families managing infant colic. *Infant Mental Health Journal*, *33*(2), 110–122. https://doi.org/10.1002/imhj.20340.

Sarasu, J. M., Narang, M., & Shah, D. (2018). Infantile colic: an update. *Indian Pediatrics*, *55*(11), 979–987. https://doi.org/10.1007/s13312-018-1423-0.

Savino, F., Garro, M., Nicoli, S., Ceratto, S., Garro, S. •, Ceratto, N. •, & Children's Hospital, M. (2015). Infantile colic: looking to old data through new eyes. *Journal of Pediatric and Neonatal Individualized Medicine (JPNIM)*, *4*(2), e040230–e040230. https://doi.org/10.7363/040230.

Sezici, E., & Yiğit, D. (2018). Comparison between swinging and playing of white noise among colicky babies: A paired randomised controlled trial. *Journal of Clinical Nursing*, *27*(3–4), 593–600. https://doi.org/10.1111/jocn.13928.

Sheidaei, A., Abadi, A., Zayeri, F., Nahidi, F., Gazerani, N., & Mansouri, A. (2016). The effectiveness of massage therapy in the treatment of infantile colic symptoms: A randomized controlled trial. *Medical Journal of the Islamic Republic of Iran*, *30*(1), 351.

Simonson, J., Haglund, K., Weber, E., Fial, A., & Hanson, L. (2021). Probiotics for the management of infantile colic: A systematic review. *MCN The American Journal of Maternal/Child Nursing*, *46*(2), 88–96. https://doi.org/10.1097/NMC.0000000000000691.

Skjeie, H., Skonnord, T., Brekke, M., Klovning, A., Fetveit, A., Landgren, K., Hallström, I. K., & Brurberg, K. G. (2018). Acupuncture treatments for infantile colic: a systematic review and individual patient data meta-analysis of blinding test validated randomised controlled trials. *Scandinavian Journal of Primary Health Care*, *36*(1), 56–69. https://doi.org/10.1080/02813432.2018.1426146.

Sung, V. (2018). Infantile colic. *Australian Prescriber*, *41*(4), 105–110. https://doi.org/10.18773/AUSTPRESCR.2018.033.

Twomey, J. E., High, P., & Lester, B. M. (2012). Colic: What's maternal mental health got to do with it? *Infant Mental Health Journal*, *33*(5), 543–552. https://doi.org/10.1002/imhj.21344.

Uysal, G., Sönmez Düzkaya, D., & Bozkurt, G. (2017). Factors affecting infantile colic with babies. *Journal of Health Sciences and Professions*, *4*(3), 221–227.

Vaziri, F., Sahebkaram, Z., Bahrami, R., Pourahmad, S., & Azima, S. (2018). Lavender oil aromatherapy on infantile colic and maternal mood: A double blind randomized clinical trial. *Pharmaceutical Sciences*, *24*(1), 38–43. https://doi.org/10.15171/ps.2018.07.

Verduci, E., Salvatore, S., Bresesti, I., Di Profio, E., Pendezza, E., Bosetti, A., Agosti, M., Zuccotti, G. V., & D'auria, E. (2021). Semi-elemental and elemental formulas for enteral nutrition in infants and children with medical complexity—thinking about cow's milk allergy and beyond. *Nutrients*, *13*(12). https://doi.org/10.3390/nu13124230.

Wessel, M. A., Cobb, J. C., Jackson, E. B., Harris, G. S., & Detwiler, A. C. (1954). Paroxysmal fussing in infancy, sometimes called colic. *Pediatrics*, *14*(5), 421–435.

Wolke, D., Bilgin, A., & Samara, M. (2019). Systematic review and meta-analysis: fussing and crying durations and prevalence of colic in infants. *Journal of Pediatrics*, *185*, 55–61. https://doi.org/10.1016/j.jpeds.2017.02.020.

Zamanillo-Campos, R., Coto Alonso, L., Fuentes Martín, M. J., Nevot Escusa, P., & Tejón Fernández, M. (2022). Nutritional counseling for cow's milk protein allergy in infants from birth to 2 y of ages: Scoping review. *Nutrition*, *98*, 1–9. https://doi.org/10.1016/j.nut.2022.111633.

Zeevenhooven, J., Browne, P. D., L'Hoir, M. P., de Weerth, C., & Benninga, M. A. (2018). Infant colic: mechanisms and management. *Nature Reviews Gastroenterology and Hepatology*, *15*(8), 479–496. https://doi.org/10.1038/s41575-018-0008-7.

Zeevenhooven, J., Koppen, I. J. N., & Benninga, M. A. (2017). The new Rome IV criteria for functional gastrointestinal disorders in infants and toddlers. *Pediatric Gastroenterology, Hepatology and Nutrition*, *20*(1), 1–13. https://doi.org/10.5223/pghn.2017.20.1.1.

Chapter 9

Evidence-Based Nursing Practices for Newborn Sleep

Mehmet Emin Düken*, PhD
and Fatma Bozdağ, PhD
Department of Nursing, Faculty of Health Sciences, Harran University, Şanlıurfa, Türkiye

Abstract

Sleep is an important physiological need for humans, but for newborn babies, who spend almost 18 hours a day asleep, it is as important as food. Sleep allows us to encode and process information and control the emotions we experience during the day. During sleep, new synaptic connections are formed in the brain and the brain development of newborn babies is completed and matures. As well as supporting brain development, sleep is important for healthy growth and strengthening the immune system. Preterm babies make up a large proportion of neonatal intensive care units. There are many factors that interrupt and shorten the sleep of preterm babies in NICUs. These factors include bright lights, painful stimuli, frequent invasive procedures, alarms, heel taps, phone rings, and noise. These factors that newborn babies are exposed to negatively affect their neurological development, and emotional and behavioral control. Both pharmacological and non-pharmacological interventions have been used to improve the quality of neonatal sleep. However, pharmacological interventions have potential adverse effects. The use of sedatives and hypnotics in newborn babies is not recommended because of their rapid growth and neurological development. In recent years, the importance of non-pharmacological methods to improve neonatal sleep has been emphasized. Non-pharmacological methods such as massage, bathing, white noise, swaddling, kangaroo care, cycled light, touch, music therapy, and non-nutritive sucking have been reported to improve sleep in preterm infants. This section highlights evidence-based non-pharmacological practices used to support sleep patterns in newborns.

Keywords: preterm, sleep, nursing, evidence-based nursing practices

---

* Corresponding Author's Email: eminduken@harran.edu.tr.

In: Evidence-Based Care Practices in Pediatric Nursing
Editors: Feyza Küçük and Serap Özdemir
ISBN: 979-8-89530-304-7

Introduction

Preterm birth and low birth weight are major health problems affecting babies worldwide. Preterm birth is defined as a live birth that occurs before the 37th week of gestation. Approximately 15 million babies are born preterm worldwide each year, accounting for about 11% of the global birth rate (Walani, 2020; WHO, 2022).

The transition of babies from the intrauterine period to incubators in the Neonatal Intensive Care Unit (NICE) often has long-term consequences, affecting many of the infant's basic development (emotional, social, physical, etc.) (De Jong et al., 2012; Hornman et al., 2016; Kerr-Wilson et al., 2012; Kerstjens et al., 2012; Walani, 2020). Preterm infants are at risk of developing lifelong health complications with behavioral deficits (Bik et al., 2022; Hornman et al., 2016; Walani, 2020). These babies are born at a very critical period of brain development. This may put preterm infants at risk, especially in terms of long-term neurodevelopmental outcomes (Bik et al., 2022; Walani, 2020). Many studies have reported that sleep has a protective effect on preterm infants whose brain development is at risk (Bennet et al., 2018; Bik et al., 2022; Walani, 2020).

Sleep is an important issue in the current practices for preterm infants in the neonatal intensive care unit (Park, 2020). Fetuses and newborns spend most of their time sleeping (Graven & Browne, 2008). Sleep in newborns consists of active sleep (AS), quiet sleep (QS), and indeterminate sleep (IS). Active sleep (AS) constitutes rapid eye movement or REM sleep, while Quiet Sleep (QS) is considered the precursor of non-rapid eye movement or NREM sleep. Indeterminate sleep (IS) is defined as a sleepless state of arousal and wakefulness (Ryan et al., 2023; Werth et al., 2017). The length and organization of sleep states change as the infant develops, and these changes are important indicators of brain development.

Sleep has an impact on many functions of babies. Sleep is considered not only as a state of rest but also as a state involving intense brain activity. Sleep allows the baby's neurons to mature, neurosensors, and cortex to develop. It supports the maturation and functioning of the central nervous system and future cognitive, psychomotor, and temperamental development. Sleep is also important in infants' growth and development, academic success, homeostatic balance, and survival (Bathory & Tomopoulos, 2017; Gregory et al., 2008; Okun, 2011; Visser et al., 2021). It contributes to the development and support of the immune system of preterm infants and energy storage (Mahmoodi et al., 2015). This makes sleep an important determinant of infants' developmental outcomes (Lan et al., 2019).

The physical and neurological development of a term baby takes place in the intrauterine environment (the baby is fed, the baby is protected from excessive light and noise, and the baby's body temperature is stabilized). This environment does not affect the baby's sleep-wake cycle (Allotey et al., 2018; Altimier et al., 2015). On the contrary, preterm babies who leave the intrauterine period early experience a disruption in the developmental process due to an early transition to the psychologically distressing and physically stressful extrauterine environment. This causes preterm infants' sleep to generally have more fragmented sleep cycles than term infants, experiencing sleep characterized by less differentiated sleep states and shorter episodes of quiet sleep (Lan et al., 2019).

Premature babies hospitalized in the NICE are exposed to many external stimuli that can seriously disrupt their sleep-wake system. According to NICE, light, noise, invasive procedures, alarms, monitor sounds, heel taps, telephone noises, and external factors that increase stress negatively affect a baby's sleep-wake cycle (Klutse et al., 2022; Sathish et al., 2019). Disruption of the sleep-wake system in preterm infants leads to increased stress, decreased oxygenation, and adverse effects on growth and neurodevelopment. Therefore, it is extremely important to improve the duration of sleep and the sleep-wake cycle of preterm infants in the neonatal intensive care unit (Firmino et al., 2022).

In the literature, pharmacological and non-pharmacological methods are used to increase the duration of sleep and regulate the sleep-wake cycle in preterm infants. However, pharmacologic interventions have potential negative effects. The use of sedative and hypnotic drugs is not recommended because of the rapid growth and neurological development of newborns. In recent years, the importance of non-pharmacological methods to improve the sleep of newborns has been emphasized (Blencowe et al., 2012; Klutse et al., 2022). Studies have reported that non-pharmacologic methods such as massage, bath, white noise, positioning, kangaroo care, cycled light, touch, and music therapy applied to preterm infants improve sleep.

Nurses have an important role in performing interventions that provide sleep quality and the sleep-wake cycle in preterm infants who leave the intrauterine environment early. Neonatal nurses divide nursing interventions to increase sleep quality and duration of preterm infants into four categories: environmental management, relaxation techniques, therapeutic positioning, and other methods. In NICE, nurses can positively affect the sleep of preterm infants by applying relaxation techniques, therapeutic positioning, and other methods in care practices and controlling environmental stimuli.

Table 1. Non-Pharmacological Methods Used in Sleep-Wake Cycles of Preterm Infants

Evidence-Based Nursing Practices for Newborn Sleep	
1.Environmental Management	Reduction of Sounds and Light Intensity,
	Use of a Looped Light System
	Music
	White Noise
2. Relaxation Techniques	Massage
	Kangaroo Care
	Bathing
3. Therapeutic Positioning	Positioning
	Nest Positioning
4. Other Methods	Dressing,
	Ear Protectors,
	Hammock Positioning
	Combined Procedural Pain Interventions

Environmental Management

Different interventions are preferred to regulate the environment to increase the duration and quality of sleep of preterm infants in NICE. These include the reduction of sounds and light intensity, the use of a looped light system, white noise, and music.

In a study developed by Varvara et al., (2016), which aimed to measure the duration of non-rapid eye movement sleep of the newborn and how it was affected by the implementation of improved nursing conditions, it was confirmed that the duration of non-rapid eye movement sleep increased significantly with the reduction of sound or light intensity. In this study, special earplugs were used to reduce the intensity of environmental sounds and minimize auditory stimuli. Incubator covers were preferred to reduce light intensity. In the study, it was reported that sleep quality and structural organization of preterm infants in the NICE unit improved at low noise and light levels (Varvara et al., 2016).

Preterm infants are highly sensitive to environmental stimuli that accelerate state change and awakening from sleep (Lehtonen & Martin, 2004). Interventions for these stimuli can contribute to the infant's early emotional processes (Graven & Browne, 2008). In the study by Stokes et al., (2018) examining the effect of music on the sleep-wake cycle, it was found that music did not increase the arousal of preterm infants and did not disrupt quiet sleep periods. It was concluded that it did not change the number, duration, or bandwidth of quiet sleep periods and was associated with fewer interruptions (Stokes et al., 2018). It was observed that music did not disrupt sleep and did not increase arousal in preterm infants. In the meta-analysis study by Costa et al., published between 2003 and 2021, it was stated that the majority of the music in 39 included studies consisted of lullabies. It was observed that music provided improvements in pain relief, cardiac and respiratory functions, weight gain, sucking and feeding behaviors, and sleep-wake cycles of preterm infants (Costa et al., 2022). In another study examining the effect of music on sleep and vital signs in preterm infants, 20 preterm infants received music therapy in two sessions per week. After music therapy, it was reported that preterm infants had decreased pulse and respiratory rate, increased oxygen saturation, and sleep duration (Kobus et al., 2021). Similarly, recent studies in the literature have shown that music therapy has a stabilizing and relaxing effect on the general behavior, sleep patterns, and vital signs of preterm infants (Bieleninik et al., 2016; Haslbeck, 2012; Loewy et al., 2013; Standley, 2012).

It was reported that a mother's voice or white noise played to preterm infants as music increased weight gain, improved physiological parameters (increased oxygen saturation, decreased pulse rate, and respiration) (Düken et al., 2023), and did not change sleep-wake cycles (Liao et al., 2021). However, in the study conducted by Düken and Yayan with preterm infants, it was observed that white noise increased sleep duration, and decreased the number of awakenings, and WASO values (Düken & Yayan, 2023a). As a result of the findings obtained in the literature, it was observed that the regulation of the environment is an important variable in the sleep-wake cycles of preterm infants.

Relaxation Techniques

In the literature, different relaxation techniques are used to improve sleep quality and duration in preterm infants. For this purpose, massage, kangaroo care, and bathing are mostly preferred. Pediatric massage is the most commonly used intervention method to promote sleep in preterm infants.

In the study by Yates et al., to determine the effect of massage on sleep in preterm infants, a massage protocol consisting of approximately ten minutes published by Field et al. was used (Field, 2014; Field et al., 2010). It was observed that preterm infants who were massaged at medium pressure fell asleep faster than those who were not massaged, but there was no difference in sleep efficiency (Yates et al., 2014). In a meta-analysis study by De

Britto Pereira et al., examining the application of massage in infants, the research included 38 articles including massage studies used in infants and children in the last decade. The study reported that massage has a positive effect on reducing pain, supporting the immune system, and mother-infant attachment. It was found to have a positive effect on infants' neuromotor development, social development, cognitive development, and sleep (de Britto Pereira et al., 2021). It has been found that long-term massage application has a positive effect on growth and development such as height, weight, and head circumference, increases the amount of daily nutrition, and shortens the discharge time (Düken & Yayan, 2023b). It was found that it decreased the pulse rate and respiratory rate and increased oxygen saturation among the physiological parameters of preterm infants (Düken et al., 2023).

In another study examining the relationship between massage therapy applied to preterm and low birth weight infants and sleep, randomization was provided between gender, gestational age, weight, and date of birth between groups. The 50 infants in the experimental group received massage therapy including light friction, stroking, passive movements of the limbs, and other kinesthetic stimulation tools by massage therapists for eight months. The infants in the control group did not receive any intervention. In the experimental group, infants were less likely to snore during sleep, needed less feeding when they woke up at night and were more energetic and alert during the day. It was reported that there was no significant difference between the sleep behaviors of term or preterm infants who received massage therapy (Kelmanson & Adulas, 2006). Again, in the study examining the effect of massage therapy and the application of white noise on sleep to preterm infants, randomization was provided according to gender and gestation week. In the massage group, 40 preterm infants received 15-minute massage therapy twice a day for three days. The infants in the control group received care. The babies in the massage group had a positive effect on sleep-wake patterns (Düken & Yayan, 2023a). Contrary to the positive effect of massage on sleep, there are also studies indicating that there is no difference between the sleep duration of infants with and without massage (Rudnicki et al., 2012; Seiiedi-Biarag et al., 2022).

Kangaroo care is one of the interventions as important as massage in the sleep-wake cycle of preterm infants. Kangaroo care provides the formation of an emotional bond between mother and baby, activating parasympathetic nerves and calming the mother and baby (Carvalho et al., 2019; Cho et al., 2016; Cleveland et al., 2017). Especially kangaroo care initiated in the early period reduces the pain of infants (Cleveland et al., 2017; Şen & Manav, 2020), reduces the development of Broncho Pulmonary Dysplasia (BPD), cholestasis and nosocomial infections (Casper et al., 2018; Cunningham et al., 2018; Karimi et al., 2019) and has a positive effect on vital signs (Butruille et al., 2017; Cho et al., 2016; Özdel & Sarı, 2020). Considering its effect on sleep; it increases the duration of quiet sleep by calming the babies, shortens the time to fall asleep, and reduces the awakening from sleep (Bastani et al., 2017; Cleveland et al., 2017). In a different study, it was determined that there was a significant difference between the deep sleep durations of infants who received kangaroo care compared to the control group, and the frequency of awakening, movement, and crying durations were less than the control group (Edraki et al., 2015). In a 10-year follow-up after kangaroo care was applied to premature infants for 14 days, it was observed that kangaroo care increased mother-baby attachment, reduced mothers' anxiety, and had a positive effect on children's cognitive activities and sleep (Feldman et al., 2014).

Similarly, another intervention that promotes sleep in preterm infants and covers the category of relaxation techniques is bathing. It is thought that routine daily bathing of preterm infants may have many negative effects on the infant's physiological responses and comfort needs. Repeated stress in preterm infants can have long-term destructive effects on brain development. In the literature, sponge baths, bathtubs, and swaddling baths are used in preterm infants. In a study, it was observed that routine bathtub bathing disrupted the sleep-wake cycle of infants and caused stressful behaviors (Liaw et al., 2006).

However, systematic studies have found that swaddling is associated with lower stress levels and temperature changes in preterm infants (Fernández & Antolín-Rodríguez, 2018). Swaddling has been shown to be the best and safest method of bathing preterm babies in the hospital and is associated with less physiological and behavioral distress in preterm babies (Fernández & Antolín-Rodríguez, 2018; Tambunan & Mediani, 2019). In another study, it was found that there was no difference between traditional and bathtub bathing in terms of body temperature, vital signs, cortisol levels, and sleep-wake states of preterm infants (de Freitas et al., 2018).

As a result of the findings obtained in the literature, it is suggested that massage, kangaroo care, and swaddling baths may be valuable approaches to improve sleep quality and sleep duration and reduce sleep-disordered breathing in low birth weight or preterm infants.

Therapeutic Positioning

Sleep is very important for infants, especially preterm infants, and is considered one of the most important behavioral states that play a role in brain development. Therefore, different interventions are performed in the NICE unit to ensure the normal sleep-wake cycle of preterm infants. Positioning (cycled light, ear protectors) is also used to regulate the sleep-wake cycle of preterm infants (Bertelle et al., 2007).

In a study, the effect of different positions (prone, supine, and right and left side) used for preterm infants admitted to NICE on non-autonomic outcomes was examined. In this meta-analysis, it was reported that preterm infants experienced less regulation behavior and less stress in prone positioning, which increased sleep duration and quality. In supine positioning, preterm infants experienced more stress and exhibited increased waking behavior due to frequent self-movement (Skelton et al., 2023). In other studies, examining positioning, the opposite is claimed. It has been stated that preterm infants have the longest sleep duration in the supine position, but it is the supine position that is exposed to the most external stimuli during sleep. It was then stated that the position methods that are effective on sleep are prone, left side, and right side, respectively (Modesto et al., 2016; Sahni, 2005).

In a meta-analysis study examining the effect of nest positioning on weight gain, motor development, and sleep patterns in preterm infants in NICE, it was found that nest positioning supported motor development, regulated sleep-wake cycle, increased weight gain, and shortened discharge time. It was also found that nest positioning in preterm infants supported flexor posture, stimulated the midline, and increased sleep duration (Carneiro et al., 2024).

Other Methods

Dressing, ear protectors, hammock positioning, and combined procedural pain interventions have been proven to be effective in the sleep-wake cycle of preterm infants.

In a study in which the duration of sleep and the time before discharge were examined by dressing preterm babies in clothes; 30 preterm babies were dressed in clothes, while 30 preterm babies were not dressed in anything. It was reported that dressing preterm babies in clothes increased sleep time and shortened discharge time (Akay Kuzey & Yildiz, 2023).

Studies investigating the effect of ear earmuffs on sleep in preterm infants found that there was no significant difference in total sleep time between preterm infants with and without ear earmuffs. The use of earmuffs was found to significantly reduce total sleep time in small-for-gestational-age preterm infants. It was found that the use of earplugs did not increase total sleep time in preterm infants (Araújo et al., 2018; Sato et al., 2020).

In the study examining the effectiveness of the hammock position in reducing pain and improving sleep-wakefulness in premature infants; it was observed that preterm infants who were positioned in the hammock position had reduced pain levels compared to those with traditional positioning. At the same time, it was revealed that it provided improvements in the sleep-wake cycles of infants, decreased pulse and respiratory rate, and increased oxygen saturation (Ribas et al., 2019).

In a study examining the effects of combined procedural pain interventions on sleep, cognitive development, and internalizing behavior in premature infants; it was observed that pain decreased, sleep duration increased, night awakenings increased and contributed positively to motor and language development (Gao et al., 2023).

Conclusion

As a result of the literature findings, it was revealed that many different interventions were used to improve sleep quality and sleep efficiency, reduce the number of awakenings, and regulate the sleep-wake cycle in preterm infants. Studies have shown that light, sound, music therapy, white noise, mother's voice, lullaby, massage, kangaroo care, swaddling bath, positioning, dressing, ear protectors, hammock position, and combined procedural pain interventions are used to regulate the sleep-wake cycle of infants.

Disclaimer

None.

References

Akay Kuzey, M., & Yildiz, S. (2023). The effects of clothing on sleep time and discharge time for preterm infants. *Journal of Neonatal Nursing*, *29*(5), 741–744. https://doi.org/10.1016/j.jnn.2023.01.009.

Allotey, J., Zamora, J., Cheong-See, F., Kalidindi, M., Arroyo-Manzano, D., Asztalos, E., van der Post, J., Mol, B., Moore, D., Birtles, D., Khan, K., & Thangaratinam, S. (2018). Cognitive, motor, behavioural and academic performances of children born preterm: a meta-analysis and systematic review involving 64 061 children. *BJOG: An International Journal of Obstetrics & Gynaecology*, *125*(1), 16–25. https://doi.org/10.1111/1471-0528.14832.

Altimier, L., Kenner, C., & Damus, K. (2015). The Wee Care Neuroprotective NICU Program (Wee Care): The Effect of a Comprehensive Developmental Care Training Program on Seven Neuroprotective Core Measures for Family-Centered Developmental Care of Premature Neonates. *Newborn and Infant Nursing Reviews*, *15*(1), 6–16. https://doi.org/10.1053/j.nainr.2015.01.006.

Araújo, F. M., Pedreira, M. da L. G., Avelar, A. F. M., Pradella-Hallinan, M. L. de C., Tsunemi, M. H., & Pinheiro, E. M. (2018). Sleep and salivary cortisol in preterm neonates: a clinical, randomized, controlled, crossover study. *Revista Brasileira de Enfermagem*, *71*(suppl 3), 1358–1365. https://doi.org/10.1590/0034-7167-2017-0546.

Bastani, F., Rajai, N., Farsi, Z., & Als, H. (2017). The Effects of Kangaroo Care on the Sleep and Wake States of Preterm Infants. *Journal of Nursing Research*, *25*(3), 231–239. https://doi.org/10.1097/JNR.0000000000000194.

Bathory, E., & Tomopoulos, S. (2017). Sleep Regulation, Physiology and Development, Sleep Duration and Patterns, and Sleep Hygiene in Infants, Toddlers, and Preschool-Age Children. *Current Problems in Pediatric and Adolescent Health Care*, *47*(2), 29–42. https://doi.org/10.1016/j.cppeds.2016.12.001.

Bennet, L., Walker, D. W., & Horne, R. S. C. (2018). Waking up too early – the consequences of preterm birth on sleep development. *The Journal of Physiology*, *596*(23), 5687–5708. https://doi.org/10.1113/JP274950.

Bertelle, V., Sevestre, A., Laou-Hap, K., Nagahapitiye, M. C., & Sizun, J. (2007). Sleep in the Neonatal Intensive Care Unit. *Journal of Perinatal & Neonatal Nursing*, *21*(2), 140–148. https://doi.org/10.1097/01.JPN.0000270631.96864.d3.

Bieleninik, Ł., Ghetti, C., & Gold, C. (2016). Music Therapy for Preterm Infants and Their Parents: A Meta-analysis. *Pediatrics*, *138*(3). https://doi.org/10.1542/peds.2016-0971.

Bik, A., Sam, C., de Groot, E. R., Visser, S. S. M., Wang, X., Tataranno, M. L., Benders, M. J. N. L., van den Hoogen, A., & Dudink, J. (2022). A scoping review of behavioral sleep stage classification methods for preterm infants. *Sleep Medicine*, *90*, 74–82. https://doi.org/10.1016/j.sleep.2022.01.006.

Blencowe, H., Cousens, S., Oestergaard, M. Z., Chou, D., Moller, A.-B., Narwal, R., Adler, A., Vera Garcia, C., Rohde, S., Say, L., & Lawn, J. E. (2012). National, regional, and worldwide estimates of preterm birth rates in the year 2010 with time trends since 1990 for selected countries: a systematic analysis and implications. *The Lancet*, *379*(9832), 2162–2172. https://doi.org/10.1016/S0140-6736(12)60820-4.

Butruille, L., Blouin, A., De Jonckheere, J., Mur, S., Margez, T., Rakza, T., & Storme, L. (2017). Impact of skin-to-skin contact on the autonomic nervous system in the preterm infant and his mother. *Infant Behavior and Development*, *49*, 83–86. https://doi.org/10.1016/j.infbeh.2017.07.003.

Carneiro, M. M. C., Ribeiro, S. N. S., Menegol, N. A., Okubo, R., Montemezzo, D., & Sanada, L. S. (2024). Nest positioning on motor development, sleep patterns, weight gain in preterm infants: systematic review. *Pediatric Research*. https://doi.org/10.1038/s41390-023-02972-w.

Carvalho, M. E. S., Justo, J. M. R. M., Gratier, M., Tomé, T., Pereira, E., & Rodrigues, H. (2019). Vocal responsiveness of preterm infants to maternal infant-directed speaking and singing during skin-to-skin contact (Kangaroo Care) in the NICU. *Infant Behavior and Development*, *57*, 101332. https://doi.org/10.1016/j.infbeh.2019.101332.

Casper, C., Sarapuk, I., & Pavlyshyn, H. (2018). Regular and prolonged skin-to-skin contact improves short-term outcomes for very preterm infants: A dose-dependent intervention. *Archives de Pédiatrie*, *25*(8), 469–475. https://doi.org/10.1016/j.arcped.2018.09.008.

Cho, E.-S., Kim, S.-J., Kwon, M. S., Cho, H., Kim, E. H., Jun, E. M., & Lee, S. (2016). The Effects of Kangaroo Care in the Neonatal Intensive Care Unit on the Physiological Functions of Preterm Infants, Maternal–Infant Attachment, and Maternal Stress. *Journal of Pediatric Nursing*, *31*(4), 430–438. https://doi.org/10.1016/j.pedn.2016.02.007.

Cleveland, L., Hill, C. M., Pulse, W. S., DiCioccio, H. C., Field, T., & White-Traut, R. (2017). Systematic Review of Skin-to-Skin Care for Full-Term, Healthy Newborns. *Journal of Obstetric, Gynecologic & Neonatal Nursing*, *46*(6), 857–869. https://doi.org/10.1016/j.jogn.2017.08.005.

Costa, V. S., Bündchen, D. C., Sousa, H., Pires, L. B., & Felipetti, F. A. (2022). Clinical benefits of music-based interventions on preterm infants' health: A systematic review of randomised trials. *Acta Paediatrica*, *111*(3), 478–489. https://doi.org/10.1111/apa.16222.

Cunningham, C., Moore, Z., Patton, D., O'Connor, T., & Nugent, L. E. (2018). Does Kangaroo care affect the weight of preterm/low birth-weight infants in the neonatal setting of a hospital environment? *Journal of Neonatal Nursing*, *24*(4), 189–195. https://doi.org/10.1016/j.jnn.2017.10.001.

de Britto Pereira, P. A. D., Mendes Abdala, C. V., Portella, C. F., Ghelman, R., & Schveitzer, M. C. (2021). Pediatrics massage evidence map. *Complementary Therapies in Medicine*, *61*, 102774. https://doi.org/10.1016/j.ctim.2021.102774.

de Freitas, P., Bueno, M., Holditch-Davis, D., Santos, H. P., & Kimura, A. F. (2018). Biobehavioral Responses of Preterm Infants to Conventional and Swaddled Tub Baths. *The Journal of Perinatal & Neonatal Nursing*, *32*(4), 358–365. https://doi.org/10.1097/JPN.0000000000000336.

De Jong, F., Monuteaux, M. C., van Elburg, R. M., Gillman, M. W., & Belfort, M. B. (2012). Systematic Review and Meta-Analysis of Preterm Birth and Later Systolic Blood Pressure. *Hypertension*, *59*(2), 226–234. https://doi.org/10.1161/HYPERTENSIONAHA.111.181784.

Düken, M. E., & Yayan, E. H. (2023a). The effects of massage therapy and white noise application on premature infants' sleep. *EXPLORE*. https://doi.org/10.1016/j.explore.2023.09.002.

Düken, M. E., & Yayan, E. H. (2023b). A follow up study on the effects of massage on preterm infants: A randomized controlled research. *EXPLORE*. https://doi.org/10.1016/j.explore.2023.10.004.

Düken, M. E., Yayan, E. H., & Arslan, Z. (2023). The effects of massage and white noise on physiological parameters of preterm infants: A randomized controlled research. *Journal of Neonatal Nursing*. https://doi.org/10.1016/j.jnn.2023.11.008.

Edraki, M., Zendehzaban, S., Beheshtipour, N., Hemmati, F., & Haghpanah, S. (2015). Comparison of the Effects of Attachment Training for Mothers on the Behavioral Responses of Premature Infants: A Randomized Clinical Trial. *Iranian Journal Of Neonatology*, *6*(2), 37–42.

Feldman, R., Rosenthal, Z., & Eidelman, A. I. (2014). Maternal-Preterm Skin-to-Skin Contact Enhances Child Physiologic Organization and Cognitive Control Across the First 10 Years of Life. *Biological Psychiatry*, *75*(1), 56–64. https://doi.org/10.1016/j.biopsych.2013.08.012.

Fernández, D., & Antolín-Rodríguez, R. (2018). Bathing a Premature Infant in the Intensive Care Unit: A Systematic Review. *Journal of Pediatric Nursing*, *42*, e52–e57. https://doi.org/10.1016/j.pedn.2018.05.002.

Field, T. (2014). Massage therapy research review. *Complementary Therapies in Clinical Practice*, *20*(4), 224–229. https://doi.org/10.1016/j.ctcp.2014.07.002.

Field, T., Diego, M., & Hernandez-Reif, M. (2010). Moderate Pressure is Essential for Massage Therapy Effects. *International Journal of Neuroscience*, *120*(5), 381–385. https://doi.org/10.3109/00207450903579475.

Firmino, C., Rodrigues, M., Franco, S., Ferreira, J., Simões, A. R., Castro, C., & Fernandes, J. B. (2022). Nursing Interventions That Promote Sleep in Preterm Newborns in the Neonatal Intensive Care Units: An Integrative Review. *International Journal of Environmental Research and Public Health*, *19*(17), 10953. https://doi.org/10.3390/ijerph191710953.

Gao, H., Li, M., Gao, H., Xu, G., Wang, D., & Lv, H. (2023). Effect of combined procedural pain interventions during neonatal intensive care on sleep, cognitive development, and internalizing behavior: a follow-up analysis of a randomized controlled trial. *Pain*, *164*(8), 1793–1800. https://doi.org/10.1097/j.pain.0000000000002877.

Graven, S. N., & Browne, J. V. (2008). Sleep and Brain Development. *Newborn and Infant Nursing Reviews*, *8*(4), 173–179. https://doi.org/10.1053/j.nainr.2008.10.008.

Gregory, A. M., Van der Ende, J., Willis, T. A., & Verhulst, F. C. (2008). Parent-Reported Sleep Problems During Development and Self-reported Anxiety/Depression, Attention Problems, and Aggressive Behavior Later in Life. *Archives of Pediatrics & Adolescent Medicine*, *162*(4), 330. https://doi.org/10.1001/archpedi.162.4.330.

Haslbeck, F. B. (2012). Music therapy for premature infants and their parents: an integrative review. *Nordic Journal of Music Therapy*, *21*(3), 203–226. https://doi.org/10.1080/08098131.2011.648653.

Hornman, J., de Winter, A. F., Kerstjens, J. M., Bos, A. F., & Reijneveld, S. A. (2016). Emotional and Behavioral Problems of Preterm and Full-Term Children at School Entry. *Pediatrics*, *137*(5). https://doi.org/10.1542/peds.2015-2255.

Karimi, F. Z., Sadeghi, R., Maleki-Saghooni, N., & Khadivzadeh, T. (2019). The effect of mother-infant skin to skin contact on success and duration of first breastfeeding: A systematic review and meta-analysis. *Taiwanese Journal of Obstetrics and Gynecology*, *58*(1), 1–9. https://doi.org/10.1016/j.tjog.2018.11.002.

Kelmanson, I. A., & Adulas, E. I. (2006). Massage therapy and sleep behaviour in infants born with low birth weight. *Complementary Therapies in Clinical Practice*, *12*(3), 200–205. https://doi.org/10.1016/j.ctcp.2005.11.007.

Kerr-Wilson, C. O., Mackay, D. F., Smith, G. C. S., & Pell, J. P. (2012). Meta-analysis of the association between preterm delivery and intelligence. *Journal of Public Health*, *34*(2), 209–216. https://doi.org/10.1093/pubmed/fdr024.

Kerstjens, J. M., De Winter, A. F., Bocca-Tjeertes, I. F., Bos, A. F., & Reijneveld, S. A. (2012). Risk of developmental delay increases exponentially as gestational age of preterm infants decreases: a cohort study at age 4 years. *Developmental Medicine & Child Neurology*, *54*(12), 1096–1101. https://doi.org/10.1111/j.1469-8749.2012.04423.x.

Klutse, K. D., Hillan, E. M., Wright, A. L., & Johnston, L. (2022). Facilitators and barriers to developmentally supportive care for preterm infants in low and middle-income countries: A scoping review. *Journal of Neonatal Nursing*, *28*(6), 388–402. https://doi.org/10.1016/j.jnn.2021.12.004.

Kobus, S., Diezel, M., Dewan, M. V., Huening, B., Dathe, A.-K., Felderhoff-Mueser, U., & Bruns, N. (2021). Music Therapy Is Effective during Sleep in Preterm Infants. *International Journal of Environmental Research and Public Health*, *18*(16), 8245. https://doi.org/10.3390/ijerph18168245.

Lan, H. Y., Yin, T., Chen, J. L., Chang, Y. C., & Liaw, J. J. (2019). Factors Associated With Preterm Infants' Circadian Sleep/Wake Patterns at the Hospital. *Clinical Nursing Research*, *28*(4), 456–472. https://doi.org/10.1177/1054773817724960.

Lehtonen, L., & Martin, R. J. (2004). Ontogeny of sleep and awake states in relation to breathing in preterm infants. *Seminars in Neonatology*, *9*(3), 229–238. https://doi.org/10.1016/j.siny.2003.09.002.

Liao, J., Liu, G., Xie, N., Wang, S., Wu, T., Lin, Y., Hu, R., & He, H.-G. (2021). Mothers' voices and white noise on premature infants' physiological reactions in a neonatal intensive care unit: A multi-arm randomized controlled trial. *International Journal of Nursing Studies*, *119*, 103934. https://doi.org/10.1016/j.ijnurstu.2021.103934.

Liaw, J. J., Yang, L., Yuh, Y. S., & Yin, T. (2006). Effects of Tub Bathing Procedures on Preterm Infants' Behavior. *Journal of Nursing Research*, *14*(4), 297–305. https://doi.org/10.1097/01.JNR.0000387589.12340.98.

Loewy, J., Stewart, K., Dassler, A. M., Telsey, A., & Homel, P. (2013). The Effects of Music Therapy on Vital Signs, Feeding, and Sleep in Premature Infants. *Pediatrics*, *131*(5), 902–918. https://doi.org/10.1542/peds.2012-1367.

Mahmoodi, N., Arbabisarjou, A., Rezaeipoor, M., & Pishkar Mofrad, Z. (2015). Nurses' Awareness of Preterm Neonates' Sleep in the NICU. *Global Journal of Health Science*, *8*(6), 226. https://doi.org/10.5539/gjhs.v8n6p226.

Modesto, I. F., Avelar, A. F. M., Pedreira, M. da L. G., Pradella-Hallinan, M., Avena, M. J., & Pinheiro, E. M. (2016). Effect of sleeping position on arousals from sleep in preterm infants. *Journal for Specialists in Pediatric Nursing*, *21*(3), 131–138. https://doi.org/10.1111/jspn.12147.

Okun, M. L. (2011). Biological consequences of disturbed sleep: Important mediators of health? 1. *Japanese Psychological Research*, *53*(2), 163–176. https://doi.org/10.1111/j.1468-5884.2011.00463.x.

Özdel, D., & Sarı, H. Y. (2020). Effects of the prone position and kangaroo care on gastric residual volume, vital signs and comfort in preterm infants. *Japan Journal of Nursing Science*, *17*(1). https://doi.org/10.1111/jjns.12287.

Park, J. (2020). Sleep Promotion for Preterm Infants in the NICU. *Nursing for Women's Health*, *24*(1), 24–35. https://doi.org/10.1016/j.nwh.2019.11.004.

Ribas, C. G., Andreazza, M. G., Neves, V. C., & Valderramas, S. (2019). Effectiveness of Hammock Positioning in Reducing Pain and Improving Sleep-Wakefulness State in Preterm Infants. *Respiratory Care*, *64*(4), 384–389. https://doi.org/10.4187/respcare.06265.

Rudnicki, J., Boberski, M., Butrymowicz, E., Niedbalski, P., Ogniewski, P., Niedbalski, M., Niedbalski, Z., Podraza, W., & Podraza, H. (2012). Recording of Amplitude-Integrated Electroencephalography,

Oxygen Saturation, Pulse Rate, and Cerebral Blood Flow during Massage of Premature Infants. *American Journal of Perinatology*. https://doi.org/10.1055/s-0032-1310529.

Ryan, M. A. J., Mathieson, S. R., Livingstone, V., O'Sullivan, M. P., Dempsey, E. M., & Boylan, G. B. (2023). Sleep state organisation of moderate to late preterm infants in the neonatal unit. *Pediatric Research*, *93*, 595–603.

Sahni, R. (2005). Sleeping position and electrocortical activity in low birthweight infants. *Archives of Disease in Childhood - Fetal and Neonatal Edition*, *90*(4), F311-f315. https://doi.org/10.1136/adc.2004.055327.

Sathish, Y., Lewis, L. E., Noronha, J. A., Nayak, B. S., Pai, M. S., & Altimier, L. (2019). Promoting developmental supportive care in preterm infants and families in a level III neonatal intensive care unit (NICU) setting in India. *Nurse Education in Practice*, *40*, 102612. https://doi.org/10.1016/j.nepr.2019.08.006.

Sato, M. H., Pedreira, M. da L. G., Avelar, A. F. M., Tsunemi, M. H., Orsi, K. C. S. C., Pradella-Hallinan, M. L. de C., Avena, M. J., & Pinheiro, E. M. (2020). Influence of Ear Protectors on the Sleep of Preterm Newborns: A Randomized Controlled Clinical Study. *Clinical Nursing Research*, *29*(4), 260–267. https://doi.org/10.1177/1054773818806171.

Seiiedi-Biarag, L., Mirghafourvand, M., & Mohammadi, A. (2022). The effect of massage therapy on sleep/awake patterns in the preterm infants: A systematic review and meta-analysis. *Journal of Neonatal Nursing*, *28*(4), 229–235. https://doi.org/10.1016/j.jnn.2021.11.005.

Sen, E., & Manav, G. (2020). Effect of Kangaroo Care and Oral Sucrose on Pain in Premature Infants: A Randomized Controlled Trial. *Pain Management Nursing*. https://doi.org/10.1016/j.pmn.2020.05.003.

Skelton, H., Psaila, K., Schmied, V., & Foster, J. (2023). Systematic Review of the Effects of Positioning on Nonautonomic Outcomes in Preterm Infants. *Journal of Obstetric, Gynecologic & Neonatal Nursing*, *52*(1), 9–20. https://doi.org/10.1016/j.jogn.2022.09.007.

Standley, J. (2012). Music Therapy Research in the NICU: An Updated Meta-Analysis. *Neonatal Network*, *31*(5), 311–316. https://doi.org/10.1891/0730-0832.31.5.311.

Stokes, A., Agthe, A. G., & El Metwally, D. (2018). Music exposure and maturation of late preterm sleep–wake cycles: a randomised crossover trial. *Acta Paediatrica*, *107*(4), 582–586. https://doi.org/10.1111/apa.14079.

Tambunan, D. M., & Mediani, H. S. (2019). Bathing Method for Preterm Infants: A Systematic Review. *KnE Life Sciences*. https://doi.org/10.18502/kls.v4i13.5220.

Varvara, B., Effrossine, T., Despoina, K., Konstantinos, D., & Matziou, V. (2016). Effects of neonatal intensive care unit nursing conditions in neonatal NREM sleep. *Journal of Neonatal Nursing*, *22*(3), 115–123. https://doi.org/10.1016/j.jnn.2015.11.004.

Visser, S. S. M., van Diemen, W. J. M., Kervezee, L., van den Hoogen, A., Verschuren, O., Pillen, S., Benders, M. J. N. L., & Dudink, J. (2021). The relationship between preterm birth and sleep in children at school age: A systematic review. *Sleep Medicine Reviews*, *57*, 101447. https://doi.org/10.1016/j.smrv.2021.101447.

Walani, S. R. (2020). Global burden of preterm birth. *International Journal of Gynecology & Obstetrics*, *150*(1), 31–33. https://doi.org/10.1002/ijgo.13195.

Werth, J., Atallah, L., Andriessen, P., Long, X., Zwartkruis-Pelgrim, E., & Aarts, R. M. (2017). Unobtrusive sleep state measurements in preterm infants – A review. *Sleep Medicine Reviews*, *32*, 109–122. https://doi.org/10.1016/j.smrv.2016.03.005.

WHO. (2022). *World Health Organization*. https://www.who.int/news-room/fact-sheets/detail/preterm-birth.

Yates, C. C., Mitchell, A. J., Booth, M. Y., Williams, D. K., Lowe, L. M., & Whit Hall, R. (2014). The Effects of Massage Therapy to Induce Sleep in Infants Born Preterm. *Pediatric Physical Therapy*, *26*(4), 405–410. https://doi.org/10.1097/PEP.0000000000000081.

Chapter 10

Evidence-Based Nursing Practices for Mother-Baby Attachment

Fatma Bozdağ*, PhD
and Mehmet Emin Düken, PhD
Department of Child Health and Disease Nursing, Faculty of Health Sciences, Harran University, Şanlıurfa Türkiye

Abstract

Attachment, defined by Bowlby and developed by Ainsworth, is a unique and emotional process established between the baby and the caregivers. In babies, the attachment figure is usually the mother, who is the primary caregiver. Mother-baby attachment begins during pregnancy and continues in the postpartum period. Many factors such as the health status of mother and baby, education level, baby's gender, number of pregnancies, the relationship status between parents, family relationships, cultural values, risky pregnancies, first pregnancy experience, planned pregnancy status, postpartum depression presence, and socio-economic status affect the attachment process. When positive interaction can be achieved between the mother and the baby, the mother enjoys physical contact with her baby, eye-to-eye communication, talking, and exploring her baby by touch. In cases where positive interaction cannot be achieved, the mother may avoid participating in the care of her baby, breastfeeding, or establishing closeness with her. Nurses are the leading members of the professional health team who strengthen the mother-baby attachment by establishing positive interactions during pregnancy, at the time of birth, and after birth. In studies, it has been proven that nurses' mother-baby-friendly interventions such as cesarean section, kangaroo care, massage, yoga, meditation, breastfeeding, gentle human touch, or yakson therapeutic touch positively affect mother-baby attachment. To ensure positive mother-baby attachment, it is necessary to screen risky groups, especially considering the factors affecting attachment, to support families during and after pregnancy, and providing necessary training. It is recommended that nurses provide appropriate interventions to the mother, considering interventions that positively affect attachment.

Keywords: mother-baby attachment, nurse, evidence-based practice

* Corresponding Author's Email: fatmabozdag@harran.edu.tr.

In: Evidence-Based Care Practices in Pediatric Nursing
Editors: Feyza Küçük and Serap Özdemir
ISBN: 979-8-89530-304-7

Introduction

Attachment

All living beings require someone who provides for their needs and offers a sense of safety and comfort after birth. Attachment is a strong emotional bond that individuals develop toward those who are important to them. The concept of attachment in infancy is defined as the emotional bond formed between a child and the caregiver. All infants have a natural tendency and need to form emotional attachments to sustain their lives (Genc and Sarıcan, 2016; Daglar and Nur, 2018; Schore, 2011).

The Attachment Theory

The Attachment Theory" is an approach that explains the reasons behind individuals' tendency to form strong emotional bonds with significant others. First proposed in 1958 by John Bowlby, a British child psychiatrist and psychoanalyst, it defines the innate connection between a baby and its mother at birth as a relationship that will influence the individual's entire life (Bowlby, 2012). It is widely accepted that every child has someone to whom they will turn and preferentially seek when they are distressed or in need. Bowlby suggests that this person is typically the mother figure, and in the absence of the mother figure, the child will ideally attach to someone familiar and trusted (Ainsworth and Wittig, 1969; Bowlby, 2012). According to attachment theory, the attachment of the baby to a caregiver, whether the mother or a substitute who provides comfort, plays a crucial role in the healthy development of the child's life (Genc and Sarıcan, 2016). Among the key figures who contributed to the development of Bowlby's theory were psychologists Robert Hinde and Mary Ainsworth. Mary Ainsworth, influenced by Bowlby's research, conducted more systematic and measurable observations. With a descriptive perspective, she clarified the emotional bond between the baby and the mother (Bowlby, 2012; Dalgar et al., 2022).

Mother-Baby Attachment

The bond between mother and baby has captivated people for centuries. It is believed that the foundation of this bond is formed during pregnancy, and even before (Zdolska-Wawrzkiewicz et al., 2020). The bond established between the mother and the unborn baby is defined as prenatal attachment (Elkin, 2015). Maternal attachment is defined as the bond established between the mother and the baby, providing high satisfaction for both parties and fostering the mother's responsibility toward the baby's physical and emotional needs. It is argued that the form of attachment a baby develops with its mother has a significant impact on its entire life. The positive establishment of the bond between mother and baby is crucial for both the physical and mental health of both (Nacar and Gokkaya, 2019).

Types of Attachment

Mary Ainsworth, in her research on Ugandan mothers and babies, developed the "Strange Situation Test" to evaluate the baby's responses to various situations. With this test, Ainsworth recorded how the babies behaved when their mother was present when they were with a stranger, and when they were alone in a new environment, as well as the type of reactions they exhibited when their mother entered the room. In early childhood, the attachment children form with their mothers is fundamentally divided into secure and insecure. Insecure attachment is further categorized as insecure/anxious and insecure/avoidant (Ainsworth et al., 1978).

Secure Attachment

The most significant indicator of secure attachment is when the child uses their mother as a secure base while exploring their surroundings. They are confident that their attachment figure will protect them under any circumstance. Securely attached children do not hesitate to engage with their environment when their mothers are present. However, they become anxious, and restless, seek their mothers, and show wariness toward unfamiliar individuals when separated from them. This distress in children is temporary; they easily seek close contact with their mothers upon their return, quickly calm down, and continue to explore their surroundings. Mothers of securely attached children are generally more sensitive to their children's needs (Dalgar et al., 2022; Sumer et al., 2016; Ozer, 2018; Comlek, 2021).

Insecure/Anxious Attachment

Anxious attachment typically begins to manifest around the age of one and is often observed in children whose parents exhibit inconsistencies in meeting their children's needs. Children with this attachment style may have mothers who are not consistently present when they cry, who are late in meeting their care needs, or who leave their care incomplete. These children cannot be sure that their mothers will be there for them when they need them, leading to feelings of unease. Even when their mothers are present, they show little interest in exploring their surroundings. When separated from their mothers, they experience intense separation anxiety and may refuse to communicate with strangers, often having crying fits. Despite experiencing intense anxiety during separation, they may not seek comfort from their mothers upon their return and may even push them away due to feelings of anger. They have difficulty calming down and may sometimes cling to their mothers instead. Children with this attachment style often have not received the love, care, and attention they expected from their mothers, leaving them feeling lonely and sometimes indifferent to separation from their mothers. They may continue to be unresponsive when their mothers return (Dalgar et al., 2022; Sumer et al., 2016; Ozer, 2018; Comlek, 2021).

Insecure/Avoidant Attachment

Children with this attachment style do not show a reaction or response when their mothers leave their side. When their mothers return, they avoid communication and closeness with them. Instead, they continue to explore their surroundings or engage in playing with their toys (Dalgar et al., 2022; Sumer et al., 2016; Ozer, 2018; Comlek, 2021).

Stages of Attachment

Bowlby divided attachment behavior into four unspecified stages (Bowlby, 1969).

Stage 1: Orientation and Signaling with Limited Discrimination of the Figure

This stage covers the first 8 weeks and can extend up to the 12th week in adverse conditions. The baby's ability to distinguish one person from others is limited during this stage and is primarily based on olfactory or auditory cues. Typically, a baby stops crying when they hear a voice (Rheingold, 1961; Bowlby, 1969).

Stage 2: Orienting to One or More Separate Figures and Directed Signals

This stage lasts until 6 months, and the baby continues to behave socially toward people. During this stage, the baby is noticeably oriented toward the mother (attachment figure) rather than other individuals (Bowlby, 1969).

Stage 3: Maintenance of Proximity to a Separate Figure Through Locomotion-Mediated Signals

The stage typically begins around the 7th month. It can extend up to the 12th month in children who spend little time with or have minimal contact with their mothers. The variety of responses from the baby increases. They begin to follow the mother, greet her when she returns, and use her as a center while exploring their surroundings. Friendly and more distinct responses to others begin to decrease. They select specific other individuals to serve as secondary attachment figures. They approach strangers with increased caution. Attachment to the mother figure becomes as apparent as everyone can discern (Bowlby, 1969).

Stage 4: Formation of a Stable Partnership with a Target

During this stage, the child begins to perceive the mother as an independent object. They cannot grasp what influences their mother's movements towards or away from them, or what measures they can take to change her behavior. The process of establishing mutual relationships begins at this stage, and the baby starts to accommodate their mother's needs during this period (Bowlby, 1969).

Stages of Mother-Baby Attachment

The psychological development of infants in their later lives is influenced by the attitudes of the mother and the relationship between the mother and the baby during the postnatal period. The behaviors of the mother after birth are of great importance in terms of mother-baby attachment (Genc and Sarıcan, 2016). There are stages that indicate healthy maternal attachment. These include preparation, acquaintance, ownership, and attachment phases (Tonkus and Muslu, 2021).

- *Preparation Phase:* The fetus has the ability to hear and respond to the emotions of the mother. During pregnancy, maternal attachment begins as the mother embraces her baby and conveys positive feelings to the baby (Tonkus and Muslu, 2021).

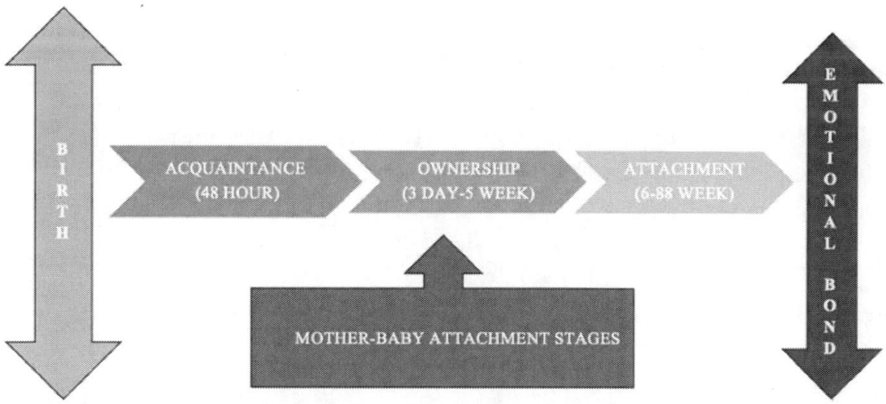

Coban, A. (2003). *Studying some of the factors affecting postnatal mother-infant interaction* (Master's Thesis, Ege University Institute of Health Sciences).

Figure 1. Mother-Baby Attachment Process.

- *Acquaintance (Identification) Phase:* This stage covers the first 48 hours after birth. After childbirth, the mother can be tired, but she can also experience happiness in being with her baby. During this phase, most of the time is spent in mutual gaze. The mother and newborn make eye contact with each other. The mother touches her baby (Tonkus and Muslu, 2021; Genc and Sarıcan, 2016).
- *Ownership (Claiming) Phase:* Begin on the third day after birth and lasts up to six weeks postpartum. During this phase, the maternal role is embraced. The mother calls her baby by name. Progress is made toward achieving mutual relationships and harmony, leading to the development of resilient bonds (Tonkus and Muslu, 2021; Genc and Sarıcan, 2016).
- *Attachment Phase:* Covers the 6th to 8th weeks after birth. During this phase, the mother is competent in caring for the baby. Mutual relationships and harmony are evident. The mother cannot bear to be separated from the baby. A deep sense of attachment and complete love between the mother and baby has developed (Tonkus and Muslu, 2021; Genc and Sarıcan, 2016).

Factors Influencing Attachment

The relationship of attachment between mother and baby is based on the prenatal period. It peaks in the first moments after birth with skin-to-skin contact and breastfeeding. Many factors during pregnancy, childbirth, and the postpartum period affect the attachment relationship. During the prenatal period, factors such as planned pregnancy, acceptance of pregnancy, the fetus's health status, feeling fetal movements, and accepting the fetus as an individual influence attachment. In the early postpartum period, factors such as depression, breastfeeding, rooming-in with the baby, skin-to-skin contact, eye contact, cuddling, and involvement in baby care affect attachment (Gunes and Isık, 2023; Basdas et al., 2022; Ozkan et al., 2020). In addition to these factors, the literature also includes variables that influence attachment, such as the mother's age, the baby's gender, the acceptance of maternal and paternal roles, the parents' childhood histories and attachment relationships with their own parents, their developmental levels, education, occupation, and temperament, marital relationships, the parents' health status, the extent to which the family fulfills its responsibilities to the child, support from extended family members and the community, relationship patterns within the family, cultural values, social security, economic status, and type of family (Karakas and Daglı, 2019; Engin and & Kuzlu-Ayyıldız, 2021; Yılmaz, 2017; Sokukcu, 2023).

Evidence-Based Nursing Practices Used to Improve Mother-Baby Attachment

Dr. Archie Cochrane's book published in 1971 laid the foundations of evidence-based medicine (Shah and Chung, 2009). The influence of this development in medical science led to the widespread adoption of evidence-based nursing research in the late 1990s (Copur et al., 2015). The translation of nursing research results into clinical practice has shaped the future of evidence-based nursing (Bagriyanik et al., 2022).

At the core of the nursing profession, the provision of high-quality and effective care is the key. The foundation of nursing care in evidence-based practices enables the establishment of standards in care, facilitates the advancement of nursing science with current knowledge, informs the creation of new policies, reduces costs in healthcare, and allows for the efficient utilization of resources (Dogan et al., 2021).

Recent years have seen an increase in evidence-based nursing research focused on mother-baby attachment. Studies indicate that implementing non-traumatic practices such as initiating breastfeeding as soon as possible, kangaroo care/skin-to-skin contact, rooming-in for mother and baby, touch and massage, yoga/meditation, and therapeutic-caring touch, as well as social support interventions, can improve mother-baby attachment (Linde, et al., 2020; Akarsu et al., 2017; Karakas and Daglı, 2019; Celebi and Cayır, 2021; Gul, 2022).

Early Initiation and Support of Breastfeeding

It is known that difficulties in breastfeeding negatively affect mother-baby attachment (Ondrušová, 2023). In a study, it was found that technology-based breastfeeding education provided to mothers positively influenced mother-infant attachment (Sarı Ozturk and Demir, 2023). In a study conducted with Spanish mothers, it was determined that breastfeeding increased maternal attachment (López-Fernández et al., 2023). Similarly, in a study conducted in Turkey, it was found that mothers who continued breastfeeding beyond the 6th month had higher levels of attachment to their babies (Yılmaz, 2017). Another study conducted with mothers of infants in the neonatal intensive care unit (NICU) reported that as the barrier to contact between mother and baby increased, mother-infant attachment was negatively affected. Therefore, practices such as breastfeeding and kangaroo care, tailored to the infant's clinical condition, are recommended to support mother-infant contact (Gunduzalp, 2023; Karakaya Suzan, 2023). A systematic review examining the relationship between mother-infant attachment and breastfeeding found that long-term breastfeeding strengthens the level of mother-baby attachment (Linde, et al., 2020). In another study, it was determined that as breastfeeding self-efficacy increased, mother-infant attachment improved (Gumussoy et al., 2020). In a study conducted with mothers in Jordan who fed their babies using three different methods (exclusive breastfeeding, formula feeding, and mixed feeding), it was reported that breastfeeding mothers had higher levels of attachment (Abuhammad and Johnson, 2021). The literature also highlights the importance of caution during the transition period when a mother attempts to wean her baby from breastfeeding. It has been noted that if this process is not managed correctly, it can negatively affect the emotional bond between the mother and the baby. Therefore, it is essential to support mothers in initiating and managing this process at an appropriate time and in a harmonious manner (Gonzales andTejero, 2022). As the results indicate, initiating breastfeeding as soon as possible, ensuring its continuity in later stages, addressing breastfeeding difficulties, and providing education on breastfeeding all contribute to strengthening the bond between mother and baby.

Kangaroo Care

In the early 1970s, researchers in Ohio, USA, began investigating the effects of immediate skin-to-skin contact between the mother and the baby right after birth. In the mid-1970s, in Bogota, Colombia, Rey, and Martinez conducted research on the same care method, and as a result of their studies, this contact was named "Kangaroo Care" (KC) (Kostandy and Ludington-Hoe, 2019). Current studies have shown that kangaroo care has positive effects not only on mother-baby attachment but also on father-baby attachment (Kucukkaya, 2022; Karakaya Suzan, 2023; Garnica-Torres et al., 2021; Yıldırım et al., 2023; Unal Toprak and Enturk Erenel, 2021).

In studies conducted in Turkey, it has been reported that kangaroo care provided to term or premature babies has a positive effect on mother-baby attachment (Cagan and Genc, 2023; Erduran, and Yaman Sozbir, 2023; Kurt et al., 2020; Zehra and Turk, 2020; Herek, 2018). Similarly, studies conducted in Iran with premature and three-month-old babies have found that kangaroo care increases mother-baby attachment (Mehrpisheh et al., 2022; Karimi et al., 2016). In another meta-analysis study, it was found that intermittent kangaroo care provided to premature babies reduces maternal depression and anxiety levels, thus improving mother-baby attachment (Pathak et al., 2023). In a study conducted in Korea, the effect of extending the duration of kangaroo care by 1 hour on postpartum depression and mother-baby attachment was examined in mothers diagnosed with postpartum depression. It was found that kangaroo care reduced postpartum depression but did not affect mother-baby attachment (Cho and Jeong, 2021). According to the research findings, providing kangaroo care to term or premature babies shortly after birth and continuing it is important to strengthen mother-baby and even father-baby attachment.

Massage

Massage is one of the oldest forms of healthcare practices in the world, involving intentional and systematic touching of the body's soft tissues. Attachment theory emphasizes the significance of physical contact between mothers and babies. Touch emerges as the initial form of communication between mothers and their infants (Yılmaz et al., 2023; Norholt, 2020). It has been proven that the body contact provided by baby massage strengthens the baby's sense of security and enhances mother-baby attachment (Zhang et al., 2023). In a study conducted in Turkey, it was reported that after receiving massage education, mothers massage their babies at least once a day, and this practice increases mother-baby attachment (Ercelik and Yılmaz, 2023). Similarly, in studies conducted with primiparous mothers in the provinces of Malatya and Erzurum in Turkey, it was found that baby massage or oxytocin massage improves mother-baby attachment (Altıparmak, 2021; Gurol and Polat, 2012). In a study where mothers of premature babies were provided with Yakson and gentle human touch training, it was reported that the Yakson touch and gentle human touch applied by mothers to their babies increased mother-baby attachment (Can and Kaya, 2022). In a study conducted with adolescent mothers in the USA, it was found that carrying their babies in a kangaroo carrier while doing daily activities up to 7 months increased attachment to the baby more than reading books to the baby (Williams and Turner, 2020).On the other hand, in a study conducted in Taiwan, where parents of premature babies were provided with massage education, the babies were evaluated 3 months after discharge. It was reported that while massage did not have a significant effect on parent-baby attachment, it did reduce parental stress and had a positive significant effect on the baby's weight gain (Hwu et al., 2023). As a result, studies in the literature suggest that baby massage should be performed due to its positive effects on infant growth and strengthening mother-baby attachment.

Music Therapy

There are promising studies regarding the ability of music interventions to increase mother-baby attachment. It is believed that mothers can use music to adapt to their babies' emotional states. For example, singing to the baby while rhythmically stroking them can strengthen the bond between them (Newman et al., 2022). In a study conducted in Switzerland, where music therapy was applied to premature babies and their parents during kangaroo care, it was determined that music therapy improved parent-baby attachment (Kehl et al., 2021). Similarly, studies conducted with mothers in Norway have found that participating in music therapy programs or singing to their babies strengthens the mother-baby attachment (Riise, 2020; Gaden and Trondalen, 2018). In Germany, a study conducted with pregnant women who participated in music therapy and singing sessions during pregnancy reported that pregnant women who sang had the highest reported levels of mother-baby attachment (Wulff et al., 2021). In a study conducted in Turkey, pregnant women were allowed to feel their babies by touching their bellies while lullabies were played to them. It was found that lullabies had a positive effect on prenatal mother-baby attachment (Baltacı and Baser, 2022). In another study conducted, involving eight neonatal intensive care units (NICUs) in Argentina, Colombia, Israel, Norway, and Poland, it was found that music therapy did not have a significant effect on mother-baby attachment at 6 and 12 months (Ghetti et al., 2023). In conclusion, there is limited research showing the positive effects of music therapy on mother-baby attachment. More studies are needed to investigate the effects of music therapy on parent-baby attachment in both the early and late stages.

Type of Birth

There is limited research on the impact of the mode of delivery on mother-baby attachment. Some studies have found that women who give birth vaginally have higher levels of mother-baby attachment compared to women who undergo a cesarean section (Doblin et al., 2023; Cankaya et al., 2017; Haratipour et al., 2021). On the other hand, there is a study indicating that the mode of delivery does not affect mother-baby attachment, but giving birth by cesarean section increases the risk of postpartum depression, which indirectly affects mother-baby attachment negatively (Tug, 2020). In a study conducted with mothers who had vaginal births in Turkey, it was found that babies who underwent delayed cord clamping had higher levels of mother-baby attachment compared to babies who underwent early cord clamping (Dinc and Kanbur, 2023). In another study conducted in Turkey, it was found that women who did not receive oxytocin induction during childbirth had higher levels of mother-baby attachment compared to women who did receive oxytocin induction (Gocen and Amanak, 2022). In conclusion, more research is needed, particularly taking into account factors such as unplanned emergency cesarean section and planned cesarean section, to determine the impact of the birth method on mother-baby attachment.

Other Studies

Many studies have reported that postpartum depression and anxiety negatively affect maternal attachment (Śliwerski et al., 2020; Cankaya et al., 2017; Aksoy Bulgurcu, 2019; Daglar, 2018). In a meta-analysis study, it was found that the likelihood of postpartum depressed mothers adopting an insecure attachment to their babies was nearly twice as high as that of healthy mothers (Barnes and Theule, 2019). In a study conducted during the pandemic, it was found that there was no significant relationship between fear of COVID-19 and mother-baby attachment (Polat and Yıldız, 2023).

In a study conducted in Turkey, it was determined that women who became pregnant through assisted reproductive techniques had higher levels of mother-baby attachment compared to women who conceived naturally (Ozdemir, 2021). In a study conducted in Turkey, it was reported that yoga practice with mothers for 8 weeks postpartum increased mother-baby attachment (Boybay Koyuncu and Yayan, 2022). In other studies conducted in Turkey, it has been proven that involving mothers in the care process in the intensive care unit, sending them a picture of their baby every day, and providing information about the baby's condition improves mother-baby attachment (Yuce, 2023; Simsek, 2023).

Conclusion

Preparing the mother for the childbirth process to strengthen the prenatal attachment between the mother and baby, providing information to mothers about the benefits of vaginal delivery and encouraging vaginal birth, initiating early breastfeeding and kangaroo care practices, providing practical breastfeeding education to mothers, ensuring that the mother and baby stay in the same room, providing mothers with baby massage training and encouraging its practice, providing training on gentle human touch and Yakson touch to mothers and facilitating their implementation, involving the mother in the baby's care, providing yoga training and encouraging its practice in the postpartum period, involving the mother in music therapy programs during pregnancy and postpartum periods, informing mothers with babies in the neonatal intensive care unit about their babies and facilitating their visitation and working to reduce factors contributing to postpartum depression and strengthening social support networks are among the main roles of nurses in strengthening the mother-baby attachment.

Disclaimer

None.

References

Abuhammad, S., & Johnson, T. (2021). Breastfeeding and maternal attachment during infancy period among Jordanian mothers: A cross-sectional study. *Annals of Medicine and Surgery, 66.* https://doi.org/10.1016/ j.amsu.2021.102395.

Ainsworth, M. D., & Wittig, B. A. (1969). Attachment and exploratory behavior of one-year-olds in a strange situation. In B. M. Foss (Ed.), *Determinants of infant behavior* (Vol. 4, pp. 113-136). London: Methuen.

Ainsworth, M. D. S., Blehar, M. C., Waters, E. & Wall, S. (1978). Patterns of attachment: *A psychological study of the strange sitiation.* Hillsdale, NJ: Erlbaum.

Akarsu, R. H., Tunca, B., & Alsac, S. Y. (2017). Evidence-based applications in mother-infant attachment. *Gumushane University Journal of Health Sciences, 6*(4), 275-279.

Aksoy Bulgurcu, R. (2019). *Evaluation of maternal-infant attachment and postpartum depression in women giving preterm and term birth* (Master's thesis, Gulhane Institute of Health Sciences).

Altıparmak, S. (2021). *The effect of hypnobreastfeeding and oxytocin massage on breastfeeding motivation, perception of insufficient milk, attachment, and uterine involution process in primiparous women* (Doctoral dissertation, Inonu University Institute of Health Sciences).

Bagriyanik, B. C., Yildiz, D., Fidanci, B. E., Pekyigit, A., Bagriyanik, T., & Asarkaya, M. Determination of the attitudes of the nurses working in children hospital on evidence-based practices. *Journal of Adnan Menderes University Health Sciences Faculty, 6*(2), 202-215. https://doi.org/10.46237/amusbfd.894471

Baltacı, N., & Baser, M. (2022). The effect of lullaby intervention on anxiety and prenatal attachment in women with high-risk pregnancy: A randomized controlled study. *Complementary Medicine Research, 29*(2), 127-135. https://doi.org/10.1159/000520139.

Barnes, J., & Theule, J. (2019). Maternal depression and infant attachment security: A meta-analysis. *Infant Mental Health Journal, 40*(6), 817-834. https://doi.org/10.1002/imhj.21812.

Basdas, O., Efe, Y. S., Erdem, E., Ozdemir, A., Gunes, T., & Ozturk, A. (2022). Factors affecting mother baby attachment. *YOBU Faculty of Health Sciences Journal, 3*(2), 130-136.

Bowlby, J. (1969). *Attachment and loss.* (Trans. T. V. Soylu). Istanbul: Pihnan Publishing.

Bowlby, J. (2012). *A secure base.* (Trans. S. Güneri). İstanbul: Psychotherapy Institute Education Publications.

Boybay Koyuncu, S., & Yayan, E. H. (2022). Effect of postpartum yoga on breastfeeding self-efficacy and maternal attachment in primiparous mothers. *Breastfeeding Medicine, 17*(4), 311-317. https://doi.org/ 10.1089/bfm.2021.0320.

Cagan, E. S., & Genc, R. (2023). The effects of kangaroo care at birth on exclusively breastfeeding, baby's growth and development according to attachment theory: A randomized controlled trial. *Early Child Development and Care*, *193*(3), 378-387. https://doi.org/10.1080/03004430.2022.2093866.

Can, S., & Kaya, H. (2022). The effects of yakson or gentle human touch training given to mothers with preterm babies on attachment levels and the responses of the baby: A randomized controlled trial. *Health Care for Women International*, *43*(5), 479-498. https://doi.org/10.1080/07399332.2021.1958817.

Cankaya, S., Yilmaz, S. D., Can, R., & Kodaz, N. D. (2017). Effect of postpartum depression on maternal attachment. *Acıbadem University Journal of Health Sciences*, (4), 232-240.

Celebi, E. Z., & Cayır, G. (2021). Factors affecting parent-infant attachment. A systematic review made by examining postgraduate theses. *Journal of Women's Health Nursing, 7*(1), 23-47.

Cho, H., & Jeong, I. S. (2021). The relationship between mother-infant contact time and changes in postpartum depression and mother-infant attachment among mothers staying at postpartum care centers: An observational study. *Nursing & Health Sciences*, *23*(2), 547-555. https://doi.org/10.1111/nhs.12847.

Coban, A. (2003). *Studying some of thr factors affecting postnatal mother-infant interaction* (Master's Thesis, Ege University Institute of Health Sciences).

Comlek, G. (2021). *Determining the relationship between mother-infant attachment and father-baby attachment* (Master's Thesis, Istanbul Medipol University Institute of Health Sciences).

Copur, E. O., Kuru, N., & Seyman, C. C. (2015). Overview of the evidence based practices in nursing. *Journal of Health and Nursing Management, 1*(2), 51-55.

Daglar, G., & Nur, N. (2018). Level of mother-baby bonding and influencing factors during pregnancy and postpartum period. *Psychiatria Danubina*, *30*(4), 433-440. https://doi.org/10.24869/psyd.2018.433.

Dalgar, G., Civil, F., Savas, E., & Sahin, A. (2022). Attachment in early childhood: An examination from John Bowlby and Mary Ainsworth. *Eurasian Journal of Health Sciences, 5*(1), 85-92. https://doi.org/10.53493/Avrasyasbd.885024.

Dinc, T., & Kanbur, A. (2023). The effect of delayed umbilical cord clamping on the infant's beta-endorphin level, mother-infant attachment and breastfeeding. *European Journal of Obstetrics & Gynecology and Reproductive Biology*, *285*, 187-192. https://doi.org/10.1016/j.ejogrb.2023.04.025.

Doblin, S., Seefeld, L., Weise, V., Kopp, M., Knappe, S., Asselmann, E., ... & Garthus-Niegel, S. (2023). The impact of mode of delivery on parent-infant-bonding and the mediating role of birth experience: A comparison of mothers and fathers within the longitudinal cohort study DREAM. *BMC Pregnancy and Childbirth*, *23*(1), 285.

Dogan, E. S., Cin, A., Demirag, H., & Ucan, M. F. (2021). Investigation of nurses' attitudes toward evidence-based nursing practices. *International Anatolian Journal of Social Sciences, 5*(2), 612-622. https://doi.org/10.47525/ulasbid.879094.

Elkin, N. (2015). Prenatal attachment levels of pregnant women and factors affecting them. *Continuing Medical Education Journal, 24*(6), 230-237.

Engin, N., & Kuzlu-Ayyıldız, T. (2021). The investigation of mother-baby attachment based on maternal perception and some variables. *Journal of Adnan Menderes University Health Sciences Faculty,5*(3), 583-596. https://doi.org/10.46237/amusbfd.947004.

Ercelik, Z. E., & Yılmaz, H. B. (2023). Effectiveness of infant massage on babies growth, mother-baby attachment and mothers' self-confidence: A randomized controlled trial. *Infant Behavior and Development*, *73*, 101897. https://doi.org/10.1016/j.infbeh.2023.101897.

Erduran, B., & Yaman Sözbir, S. (2023). Effects of intermittent kangaroo care on maternal attachment, postpartum depression of mothers with preterm infants. *Journal of Reproductive and Infant Psychology*, *41*(5), 556-565. https://doi.org/10.1080/02646838.2022.2035703.

Gaden, T. S., & Trondalen, G. (2018). Bonding through music: Music therapy as health promotion for mothers and children at a public health clinic. *Music and Public Health: A Nordic Perspective*, 151-166..

Garnica-Torres, Z., Gouveia Jr, A., & da Silva Pedroso, J. (2021). Attachment between father and premature baby in kangaroo care in a neonatal unit of a public hospital. *Journal of Neonatal Nursing*, *27*(5), 334-340. https://doi.org/10.1016/j.jnn.2020.12.005.

Genc, R. E., & Sarıcan, E. S. (2016). For midwives, newborn health and diseases. Genc, R.E., & Ozkan, H. (Ed.), *Mother baby attachement* (ss.643-649). Elazıg: Nobel Medical Bookstores.

Ghetti, C. M., Gaden, T. S., Bieleninik, Ł., Kvestad, I., Assmus, J., Stordal, A. S., ... & Gold, C. (2023). Effect of music therapy on parent-infant Bonding among infants born preterm: A randomized clinical trial. *JAMA Network Open*, *6*(5), e2315750-e2315750. https://doi.org/10.1001/jamanetworkopen.2023.15750.

Gocen, N. N., & Amanak, K. (2022). The effects of labor induction on postpartum mother-infant bonding and anxiety levels. *Jurnal Medical Brasovean*, (1), 17-25. https://doi.org/10.31926/jmb.2022.1.1.

Gonzales Jr, A. M., & Tejero, L. M. S. (2022). Concept analysis of maternal-infant attachment during the weaning process. *Belitung Nursing Journal*, *8*(5), 381. https://doi.org/10.33546/bnj.2178.

Gul, F. (2022). *Applications in postpartum depression counseling strengthening mother-infant attachment and increasing mother's self-recovery power* (Master's thesis, Karatay University Institute of Graduate Education).

Gumussoy, S., Celik, N. A., Guner, O., Kıratlı, D., Atan, S. U., & Kavlak, O. (2020). Investigation of the relationship between maternal attachment and breastfeeding self-efficacy and affecting factors in Turkish sample. *Journal of Pediatric Nursing*, *54*, e53-e60. https://doi.org/10.1016/j.pedn.2020.04.022.

Gunduzalp, R. (2023). *Determination of the relationship between stress levels of mothers with babies in the neonatal intensive care unit and barriers to mother-infant contact with mother-infant attachment* (Master's thesis, Erzurum Technical University Institute of Health Sciences).

Gunes, E., & Isık, C. (2023). Factors affecting maternal - paternal attachment and midwifery approaches. *Journal of Health Professions Research*, *5*(1), 89-95. https://doi.org/10.57224/jhpr.1158640.

Gurol, A., & Polat, S. (2012). The effects of baby massage on attachment between mother and their infants. *Asian Nursing Research*, *6*(1), 35-41. https://doi.org/10.1016/j.anr.2012.02.006.

Haratipour, H., Partash, N., Ebrahimi, E., Zadeh, M. D., & Bolbolhaghighi, N. (2021). Non-physiological and physiological delivery method: Comparison of maternal attachment behaviors and anxiety. *Journal of Caring Sciences*, *10*(1), 37. https://doi.org/10.34172/jcs.2021.011.

Herek, B. (2018). *Maternal attachment and postpartum depression in kangaroo cared mothers of prematüre infants treated in newborn* (Master's thesis, Gazi University Institute of Health Sciences).

Herek, B. (2018). *Maternal attachment and postpartum depression in kangaroo cared mothers of prematüre infants treated in newborn* (Master's thesis, Gazi University Institute of Health Sciences) .

Hwu, L. J., Tzeng, Y. L., Teng, Y. K., & Liu, S. J. (2023). Effects of massage intervention on discharged premature infants' weight, parental stress, and parent–child attachment: A randomized controlled trial. *Infant Behavior and Development*, *72*, 101867. https://doi.org/10.1016/j.infbeh.2023.101867.

Karakas, N. M., & Daglı, F. S. (2019). The importance of attachment in infant and influencing factors. *Turkish Archives of Pediatrics, 54*(2), 76-81. https://doi.org/10.14744/TurkPediatriArs.2018.80269.

Karakaya Suzan, O. (2023). *Investigation of the effect of attachment-based support given during the perinatal period on prenatal attachment, early mother and baby bonding and maternal attachment* (Doctoral dissertation, Sakarya University Institute of Health Sciences).

Karimi, F. Z., Khadivzadeh, T., Saeidi, M., & Bagheri, S. (2016). The effect of kangaroo mother care immediately after delivery on mother-infant attachment 3 months after delivery. *International Jornal of Pediatrics*, *4*(9), 3561-70. https://doi.org/10.22038/ijp.2016.7430.

Kehl, S. M., La Marca-Ghaemmaghami, P., Haller, M., Pichler-Stachl, E., Bucher, H. U., Bassler, D., & Haslbeck, F. B. (2021). Creative music therapy with premature infants and their parents: A mixed-method pilot study on parents' anxiety, stress and depressive symptoms and parent–infant attachment. *International Journal of Environmental Research and Public Health*, *18*(1), 265. https://doi.org/10.3390/ijerph18010265.

Kucukkaya, B. (2022). *The effect of early initiation of swaddling and kangaroo care practices in preterm infants on breastfeeding, mother-infant bonding, maternal sleep quality, and postpartum depression* (Doctoral dissertation, Sakarya University Institute of Health Sciences).

Kurt, F. Y., Kucukoglu, S., Ozdemir, A. A., & Ozcan, Z. (2020). The effect of kangaroo care on maternal attachment in preterm infants. *Nigerian Journal of Clinical Practice*, *23*(1), 26-32. https://doi.org/10.4103/njcp.njcp_143_18.

Linde, K., Lehnig, F., Nagl, M., & Kersting, A. (2020). The association between breastfeeding and attachment: A systematic review. *Midwifery*, *81*, 102592. https://doi.org/10.1016/j.midw.2019.102592.

López-Fernández, G., Barrios, M., & Gómez-Benito, J. (2023). Breastfeeding and maternal attachment: The moderating roles of maternal stress and child behavior. *Journal of Pediatric Nursing*, *69*, e80-e87. https://doi.org/10.1016/j.pedn.2022.12.011.

Mehrpisheh, S., Doorandish, Z., Farhadi, R., Ahmadi, M., Moafi, M., & Elyasi, F. (2022). The Effectiveness of kangaroo mother care (KMC) on attachment of mothers with premature infants. *European Journal of Obstetrics & Gynecology and Reproductive Biology: X*, *15*, 100149. https://doi.org/10.1016/j.eurox.2022.100149.

Nacar, E. H., & Gokkaya, F. (2019). A review article on attachment and maternal attachment. *Cyprus Turkish Journal of Psychiatry & Psychology*, *1*(1), 50-56. https://doi.org/10.35365/ctjpp.19.1.06.

Newman, L. J., Stewart, S. E., Freeman, N. C., & Thompson, G. (2022). A systematic review of music interventions to support parent–child attachment. *Journal of Music Therapy*, *59*(4), 430-459. https://doi.org/10.1093/jmt/thac012.

Norholt, H. (2020). Revisiting the roots of attachment: A review of the biological and psychological effects of maternal skin-to-skin contact and carrying of full-term infants. *Infant Behavior and Development*, *60*, 101441. https://doi.org/10.1016/j.infbeh.2020.101441.

Ondrušová, S. (2023). Breastfeeding and bonding: A surprising role of breastfeeding difficulties. *Breastfeeding Medicine*, *18*(7), 514-521. https://doi.org/10.1089/bfm.2023.0021.

Ozdemir, E. (2021). Evaluation of mother-infant attachment and postpartum depression levels in women conceiving naturally and through assisted reproductive techniques (Doctoral dissertation, Ankara Yıldırım Beyazıt University Institute of Health Sciences).

Ozer, I. O. (2018). Natural result of attachment: Separation anxiety. *COMU International Journal of Social Sciences, 3*(1), 125-134. https://doi.org/10.31454/usb.419854.

Ozkan, T. K., Kucukkelepce, D. S., & Ozkan, S. A. (2020). Relationship between prenatal attachment and body sense in pregnancy and affecting factors. *Manisa Celal Bayar University Journal of Institute of Health Science, 7*(1), 49-54. https://doi.org/10.34087/cbusbed.587467.

Pathak, B. G., Sinha, B., Sharma, N., Mazumder, S., & Bhandari, N. (2023). Effects of kangaroo mother care on maternal and paternal health: systematic review and meta-analysis. *Bulletin of the World Health Organization*, *101*(6), 391. https://doi.org/10.2471/BLT.22.288977.

Polat, M., & Yıldız, I. (2023). The relationships between the COVID-19 fears of mothers and their mother-infant bonding and breastfeeding self-efficacy in the postpartum period. *Early Child Development and Care*, *193*(15-16), 1517-1529. https://doi.org/10.1080/03004430.2023.2257003.

Rheingold, H .L. (1961). "The effect of environmental stimulation upon social and exploratory behavior in the human infant." *In Determinants of Infants Behavior (*Vol. 1, ed. B. M. Foss). London: Methuen; New York: Wiley.

Riise, K. M. (2020). *Music therapy as a means for increased bonding and attachment between mother and infant A qualitative literature review exploring how music therapy, or the use of music could promote bonding and attachment between mothers with postpartum depression and their infants* (Master's thesis, The University of Bergen).

Sarı Ozturk, C., & Demir, K. (2023). The effect of mandala activity and technology-based breastfeeding program on breastfeeding self-efficacy and mother-infant attachment of primiparous women: A randomized controlled study. *Journal of Medical Systems*, *47*(1), 44. https://doi.org/10.1007/s10916-023-01942-3.

Schore, A .N. (2011). *Developmental neurobiology and attachment theory.* Istanbul: Ozak Publishing House.

Shah, H. M., & Chung, K. C. (2009). Archie Cochrane and his vision for evidence-based medicine. *Plastic and Reconstructive Surgery*, *124*(3), 982-988. https://doi.org/10.1097/PRS.0b013e3181b03928.

Simsek, K. N. (2023). *The effect of different communication methods established with mothers with babies in the neonatal intensive care unit on the level of hopelessness and mother-infant attachment* (Master's thesis, Biruni University Üniversitesi Graduate School of Education).

Śliwerski, A., Kossakowska, K., Jarecka, K., Świtalska, J., & Bielawska-Batorowicz, E. (2020). The effect of maternal depression on infant attachment: A systematic review. *International Journal of Environmental Research And Public Health*, *17*(8), 2675. https://doi.org/10.3390/ijerph17082675.

Sokukcu, E. (2023). *Examination of comfort level of mothers in the postpartum period and mother-infant attachment* (Master's thesis, Ege University Institute of Health Sciences).

Sumer, N., Sayıl, M. ve Berument, S. K. (2016). *Maternal sensitivity and attachment in children.* (1st Edition). Istanbul: Koc University Publications.

Tonkus, M. B., & Muslu, S. N. (2021). Maternal Attachment and Related Factors. *Journal of Medical Sciences*, *2*(2), 32-40. https://doi.org/10.46629/JMS.2021.39.

Tug, E. (2020). *Evaluation of the effect of delivery mode on postpartum depression risk and mother-infant attachment* (Medical Specialization Thesis, Health Sciences University Ankara Dıskapı Yıldırım Beyazıt Health Practice and Research Center).

Unal Toprak, F., & Senturk Erenel, A. (2021). Impact of kangaroo care after caesarean section on paternal–infant attachment and involvement at 12 months: A longitudinal study in Turkey. *Health & Social Care in the Community*, *29*(5), 1502-1510. https://doi.org/10.1111/hsc.13210.

Williams, L. R., & Turner, P. R. (2020). Infant carrying as a tool to promote secure attachments in young mothers: Comparing intervention and control infants during the still-face paradigm. *Infant Behavior and Development*, *58*, 101413. https://doi.org/10.1016/j.infbeh.2019.101413.

Wulff, V., Hepp, P., Wolf, O. T., Balan, P., Hagenbeck, C., Fehm, T., & Schaal, N. K. (2021). The effects of a music and singing intervention during pregnancy on maternal well-being and mother–infant bonding: a randomised, controlled study. *Archives of Gynecology and Obstetrics*, *303*, 69-83. https://doi.org/10.1007/s00404-020-05727-8.

Yildirim, F., Duman, N. B., Şahin, E., & Vural, G. (2023). The effect of kangaroo care on paternal attachment: A Randomized Controlled Study. *Advances in Neonatal Care*, *23*(6), 596-601. https://doi.org/10.1097/ANC.0000000000001100.

Yılmaz, F. (2017). *Factors cause to quit feeding with breast milk and effect of breastfeeding duration to mother child bonding* (Master's Thesis, Maltepe University Institute of Health Sciences).

Yilmaz, H. B., Kucuk, S., Ugur, S., Onel, A. E., & Giynas, T. (2023). Investigation of the effects of infant massage in postgraduate theses in Turkey: A systematic review. Journal of Health Academicians, *10*(2), 291-301. https://doi.org/10.52880/sagakaderg.1192374.

Yuce, C. M. (2023). *The effect of involving mothers in the care of newborns in surgical intensive care on self-confidence and mother-infant attachment* (Master's thesis, Tokat Gaziosmanpasa University Graduate School of Education).

Zdolska-Wawrzkiewicz, A., Chrzan-Dętkoś, M., Pizuńska, D., & Bidzan, M. (2020). Attachment styles, various maternal representations and a bond to a baby. *International Journal of Environmental Research and Public Health*, *17*(10), 3363. https://doi.org/10.3390/ijerph17103363.

Zehra, C. & Turk, R. (2020). The effect of early kangaroo care provided to term babies on the maternal-fetal attachment. *International Journal of Caring Sciences*, *13*(1), 24-34.

Zhang, Y., Duan, C., Cheng, L., & Li, H. (2023). Effects of massage therapy on preterm infants and their mothers: A systematic review and meta-analysis of randomized controlled trials. *Frontiers in Pediatrics*, *11*. https://doi.org/10.3389/fped.2023.1198730.

Chapter 11

Evidence-Based Nursing Practices in Children Suffering from Asthma

Emine Gunes San*, **MSc**
Department of Child Health, and Disease Nursing, Faculty of Health Science, Bartin University, Bartin, Türkiye

Abstract

Asthma is a chronic disease that affects millions of children worldwide. Despite improving nursing care, the prevalence of childhood asthma continues to rise. Asthma can have a negative impact on the quality of life. Children who have been diagnosed with asthma can experience physical, psychological, and social problems. Recurrent and uncontrolled asthma attacks in children can be a cause of breathlessness, activity limitation, school absenteeism, and less participation in school activities. These problems can cause the child to experience feelings such as fear of rejection, low self-esteem, feelings of inadequacy, helplessness, and depression. The Global Initiative for Asthma (GINA) guidelines support the implementation of nursing interventions to manage childhood asthma. These interventions support and guide children's efforts to manage their asthma. Therefore, the primary focus of nurses should be on the provision of preventive care rather than on the care of children with asthma exacerbation. Nurses and health professionals aim to ensure that children's asthma is controlled, with fewer symptoms, no problems sleeping, and no restrictions on exercise. Additionally, the maintenance of normal lung function and the prevention of side effects related to medical conditions should be among their main goals. Knowledge of evidence-based practices is essential for this purpose.

This section discusses evidence-based practices for children with asthma, which are presented under four headings: (1) evaluating asthma, (2) education in asthma care, (3) controlling environmental factors and co-morbidities, and (4) pharmacological treatment.

Keywords: asthma, child, chronic disease, evidence-based nursing

* Corresponding Author's Email: esan@bartin.edu.tr.

In: Evidence-Based Care Practices in Pediatric Nursing
Editors: Feyza Küçük and Serap Özdemir
ISBN: 979-8-89530-304-7

Introduction

Asthma is a common chronic condition that is characterized by bronchial hyperresponsiveness and airway obstruction (Jia et al., 2023; Tao et al., 2023). In many countries, its prevalence is increasing, particularly in children and adolescents (Ferrante and La Grutta 2018; Reddel et al., 2022). It is estimated to affect more than 334 million people (Farzandipour et al., 2024). This number is expected to reach 400 million by 2025 (Alharbi et al. 2020). Asthma in children can progress differently (NHLBI, 2007).

Children with asthma may experience physical, psychological, and social problems, when compared to children without an asthma diagnosis (de Assis et al., 2019; Dharmage, Perret, and Custovic, 2019). Recurrent and uncontrolled asthma attacks in children can lead to respiratory distress, restrictions on physical activity, school absences (Vazquez-Ortiz et al. 2020), less participation in school-related activities, increased emergency room visits, and hospital admissions (Guttmann et al., 2007; Massie et al., 2004; Rosychuk et al. 2010). Because of this children can experience feelings such as fear of rejection, low self-esteem, inadequacy, helplessness, and depression (Merianos et al., 2015; Teymouri et al., 2017). Therefore, it is important to improve the self-care and self-management skills of children diagnosed with asthma and to offer a holistic care approach (de Benedictis & Bush, 2017; Mosnaim et al., 2016).

Nurses play a critical role in the treatment and management of asthma in children (Abd et al., 2018). They collaborate with parents, primary caregivers, and healthcare professionals to ensure optimal asthma management. To effectively manage asthma, healthcare professionals must provide a consistent message that helps families fully understand the clinical situation and adhere to treatment regimens. In summary, nurses are a valuable asset in the management of chronic diseases. With appropriate training, they can provide high-quality care to children with asthma and their families (Wooler, 2001).

To provide evidence-based care and management of asthma, up-to-date guidelines for asthma are necessary. Guides can be a useful tool to ensure that children receive the best and most accurate care possible (Bousquet et al., 2007). The literature has developed evidence-based guidelines for asthma in children (GINA 2023; Trottier et al., 2021), which summarize research findings and contribute to care. Evidence suggests that evidence-based therapies can lessen emergency visits and hospital admissions while also improving asthma management (Higuchi et al., 2011; Massie et al., 2004). Implementation of asthma care guidelines has been shown to improve nurses' knowledge and practice (Abd et al., 2018). Therefore, it is recommended that evidence-based nursing guidelines for asthma be published nationally and internationally. This section discusses evidence-based practices for children with asthma, which are presented under four headings: (1) evaluating asthma, (2) education in asthma care, (3) controlling environmental factors and co-morbidities, and (4) pharmacological treatment (NHLBI, 2007; Sun, Sun, and Wang, 2023).

Most asthma guidelines recommend retrospective evaluation of asthma severity and control. Guidelines have been established for assessing, preventing, and managing asthma attacks (GINA, 2023; National Heart Lung and Blood Institute, 2007, 2020; SIGN, 2019; Royal Children's Hospital, 2018). Evidence levels for recommendations from these guidelines will be presented in the relevant sections (see Table 1).

Table 1. Evidence Levels

Level of Evidence	Type of Evidence
A	RCTs, systematic reviews, and observational evidence (Rich data)
B	RCTs and systematic reviews (Limited amount of data).
C	Non-randomized controlled studies or observational studies.
.D	Panel consensus decision
I	High-quality data from at least one systematic review of RCTs
II	High-quality data from at least one RCT of appropriate size
III	Non-randomized, single-group pre-post evaluation, cohort, time series, and case-control studies
IV	Evidence from non-experimental designs
V	Evidence-based on the opinions of respected authorities, descriptive studies of expert committees

Abbreviations: Randomized controlled trials (RCTs).
Reference: GINA, 2023; NHLBI, 2007, Rogers and Berry 2018.

Evaluation of Asthma

When evaluating asthma in children and adolescents, it is important to assess asthma control and current condition (see Table 1) (GINA, 2023). To accurately evaluate asthma and determine its severity, a thorough history should be taken, and a comprehensive clinical examination should be performed (Sun et al., 2023). The clinical examination should be thorough, encompassing the children's family history of asthma and exposure to secondary tobacco or other environmental smoke. It is essential to identify any conditions that may impact treatment compliance and quality of life, particularly the inhaler technique (Fraser et al., 2017; GINA, 2023). When dealing with young children, it is crucial to rule out whooping cough, bronchiolitis, or pneumonia as potential causes of symptoms (Fraser et al., 2017). Additionally, it is important to consider the possibility of aspiration.

Table 2. Evaluation of Asthma in Years 6-11

Evaluation of Asthma Control
- Symptom control is assessed over the last four weeks. - Lung function is measured at the beginning, three to six months after treatment, and then at least once or twice a year.
Evaluation of Treatment Problems

- The evaluation of current treatment
    - Assessment of inhaler technique,
    - Medication compliance,
    - Side effects,
    - The existence of an action plan.
- Questions about children's attitudes and goals regarding asthma and medication use.

Evaluation of Comorbid Diseases
- Rhinitis, gastroesophageal reflux, obesity, depression, and anxiety can have a negative impact on an individual's quality of life, symptoms, and asthma control.

Reference: GINA, 2023.

Table 3. Evaluation of Asthma Severity in Years 0-11

Severe Asthma
Symptoms that continue throughout the day
Common night symptoms
PEF: less than 60%
FEV1 is less than 75% of the predicted value.
Extremely limited activity
Several times a day, short-acting β-agonists are used for symptom control.
Moderate Asthma
Daily symptoms
Night-time symptoms occur three or four times a month in children aged zero to four years, and more than once a week but not each night for ages 5 to 11.
The PEF values range from 60% to 80% of the predicted value.
FEV 1: 75%-80%
PEF variability is more than 30%.
Activity: Some limitations
Short-acting β-antagonists are used for symptom control on a daily basis.
Mild Asthma
Symptoms occur between two and six times per week.
The frequency of nighttime symptoms is once or twice a month for children aged 0-4 years and three or four times a month for children aged 5- 11 years.
PEF or FEV1 should be equal to or greater than 80% of the predicted value.
PEF variability ranges from 20% to 30%.
Activity: Minor limitations
The use of short-acting β-agonists more than two days a week, but not daily.
Intermittent Asthma
Have symptoms less than 2 days a week
Nocturnal symptoms (awakenings): None (0-4 years); less than twice a month (ages 5 to 11)
PEF or FEV1 equal to or greater than 80% of the predicted value.
PEF variability: less than 20%
No limitation activity
The use of short-acting β-agonists for symptoms less than 2 days a week.

Abbreviations: Forced expiratory volume in 1 second (FEV1); Peak expiratory flow (PEF).
Reference: Available at www.nhlbi.nih.gov/guidelines/asthma/index.htm.

Asthma control can be provided or eliminated by treatment. Nurses should assess whether children's asthma is well controlled before starting treatment (GINA, 2023; Sun et al. 2023). Controlling asthma focuses on two main areas: managing symptoms and reducing the risk of future adverse events. Assessment of lung function is important for evaluating future outcomes. Measurements should be taken at the beginning of treatment, 3-6 months after treatment, and periodically thereafter to assess the ongoing risk (GINA, 2023). To evaluate asthma control, there are several popular questionnaires that have been validated and their reliability has been studied in many countries. These are the Asthma Control Questionnaire (ACQ) (for ages 6-11), Childhood ACT (C-ACT) (for ages 4-11 years old), Paediatric Asthma Quality of Life Questionnaire (PAQLQ) (for ages 7-11 years old) (GINA, 2023; SIGN, 2019). Furthermore, asthma diaries are crucial in evaluating asthma control. They give information about respiratory symptoms as well as daily routines including sleeping, eating, and exercising. Additionally, the diary should contain data on medication use, peak flow meter monitoring values, and respiratory functions assessed using a spirometer (Arakawa et al., 2017).

Asthma severity can be assessed by evaluating symptoms and current lung function after at least 2-3 months of treatment with a controller medication. Table 3 shows the four levels of asthma (Arakawa et al., 2017).

If a child has asthma, nurses may observe the following indicators: the lungs of children with asthma produce a louder and hollower sound on percussion than those of healthy children. Additionally, during an asthma attack, the expiratory phase of breathing is longer than the inspiratory phase, whereas in normal breathing, the inspiratory phase is longer. Furthermore, children with asthma may exhibit movement of the inward chest wall while breathing. As the airways become more constricted, the wheezing sound may decrease as very little air can escape from the lungs. Children with asthma often prefer to sit or stand during attacks, rather than lie down. When sitting, they can lean forward and lift their shoulders to make breathing easier. According to Flagg and Pilitteri (2018), children who agree to lie down can do so because they are either at the end of an attack and feel less threatened by shortness of breath, or because they are so exhausted from coughing that they do not have the strength to sit upright (Flagg and Pilitteri, 2018).

The guidelines for evaluating asthma recommend the following:

NHLBI Recommendations, 2007

- Predisposing factors should be identified (e.g. exposure to inhaled allergens, cigarette smoke, irritants, or viral respiratory infections at home, work, daycare, or school) (Evidence A).
- Diseases accompanying asthma should be identified
- Asthma severity should be classified (Evidence B, Evidence C).
- Pulmonary function measurements should be performed using spirometry to assess the severity of asthma. FEV1 is an indicator of current obstruction and predicts future exacerbations (Evidence C).

British Guideline (SIGN) Recommendations, 2019

- The severity of asthma attacks should be assessed by asking about the history of previous attacks, objectively assessing current asthma control, and reviewing reliever use at every asthma visit (Evidence D, <5 years; Evidence B, 5-12 years; Evidence D, >12 years).
- When evaluating a child with severe asthma, it is important to consider the risk of recurrent asthma attacks. This can be done by assessing the child's history of previous asthma attacks, checking lung function, and asking structured questions about control asthma (Evidence D for ages 5-12 years and >12 years) (SIGN, 2019).

Global Initiative for Asthma (GINA) Recommendations, 2023

- Lung function in children with asthma should be monitored more frequently (Evidence D).
- It is important to note that spirometry may not provide reliable results in children until the age of 5 and is even less useful than in adults. Additionally, many children

with uncontrolled asthma may have normal lung function during exacerbation's (GINA, 2023).

Education in Asthma Care

Nurses have a crucial role in asthma care programs. They can establish an active partnership with children and their families by encouraging open communication, addressing children and family concerns about asthma and its treatment, and creating treatment goals (Sun et al., 2023). Asthma training should provide information about asthma, improve inhaler device usage skills, increase health literacy levels, and create written action plans (Conlon and Wilson, 2015). The Nurse Asthma Care Education (NACE) program was developed in 2011 in collaboration with the Chronic Disease Management Center at the University of Michigan and the National Respiratory Education Center. The program aims to provide evidence-based education about asthma to nurses. The program is designed for nurses to achieve the following objectives: (1) enhance clinical skills, (2) improve communication and counseling skills, and (4) enhance competencies as practitioners. The article focuses on enhancing individuals' health perceptions and self-confidence. It also aims to promote leadership in asthma control activities, increase nurses' job satisfaction, and equip them with new asthma-related skills (Policicchio, Nelson, and Duffy, 2011). It has been shown that self-management training provided under the leadership of nurses improves the condition and quality of life of asthma. As seen in the evidence-based studies in Table 4, training on asthma management caused reductions in emergency room and hospital admissions, school absences, sleep loss, and health expenditures. Furthermore, these training programs resulted in improvements in asthma control test (ACT) scores, medication compliance, knowledge, attitude, and behavior.

The guideline on education in asthma care offer the following recommendations:

Royal Children's Hospital Recommendations, 2018

- Action plans have been shown to be effective (Evidence IV).
- Educating parents about the severity of asthma exacerbations at discharge has been shown to improve hospital admission rates (Evidence IV).
- Asthma education has been shown to reduce emergency visits and hospitalizations in children and their primary caregivers (Evidence I).
- When guiding inhaler technique to children and their primary caregivers, it is important to ensure that any mistakes are corrected (Evidence I).
- Additionally, it is crucial to consider the health literacy level of parents and caregivers, as poor health literacy can hinder the acquisition of asthma self-management skills (Evidence IV) (Rogers and Berry 2018).

Table 4. Evidence-Based Nursing Studies in Children with Asthma Management

Author, Year	Research Type	Sample Size	Application	Result/Evidence Level
(Chen and Chen 2021)	RCT	n=120	Web-based application: A nurse-led educational application outside the hospital	The intervention group showed a significant reduction in the number of acute asthma attacks, emergency medical treatment, and hospitalization rates ($P<0.05$). Additionally, they exhibited better ACT scores, daily PEF change rates, respiratory function, serum inflammatory factors, and asthma medication compliance compared to the control group. Quality of life scores were also higher in the intervention group.
(Gao et al. 2020)	RCT	n=125	mHealth application: Structured training was provided under nurse leadership.	The intervention group demonstrated significantly higher scores on health-related quality of life, inhaler technique, and asthma control tests. Additionally, the intervention group had fewer unplanned doctor visits and school absences compared to the control group. However, there was no significant difference observed in emergency department visits and hospitalizations.
(Harrington et al., 2018)	RCT	n=44	School-based practice: updated asthma action plan, daily ICS check (provided by school nurse).	In the intervention group, the patients received 91.7% (95% CI [87.7, 95.5]) of their expected morning ICS doses during treatment. The intervention significantly improved patients' family life (23.8% vs. 56.5%, $p=0.03$) and reduced sleep loss (1.7 vs. 4.1 nights in the last 2 weeks).
(Horner et al., 2016)	RCT	n=196	School-based implementation: curriculum for asthma plans in children	Asthma severity decreased significantly, resulting in fewer emergency room and office visits, as well as significantly lower hospitalization rates.
(Lv et al., 2019)	RCT	n=152	Mobile app: a nurse-led program	The frequency of asthma exacerbations decreased due to better compliance, higher ACT scores, reductions in respiratory infections, days of antibiotic use, days absent from school, parental job loss, and reduced healthcare expenses.
(Ng et al., 2021)	RCT	n=112	Web-based application: nurse-led home asthma education program. It was administered under the nurse's leadership before discharge.	Differences were found in the intervention group regarding parents' knowledge, attitudes, and practices regarding asthma, as well as the frequency of unplanned visits and readmissions in children.

Abbreviations: ACT, asthma control test; ICT, inhaled corticosteroids; mHealth, mobile health; PEF, the peak expiratory flow; RCT, randomized controlled trial.

Controlling Environmental Factors and Comorbidities

Controlling environmental factors and comorbidities, non-pharmacologic interventions should be considered to improve quality of life and reduce symptoms in children. They can be provided not to use cigarettes, avoidance of triggers, and avoidance of pollution and irritants. Weight loss should also be recommended. Children who have been diagnosed with asthma are recommended to take part in a program of breathing exercises to help them manage their condition (Tesse et al., 2018).

Asthma attacks can be triggered by various factors, including comorbid diseases and exposure to asthma triggers. It is important to identify and avoid triggers, which can vary between individuals. Asthma can be triggered by a variety of factors, including tobacco smoke, dust mites, pesticides, cleaning or disinfection products, comorbid diseases, emotions, odors, and physical exercise (Centers for Disease Control and Prevention (CDC) 2022).

The guidelines for the control of environmental factors and comorbid conditions recommend the following:

Royal Children's Hospital Recommendations, 2018

- Reduce exposure to smoke is associated with asthma attacks, respiratory emergency room visits, and hospitalizations (Evidence II) (Rogers and Berry 2018).

Japanese Guidelines Recommendations, 2020

- Reducing exposure to smoke, pollutants, and smoking is recommended to improve the health of children and adolescents with asthma (Evidence C).
- It is advisable to wash bed linens frequently and hang them outside to dry in the sun.
- It is recommended to use sofas made of leather or artificial leather.
- It is recommended to use washable toys instead of stuffed toys.
- Using window shades instead of curtains, not keeping pets or plants indoors, and not hanging out laundry are all good ways to maintain a clean and healthy indoor environment.
- Additionally, it is advisable to persuade family members to avoid smoking in the rooms (Arakawa et al., 2020).

SIGN Recommendations, 2019

- It is important to recognize co-morbidities, obesity, and exposure to smoke to avoid asthma attacks (Evidence B for ages 5-12 years; Evidence D for ages under 5 years).
- Healthcare professionals should not recommend pet ownership as a strategy to prevent childhood asthma (Evidence B).
- Encouragement of breastfeeding is recommended, as it has many benefits, including its potential protective effect against asthma (Evidence C).
- Children who are overweight or obese and display signs of asthma should be offered weight loss programs to reduce the likelihood of respiratory symptoms (Evidence C).

- Parents should be informed about the various harmful effects of smoking during infancy, including increased wheezing and a higher risk of persistent asthma (Evidence B).
- Individuals with asthma and parents/caregivers of children with asthma should be educated about the hazards of smoking and exposure to second-hand smoke. They should also be offered appropriate assistance to quit smoking (Evidence B).
- Childhood vaccinations should be administered as usual, as there is no evidence of a detrimental impact on asthma incidence (Evidence C) (SIGN 2019).

Pharmacological Treatment

Children who suffer from asthma can have variable exacerbations, ranging in severity from wheezing to life-threatening conditions. All family members should recognize the early signs of asthma and monitor for symptoms. To assess the severity of exacerbations and treatments response, children with moderate to severe asthma should learn to monitor their peak flow rates. Furthermore, it is recommended that all children receive an action plan to follow in case of symptoms or flare-ups. This plan should include instructions about response to signs, symptoms, and PEF measurements, as well as when to seek medical attention (Conlon and Wilson, 2015). The main goals of treating children with asthma are to manage their symptoms, reduce exacerbations, and enable them to maintain their daily activities. To effectively manage asthma and provide appropriate treatment advice, nurses must maintain up-to-date knowledge and skills. Their responsibilities include overseeing self-management programs, educating children on inhaler techniques, and managing acute exacerbations. Asthma control refers to the degree to which a children's symptoms are reduced or eliminated (Sun et al., 2023).

The treatment of asthma is personalized and primarily depends on the severity of the attack. Typically, it involves the use of a symptom-controlling medication, such as an inhaled bronchodilator, and a preventive medication, usually a low-dose corticosteroid or long-acting bronchodilator. In acute attacks, oral steroids and other inhibitory drugs may also be used. In cases of severe, acute asthma attacks, intravenous administration of bronchodilators (such as salbutamol, aminophylline, or magnesium sulfate) and corticosteroids (such as hydrocortisone or methylprednisolone) is recommended as nebulized treatment may not be effective (Fraser et al., 2017). Pharmacological treatment should be approached in phases, depending on the asthma severity. Long-term asthma treatment can be provided with controller and reliever medications. Controlling medications are used to reduce inflammation in the airway, control symptoms, and reduce exacerbations. It is important to note that these medications should only be taken as prescribed by a healthcare professional. On the other hand, reliever medications are used to alleviate immediate symptoms, including worsening asthma or flares. Relief inhalers are recommended to prevent exercise-induced bronchoconstriction. They are also known as rescue inhalers and can be used to relieve symptoms as well as to prevent exercise-induced asthma symptoms. It is important to note that these inhalers should only be used as directed by a healthcare professional (GINA, 2023).

The guidelines for pharmacological treatment recommend the following:

SIGN Recommendations, 2019

- Children with life-threatening asthma or SpO2 less than 94% should receive high-flow oxygen through a well-fitted face mask or nasal cannula at flow rates that achieve normal saturation of 94-98 %.
- Inhaled β2-agonists are the first-line treatment for acute asthma in children (Evidence A).
- Administering oral steroids early in the treatment of acute asthma attacks in children is also recommended (Evidence A).

Turkish National Allergy and Clinical Immunology Association Recommendations, 2020

- During the first year of treatment, monthly checks should be conducted until control is achieved (Evidence A). Afterward, checks should be performed at regular intervals, such as every 3-6 months, and increased, if necessary, based on the children's needs.
- A Respiratory Function Test (PFT) should be conducted 3 months after treatment.
- Before proceeding with treatment, it is essential to assess the child's compliance with medication, the use of appropriate techniques, and whether any comorbid diseases are under control.
- Parents should have written action plans to help them recognize asthma attacks, initiate treatment, and understand when they become severe and require hospital admission (Evidence D, <5 years).
- If the child does not experience severe attacks and can use the mediator tube effectively at home, they prefer it to the nebulizer (Evidence A) (Turkish National Allergy and Clinical Immunology Association, 2020).

Nursing Interventions in Children with Asthma

Nurses should take a comprehensive health history to begin assessing children with asthma. A comprehensive physical assessment is then conducted, with a focus on the attitudes of both the parents and the child toward the child's condition and respiratory system. Nursing care for children with asthma encompasses both acute and long-term care. Nurses have a crucial role in helping children and their families learn to live with asthma, whether they are being cared for at home, in the hospital, at school, or in outpatient clinics. It is possible to manage the disease without the need for emergency room visits or hospitalization, and without affecting family life, physical activity, or school attendance. The following nursing interventions should be applied in the case of asthma:

- The necessary practices are carried out in collaboration with the child and/or caregiver, ensuring their competence.
- The child's privacy and individuality are respected.

- The child is allowed to assume a comfortable position to ensure maximum ventilation.
- Humidified oxygen is applied to increase tissue oxygenation and maintain oxygen saturation above 90%.
- The child and the parent are provided with clear explanations to reassure them that symptoms will be controlled, and airway starvation will be prevented.
- Medications are administered as prescribed to reduce anxiety caused by hypoxia.
- The child's response to medication is evaluated.
- Preventive medications are administered appropriately to determine the optimal response intensity.
- To manage asthma symptoms, it is important to monitor any exacerbations.
- Encourage the children to drink small amounts of fluids frequently to maintain hydration. In cases of severe and unresponsive asthma exacerbations, a peripheral intravenous line should be initiated to maintain hydration and administer medications.
- The oxygen concentration should be adjusted based on the children's response to their medications, as indicated by their oxygen saturation levels.
- The cause of the asthma exacerbation should be evaluated.
- Nursing practice should be documented appropriately, and any after-effects should be monitored. Any abnormal findings should be reported promptly to ensure safe practice.
- Provide appropriate discharge education to ensure continued control of asthma symptoms and to prevent recurrence. Review information regarding home medication use, written action plan, signs and symptoms requiring urgent medical attention, allergens and other triggering factors, and inhaler or nebulizer use.
- Training is provided to enhance individuals' sense of control, boost self-esteem, manage symptoms, and prevent exacerbations (Conlon and Wilson 2015; Jamieson, McCall, and Whyte 2003; Kılıçarslan Törüner and Büyükgönenç 2023).

Conclusion

Millions of children worldwide are thought to have suboptimal asthma control, despite significant advances in childhood asthma and the availability of high-quality guidelines to support asthma management. It is thought that this may be due to a lack of adherence to the guidelines. The guidelines cover best clinical practices for managing pediatric asthma and are generally agreed. Numerous guidelines have been published for the diagnosis, treatment, and management of asthma. As stated in these guidelines, educating the children and their families is a crucial step. It is important to educate children on inhaler use techniques, asthma action plans, and treatment compliance for effective management. Furthermore, children require support to control their asthma, cope with the condition, and maintain a normal lifestyle. Nurses often have the final opportunity to provide support to children with asthma and their families before discharge from the ward. Therefore, nurses play a crucial role in evidence-based asthma education programs that can improve self-esteem, knowledge, and self-management behaviors.

References

Abd, Abeerahmed, El-Neam El-Adel, Rahmabahgat Soliman, Fatenshafikmohmoud Nassar, and Basmarabeeabdel Sadek. 2018. "Evidence Based Guidelines For Nurses Caring For Children Suffering From Bronchial Asthma." *Mansoura Nursing Journal* 5(1):18235–2018.

Alharbi, Saleh A., Sumayyah A. N. Kobeisy, Suzan A. Alkhater, Adel S. Alharbi, Mansour M. Alqwaiee, Faisal N. Alotaibi, Khalid A. Alawam, Turki S. Alahmadi, Faisal M. Al-Somali, Talal M. Almaghamsi, and Abdullah A. Yousef. 2020. "Childhood Asthma Awareness in Saudi Arabia: Five-Year Follow-up Study." *Journal of Asthma and Allergy* 13:399–407. doi: 10.2147/JAA.S272850.

Arakawa, Hirokazu, Yuichi Adachi, Motohiro Ebisawa, Takao Fujisawa, ... and Sankei Nishima. 2020. "Japanese Guidelines for Childhood Asthma 2020." *Allergology International : Official Journal of the Japanese Society of Allergology* 69(3):314–30. doi: 10.1016/J.ALIT.2020.02.005.

Arakawa, Hirokazu, Yuhei Hamasaki, Yoichi Kohno, Motohiro Ebisawa, Naomi Kondo, Sankei Nishima, Toshiyuki Nishimuta, and Akihiro Morikawa. 2017. "Japanese Guidelines for Childhood Asthma 2017." *Allergology International* 66(2):190–204. doi: 10.1016/J.ALIT.2016.11.003.

de Assis, Elisangela Vilar, Milana D. R. Santana, Ankilma do N. A. Feitosa, Milena N. Alve. de Sousa, Ubiraídys de A. Isidório, Vitor E. Valenti, and Fernando Luiz Affonso Fonseca. 2019. "Prevalence of Asthma Symptoms and Risk Factors in Adolescents." *Journal of Human Growth and Development* 29(1):110–16. doi: 10.7322/jhgd.157758.

Bousquet, J., T. J. H. Clark, S. Hurd, N. Khaltaev, C. Lenfant, P. O'Byrne, and A. Sheffer. 2007. "GINA Guidelines on Asthma and Beyond." *Allergy: European Journal of Allergy and Clinical Immunology* 62(2):102–12. doi: 10.1111/J.1398-9995.2006.01305.X.

Centers For Disease Control and Prevention (CDC). 2022. "Common Asthma Triggers." Retrieved (https://www.cdc.gov/asthma/triggers.html).

Chen, J., and Y. Chen. 2021. "A Nurse-Led Hierarchical Management Model for the out-of-Hospital Management of Children with Bronchial Asthma: A Prospective Randomized Controlled Study." *American Journal of Translational Research* 13(6):6488–6497.

Conlon, P., and D Wilson. 2015. "The Child with Respiratory Dysfunction." P. 1164 in *Wong's nursing care of infants and children*, edited by M. Hockenberry and David Wilson. Canada.

Dharmage, Shyamali C., Jennifer L. Perret, and Adnan Custovic. 2019. "Epidemiology of Asthma in Children and Adults." *Frontiers in Pediatrics* 7:246. doi: 10.3389/FPED.2019.00246.

Farzandipour, M., MH Arani, R. Sharif, … E. Nabovati-Respiratory, and Undefined 2024. 2024. "Improving Asthma Control and Quality of Life via a Smartphone Self-Management App: A Randomized Controlled Trial." *Respiratory Medicine* 107539.

Ferrante, Giuliana, and Stefania La Grutta. 2018. "The Burden of Pediatric Asthma." *Frontiers in Pediatrics* 6:394966. doi: 10.3389/FPED.2018.00186/BIBTEX.

Flagg, J. S., and A. Pilitteri. 2018. *Maternal & Child Health Nursing : Care of the Childbearing & Childrearing Family*. Eighth Ed. Philadelphia: Wolters Kluwer.

Fraser, J., D. Waters, E. Forster, and N. Brown. 2017. *Paediatric Nursing in Australia*. 2 th. Cambridge University Press.

Gao, Guozhen, Yaoji Liao, | Lulu Mo, Yucui Gong, | Xia, Shao Rn, and Jinying Li. 2020. "A Randomized Controlled Trial of a Nurse-led Education Pathway for Asthmatic Children from Outpatient to Home." *International Journal of Nursing Practice* 26(3). doi: 10.1111/ijn.12823.

GINA. 2023. *Global Initative ForAsthma 2023: Difficult-to-Treat & Severe Asthma: Diagnosis and Management*.

Guttmann, Astrid, Brandon Zagorski, Peter C. Austin, Michael Schull, Asma Razzaq, Teresa To, and Geoff Anderson. 2007. "Effectiveness of Emergency Department Asthma Management Strategies on Return Visits in Children: A Population-Based Study." *Pediatrics* 120(6). doi: 10.1542/peds.2007-0168.

Harrington, Cherise B., Eric Langhans, Deborah Q. Shelef, Molly Savitz, Colleen Whitmore, and Stephen J. Teach. 2018. "A Pilot Randomized Trial of School-Based Administration of Inhaled Corticosteroids for at-Risk Children with Asthma." *Journal of Asthma* 55(2):145–51. doi: 10.1080/02770903.2017.1323915.

Higuchi, Kathryn Smith, Barbara L. Davies, Nancy Edwards, Jenny Ploeg, and Tazim Virani. 2011. "Implementation of Clinical Guidelines for Adults with Asthma and Diabetes: A Three-Year Follow-up Evaluation of Nursing Care." *Journal of Clinical Nursing* 20(9–10):1329–38. doi: 10.1111/J.1365-2702.2010.03590.X.

Horner, Sharon D., Adama Brown, Sharon A. Brown, and D. Lynn Rew. 2016. "Enhancing Asthma Self-Management in Rural School-Aged Children: A Randomized Controlled Trial." *The Journal of Rural Health : Official Journal of the American Rural Health Association and the National Rural Health Care Association* 32(3):260–68. doi: 10.1111/JRH.12150.

Jamieson, E. M., J. M. McCall, and L. Whyte. 2003. *Clinical Nursing Practices*. 4 th. China: Churchill Livingstone.

Jia, Yuanmin, Haixia Wang, Zeyi Zhang, Jingjing Wang, Mo Yi, and Ou Chen. 2023. "Parenting Style and Child Asthma Control in Families of School-Age Children with Asthma: The Mediating Effects of Children's General Self-Efficacy and Medication Adherence." *Journal of Pediatric Nursing* 73:e293–301. doi: 10.1016/J.PEDN.2023.09.025.

Kılıçarslan Törüner, E., and L. Büyükgönenç. 2023. *Child Health Basic Nursing Approaches*. 3. Edition. Ankara (Turkey): Ankara Nobel Bookstores.

Lv, S., X. Ye, Z. Wang, W. Xia, … Y. Qi-Journal of advanced, and Undefined 2019. 2019. "A Randomized Controlled Trial of a Mobile Application-assisted Nurse-led Model Used to Improve Treatment Outcomes in Children with Asthma." *Journal of Advanced Nursing* 75(11):3058–67. doi: 10.1111/jan.14143.

Massie, J., D. Efron, B. Cerritelli, M. South, C. Powell, M. M. Haby, E. Gilbert, S. Vidmar, J. Carlin, and C. F. Robertson. 2004. "Implementation of Evidence Based Guidelines for Paediatric Asthma Management in a Teaching Hospital." *Archives of Disease in Childhood* 89(7):660–64. doi: 10.1136/ADC.2003.032110.

National Heart Lung and Blood Institute. 2007. *National Asthma Education and Prevention Program.Expert Panel Report 3: Guidelines for the Diagnosis and Management of Asthma Full Report 2007*.

National Heart Lung and Blood Institute (NHLBI). 2020. *2020 Focused Updates to the Asthma Management Guidelines: National, A Report from the Prevention, Asthma Education and Committee, Program Coordinating Group, Expert Panel Working*.

Ng, JSK, JPC Chau, AWK Chan, … JKC Lui-Journal of Pediatric, and Undefined 2021. 2021. "A Nurse-Led Web-Based Home Asthma Education Program for Children and Their Families: A Randomized Controlled Trial." *Journal of Pediatric Nursing* 59:158–63. doi: https://doi.org/10.1016/j.pedn.2021.04.014.

Policicchio, J., B. Nelson, and S. Duffy. 2011. "Bringing Evidence-Based Continuing Education on Asthma to Nurses." *Clinical Nurse Specialist* 25(3):125–32.

Reddel, Helen K., Leonard B. Bacharier, Eric D. Bateman, Christopher E. Brightling, Guy G. Brusselle, Roland Buhl, Alvaro A. Cruz, Liesbeth Duijts, Jeffrey M. Drazen, J. Mark Fitzgerald, Louise J. Fleming, Hiromasa Inoue, Fanny W. Ko, Jerry A. Krishnan, Mark L. Levy, Jiangtao Lin, Kevin Mortimer, Paulo M. Pitrez, Aziz Sheikh, Arzu A. Yorgancioglu, and Louis-Philippe Boulet. 2022. "Global Initiative for Asthma Strategy 2021: Executive Summary and Rationale for Key Changes." *Atsjournals.Org* 205(1):17–35. doi: 10.1164/rccm.202109-2205PP.

Rogers, K., and A. Berry. 2018. "Asthma Inpatient Discharge Education: Nursing Guideline." Retrieved (https://www.rch.org.au/rchcpg/hospital_clinical_guideline_index/Asthma_inpatient_discharge_education/).

Rosychuk, Rhonda J., Donald C. Voaklander, Terry P. Klassen, Ambikaipakan Senthilselvan, Thomas J. Marrie, and Brian H. Rowe. 2010. "Asthma Presentations by Children to Emergency Departments in a Canadian Province: A Population-based Study." *Pediatric Pulmonology* 45:985–92. doi: 10.1002/ppul.21281.

SIGN. 2019. *British Guideline on the Management of Asthma: A National Clinical Guideline*. Scotland.

Sun, D., P. Sun, and Z. Wang. 2023. "Assessment and Therapeutic Management of Acute Asthma: The Approaches of Nursing Staff in Patient Care." *Advances in Clinical and Experimental Medicine*. doi: https://doi.org/10.17219/acem/161156.

Tao, Shuai, Qiuhua Fan, Head Nurse, Vishnu Shankar Hariharan, Haoliang Zhi, and Correspondence Haoliang Zhi. 2023. "Effectiveness of Nursing Interventions for Management of Children with Bronchial Asthma: A Systematic Review and Meta-analysis." *Wiley Online Library*. doi: 10.1111/ijn.13139.

Tesse, Riccardina, Giorgia Borrelli, Giuseppina Mongelli, Violetta Mastrorilli, and Fabio Cardinale. 2018. "Treating Pediatric Asthma According Guidelines." *Frontiers in Pediatrics* 6:234. doi: 10.3389/FPED.2018.00234.

Trottier, ED, K. Chan, … D. Allain-Paediatrics &. Child, and Undefined 2021. 2021. "Managing an Acute Asthma Exacerbation in Children." *Paediatrics & Child Health* 26(7):438. doi: https://doi.org/10.1093/pch/pxab058.

Türkiye Ulusal Allerji ve Klinik İmmünoloji Derneği. 2020. *Çocukluk Çağı Astım Tanı ve Tedavi Rehberi El Kitapçığı 2020*. Ankara.

Vazquez-Ortiz, Marta, Elizabeth Angier, Katharina Blumchen, Pasquale Comberiati, Bettina Duca, Audrey DunnGalvin, Claudia Gore, Valérie Hox, Britt Jensen, Helena Pite, Alexandra F. Santos, Silvia Sanchez, Cherry Alviani, Teresa Garriga-Baraut, Rebecca Knibb, Charlotte G. Mortz, M. Hazel Gowland, Frans Timmermans, and Graham Roberts. 2020. "Understanding the Challenges Faced by Adolescents and Young Adults with Allergic Conditions: A Systematic Review." *Allergy* 75(8):1850–80. doi: 10.1111/ALL.14258.

Wooler, E. 2001. "The Role of the Nurse in Paediatric Asthma Management." *Paediatric Respiratory Reviews* 2(1):76–81. doi: 10.1053/PRRV.2000.0105.

Chapter 12

Evidence-Based Nursing Practices in Type 1 Diabetes Mellitus

Emine Çubukcu*, MSc
Hatay Mustafa Kemal Universty Hospital, Hatay, Türkiye

Abstract

Type 1 Diabetes Mellitus (T1DM) is an important public health problem with increasing prevalence. It is an autoimmune disease that causes hyperglycemia and related symptoms and leads to insulin deficiency. T1DM, which damages various organs and tissues of the body in the long term, is a social and economic health problem frequently seen all over the world because it causes high treatment and care costs and negatively affects the quality of life. T1DM directly affects many areas of the daily life of children and adolescents such as nutrition, physical activity, academic performance, mental status, and social relationships. Pediatric nurses, physicians, and all health professionals working with children and adolescents with T1DM play an important role in the care and support of the child. In the management of diabetes, to prevent acute complications and prevent chronicity, blood glucose levels should be maintained under control and specific plans and training should be organized for the needs of the child and parents on issues such as nutrition, physical activity, insulin treatment, and management of complications. In adapting to the diabetes management process and gaining care skills, all health professionals, especially nurses, should address the child and family with a holistic and supportive approach. In the diabetes management process, nurses play an important role in supporting the child and the family by using education and counseling roles at the point of adapting to changes and maintaining health. In the treatment and control of T1DM, which is the subject of many national and international studies, it is extremely important to adopt nursing practices with a high level of evidence. In this section, evidence-based nursing practices applied in the treatment and control of children with type 1 diabetes are examined in line with the literature. Activities via a mobile device can have limited effectiveness. Future studies could focus on their further applicability to various contexts in medical education.

Keywords: type 1 diabetes mellitus, evidence-based practices, pediatric nursing, child

* Corresponding Author's Email: eminacubukcu@gmail.com.

In: Evidence-Based Care Practices in Pediatric Nursing
Editors: Feyza Küçük and Serap Özdemir
ISBN: 979-8-89530-304-7

Introduction

Type 1 Diabetes Mellitus (T1DM) is a chronic disease that results in insufficient insulin secretion and hyperglycemia as a result of the destruction of pancreatic beta cells, and its care and management require attention and care (Bideci and Döğer, 2021; Dai et al., 2022; Giwa et al., 2020). T1DM is one of the most common pediatric endocrine and metabolic disorders (Dai et al., 2022). T1DM may present with symptoms such as polydipsia, polyuria, nocturia, polyphagia, and inability to gain weight despite polyphagia, anorexia, unexplained weight loss, weakness, fatigue, dry mouth, and frequent recurrent infections (Güzel and Gülşen, 2023). Acute complications include diabetic ketoacidosis requiring urgent intervention, while chronic complications include micro/macrovascular diseases. Patients with T1DM are at higher risk for other autoimmune diseases and psychosocial problems (Syed, 2022).

Diagnosis of T1DM according to the American Diabetes Association (ADA); fasting blood glucose level ≥126 mg/dL (7.0 mmol/L) or 2-hour plasma glucose level ≥200 mg/dL (11.1 mmol/L), during oral glucose tolerance test (OGTT) or HbA1C ≥6% in a child or adolescent, 5 (48 mmol/mol) or a random blood glucose of ≥200 mg/dL (11.1 mmol/L) in a patient with classic symptoms of hyperglycemia or hyperglycaemic crisis (Bekele et al., 2022).

The prevalence of diabetes is increasing day by day in children (Akbarizadeh et al., 2022). The prevalence varies worldwide with the effect of environmental factors as well as genetic factors (Demir et al., 2022). T1DM peaks in the preschool period (around 6 years of age), puberty (around 13 years of age), and late adolescence (around 20 years of age) (Güzel & Gülşen, 2023; Pedrosa et al., 2023). According to the International Diabetes Federation (IDF) Diabetes Atlas 10th Edition, Type 1 Diabetes affects more than 1.52 million children and adolescents under 20 years of age worldwide according to 2022 data (IDF, 2023). Studies have concluded that the greatest increase occurs in children under 6 years of age (Nevo-Shenker et al., 2020).

Type 1 diabetes, which requires changes in lifestyle and causes damage and loss of function in various organs and systems of the body in the long term (Binay-Yaz and Cinar, 2023), is a social and economic health problem that is frequently seen all over the world because it also causes a decrease in quality of life, treatment, and high care costs (Demirdağ, 2022). Children with type 1 diabetes and their families need intensive diabetes education by a multidisciplinary team including specialized endocrinologists, dieticians, and diabetes nurses. This education should include topics such as the effect of insulin, dose adjustment and application techniques, blood glucose, and ketone monitoring, prevention of ketoacidosis, nutritional therapy, physical activity, and prevention of hypoglycemia (Aslan, 2019) and should be planned individually. With these plans, individuals with diabetes can lead a healthy life and delay possible complications (Demirdağ, 2022). Diabetes management should focus on optimizing glucose control to reduce acute and chronic complications (Syed, 2022).

It may be more difficult to plan diabetes management in children due to their growth, physical activity, and eating habits. The child and his/her family may experience physical and psychological difficulties in the process of adaptation to the planned changes. All health professionals, especially nurses (due to their education and counseling roles), should take an active role in adapting to the diabetes management process and gaining care skills (Demirdağ, 2022).

Nurses should support the child and the family by using evidence-based practices in diabetes management using their educational and counseling roles. Evidence-based practice is a clinical problem-solving method that includes the process of literature review, research/evaluating the results, and deciding on the applications to be made based on these results (Alqahtani et al., 2020; Çalık-Bağrıyanık et al., 2022). The aim of evidence-based practices is to integrate the best evidence from scientific research into the clinic and care in line with the patient's preferences and needs, as well as existing clinical expert experiences (Halili et al., 2022). These practices also help healthcare professionals stay up-to-date and make better healthcare decisions (Rahmayanti et al., 2020).

Evidence-based nursing practices are the use of the evidence obtained from these researches in health care services, taking into account the needs and preferences of the person receiving care. Evidence-based nursing research increased rapidly toward the end of the 90s (Çalık-Bağrıyanık et al., 2022). In the literature, it is emphasized that with evidence-based practices, resources are used more efficiently, patient care is improved, costs and length of hospital stay are reduced, patient satisfaction is increased, and unnecessary and ineffective practices are eliminated (Alqahtani et al., 2020; Karakoç-Kumsar et al., 2020). In this direction, nurses need to know and implement interventions whose usefulness has been proven by scientific studies both in the treatment and control of diabetes (Taşkın-Yılmaz, 2015). In this section, evidence-based nursing practices applied in the treatment and control of children with type 1 diabetes are examined in line with the literature.

Evidence-Based Nursing Practices in the Treatment of Type 1 Diabetes

In the treatment and control of T1DM, which is the subject of many national and international studies, it is extremely important to adopt nursing practices with a high level of evidence. There are four important steps in the management of type 1 diabetes: an effective and correct dose of insulin therapy, a balanced and healthy diet, regular exercise, and patient and family education. The main aim of treatment is to improve the quality of life, to ensure glycaemic control, to protect the child from acute and chronic complications, and to maintain growth and development according to age peers (Danne et al., 2018)

Insulin Therapy

Insulin is the main component of T1DM treatment (Kardaş & Gürol, 2022). Today, different tools and methods are used in insulin applications with the development of technology (Demir et al., 2022). Multiple doses or continuous subcutaneous insulin infusion is used in the treatment of T1DM (A) (ADA, 2021). When used correctly, real-time continuous glucose monitoring in combination with insulin therapy is a useful tool to lower and/or maintain A1c levels and/or reduce hypoglycemia (A) (ADA, 2021). Insulin in children with T1DM is administered via injector, pen, and pump. The insulin treatment to be used should be planned by considering factors such as the child's age, nutritional characteristics, physical activity status, lifestyle, and skill in injection applications (Kardaş and Gürol, 2022).

Nutrition Therapy

In 1994, the ADA recommended the use of the term "medical nutrition therapy" instead of diet therapy due to its negative connotations (Yılmaz, 2017). In T1DM, medical nutrition therapy is one of the main components of diabetes care and education (Altınok, 2019). Individualized nutrition therapy is recommended for type 1 diabetes (A) (ADA, 2021). Individualized nutrition therapy should be planned to consider family habits, religious or cultural beliefs, economic status, programs, physical activity, educational status of the family and children, and skills in diabetes self-management. In dietitian or nutritionist controls, the individual should be evaluated in terms of cardiovascular risk, growth and development, weight, dietary preferences changing over time, access to food, and the potential for disordered eating. Adherence to recommended diet plans is associated with better glycemic outcomes in individuals with type 1 diabetes (Elyased et al., 2023).

Medical nutrition is of great importance in ensuring metabolic control, preventing complications (hyperglycemia, and severe hypoglycemia), healthy growth and development of children, and gaining adequate and balanced eating habits (Caferoğlu & Şahin, 2020; Shorey et al., 2022).

Medical nutrition therapy for type 1 diabetes should be arranged by taking into account the socioeconomic status, lifestyle, physical activity level, eating habits, type, and dose of insulin used, laboratory results, age, and anthropometric measurements (Yılmaz, 2017). With medical nutrition therapy, the A1c levels of individuals with type 1 diabetes are reduced by 0.3-1% (Koç et al., 2018).

Physical Activity and Exercise

In diabetes management and care, both physical activity and exercise, along with insulin and a healthy diet, are the main components of treatment that should be maintained in balance (Adolfsson et al., 2022). For individuals with T1DM, physical activity provides many benefits, including glycaemic control, blood lipid levels, cardiovascular function, and psychological well-being (Chetty et al., 2019; Cockcroft et al., 2023; Dash et al., 2020; Kenger and Ergün, 2019; Pulungan et al., 2021; Özgül et al., 2022).

Exercise management in children with type 1 diabetes is affected by many factors, such as the type, intensity, duration of the activity, the amount of insulin in the body, and the emotional effects of the activity on the individual with diabetes (Chetty et al., 2019). ADA recommends that all children and adolescents should exercise for at least 60 minutes a day among the basic measures aimed at providing metabolic control in Type 1 diabetes. It recommends 3 days of moderate to vigorous aerobic physical activity in addition to vigorous exercise and bone and muscle strengthening activities (C) (ADA, 2022; Elyased et al., 2023). Individual-specific plans should be made on exercise and its management; the points in blood glucose management in exercise (exercise intensity, duration, and intensity, interventions to be made in insulin dose before exercise, additional carbohydrates to be taken during exercise) should be explained in detail to children, adolescents, and family members, and continuity of education should be ensured (Adolfsson et al., 2022).

Education

Education, which is the key to successful diabetes management (Olinder et al., 2022; Phelan et al., 2018; Zhao et al., 2021), should include children, adolescents, and parents. The aim of education is to provide individuals with the self-care behaviors and coping skills they need to improve their clinical outcomes, health status, and quality of life and at the same time to manage their lives well in the best and least costly possible under their own conditions (Phelan et al., 2018).

The multidisciplinary team responsible for diabetes education should use patient-centered, interactive teaching methods planned to meet the different needs of children, adolescents, and parents with diabetes, their personal choices, perceptions, and learning models according to the sociocultural and socioeconomic situation they are in (ADA, 2021). The content and curriculum of structured diabetes education have a planned, tailor-made, agreed upon, written, and evaluated curriculum (Olinder et al., 2022). In this context, individuals diagnosed with diabetes should receive self-management skills training in line with national standards from the moment of diagnosis (B) (ADA, 2021).

In the literature, it has been concluded that diabetes education generally positively affects the psychosocial and clinical parameters of individuals with diabetes, increases diabetes knowledge, reduces the need for medication, enables the patient to focus on self-management, and is effective in reducing the risk of developing complications (Al Ksir et al., 2022; D'Souza et al., 2021; Skinner et al., 2018; Yoo et al., 2022).

Use of Digital Technologies in Treatment

Developing technology and innovative approaches facilitate diabetes management day by day (Tauschmann and Hovorka, 2018). The use of technology should be individualized according to the patient's needs, wishes, skill level, and availability of devices (E) (ADA, 2020). Technology-based tools include smartphone apps, insulin pumps, continuous glucose monitoring (CGM), sensor-enhanced pump therapy, and closed-loop technology. Smartphone apps can also help individuals record exercise management and make exercise management decisions (Chetty et al., 2019).

To maximize the effectiveness of diabetes treatment and advances in diabetes management and technology, including continuous subcutaneous insulin infusion (CSII) and CGM, it is recommended that all individuals with diabetes and their families receive structured education according to quality standards (e) (Olinder et al., 2022).

The use of technology and blood glucose monitoring in diabetes; lowers A1c value, better metabolic control, reduction of total daily insulin doses, ease insulin dose calculation, as well as significantly reduces stress (Gülen et al., 2023).

Prevention of Complications

Optimal glycemia should be maintained to prevent or delay the progression of T1DM complications (A) (ADA, 2021). Regular health checks are recommended to prevent complications. Health checks include general diabetes control once every three months, physical examination and foot examination, ophthalmological examination, and laboratory tests once a year, blood glucose level (self-measurement) 1 day 4 times a week, A1c follow-up at least twice a year (Taşkın-Yılmaz, 2015).

Psychosocial Care

In addition to the impact of diabetes on quality of life, it is important to consider the development of mental health problems related to diabetes stress, fear of hypoglycemia/hyperglycemia, anxiety and depression symptoms, and eating disorders (Elyased et al., 2023). At the time of diagnosis and during routine follow-up care, it is recommended that psychosocial problems and familial stresses that can affect diabetes management should be screened and referred to psychiatrists experienced in childhood diabetes (C) (Elyased et al., 2023). The presence of psychiatrists in pediatric multidisciplinary teams is important in terms of dealing with the psychosocial problems of diabetes. These psychosocial problems are significantly associated with difficulties in self-management, poor quality of life, high A1c, and increased rates of acute/chronic diabetes complications (Elyased et al., 2023).

Conclusion

In the management process of diabetes managed by a multidisciplinary team, all health professionals, especially nurses, should support the child and his/her family in adapting to the disease and providing care skills to individuals. In the diabetes management process, nurses play an important role in supporting the patient and his/her family with their education and counseling roles at the point of adapting to changes and maintaining health. T1DM, which is the subject of many national and international studies, is extremely important in terms of the adoption of evidence-based practices in nursing practices, the management of the disease, and the satisfaction of the patient and the family.

References

Adolfsson, P., Taplin, C. E., Zaharieva, D. P., Pemberton, J., Davis, E. A., Riddell, M. C., ... & DiMeglio, L. A. (2022). ISPAD Clinical Practice Consensus Guidelines 2022: Exercise in children and adolescents with diabetes. *Pediatric Diabetes*, 23(8), 1341-1372. https://doi.org/10.1111/pedi.13452

Alqahtani, N., Oh, K. M., Kitsantas, P., & Rodan, M. (2020). Nurses' evidence-based practice knowledge, attitudes and implementation: A cross-sectional study. *Journal of clinical nursing*, 29(1-2), 274-283. https://doi.org/10.1111/jocn.15097

Al Ksir, K., Wood, D. L., Hasni, Y., Sahli, J., Quinn, M., & Ghardallou, M. (2022). Motivational interviewing to improve self-management in youth with type 1 diabetes: A randomized clinical trial. *Journal of Pediatric* Nursing, 66, e116-e121. https://doi.org/10.1016/j.pedn.2022.05.001

Akbarizadeh, M., Naderi far, M., & Ghaljaei, F. (2022). Prevalence of depression and anxiety among children with type 1 and type 2 diabetes: a systematic review and meta-analysis. *World Journal of Pediatrics*, 1-11. https://doi.org/10.1007/s12519-021-00485-2

American Diabetes Association Professional Practice Committee, & American Diabetes Association Professional Practice Committee. (2022). 3. Prevention or delay of type 2 diabetes and associated comorbidities: Standards of Medical Care in Diabetes—2022. *Diabetes Care*, 45(1), S39-S45.

American Diabetes Association. (2021). 13. Children and adolescents: standards of medical care in diabetes—2021. *Diabetes care*, 44(1), S180-S199. https://doi.org/10.2337/dc21-S013

American Diabetes Association. (2020). 7. Diabetes technology: standards of medical care in diabetes—2020. *Diabetes Care*, 43(1), S77-S88. https://doi.org/10.2337/dc20-ad08c

Altınok, Y. A. (2019). Tip 1 Diyabetli Çocuk ve Adölesanların Beslenme Sorunlarına Yaklaşım ve Yetişkin Kliniğe Devri. *Beslenme ve Diyet Dergisi*, 47, 52-59. https://doi.org/10.33076/2019.BDD.1315

Aslan, B. (2019). Tip 1 diyabetli adölesan bireylerde uyku kalitesi ve beslenme durumu arasındaki ilişkinin belirlenmesi (Yüksek Lisans Tezi, Başkent Üniversitesi Sağlık Bilimleri Enstitüsü).

Bideci, A., & Döğer, E., (2021). *Insulin treatment and long-term monitoring in type 1 diabetes. Innovations in diabetes of children and adolescents* (pp.33-40), Ankara: Türkiye Klinikleri Yayınevi.

Bekele, B. T., Demie, T. G., & Worku, F. (2022). Health-related quality-of-Life and associated factors among children and adolescents with type 1 diabetes mellitus: A cross-sectional study. *Pediatric Health, Medicine and Therapeutics*, 243-256. https://doi.org/10.2147/PHMT.S364454

Caferoğlu, Z., Şahin, G. A., Hatipoğlu, N., & İnanç, N. (2020). Tip 1 Diyabetli Çocuk ve Adölesanların Diyet Kalitesi, Diyet asit yükü ve glisemik kontrol ile ilişkisi. *Beslenme ve Diyet Dergisi*, 48(1), 31-42. https://doi.org/10.33076/2020.BDD.1229

Chetty, T., Shetty, V., Fournier, P. A., Adolfsson, P., Jones, T. W., & Davis, E. A. (2019). Exercise management for young people with type 1 diabetes: a structured approach to the exercise consultation. *Frontiers in Endocrinology,* 10, 326. https://doi.org/10.3389/fendo.2019.00326

Cockcroft, E. J., Wooding, E. L., Narendran, P., Dias, R. P., Barker, A. R., Moudiotis, C., ... & Andrews, R. C. (2023). Factors affecting the support for physical activity in children and adolescents with type 1 diabetes mellitus: a national survey of health care professionals' perceptions. *BMC pediatrics*, 23(1), 131. https://doi.org/10.1186/s12887-023-03940-3

Çalık Bağrıyanık, B., Yıldız, D., Eren Fidancı, B., Pekyiğit, A., Et Al. (2022). Çocuk hastanesinde çalışan hemşirelerin kanıta dayalı uygulamalara ilişkin tutumlarının belirlenmesi. Adnan Menderes Üniversitesi *Sağlık Bilimleri Fakültesi Dergisi,* 6(2), 202-215. https://doi.org/10.46237/amusbfd.894471

Dai BD, H., Huang, H., & Yang, X. (2022). The role of nurses in taking care of children with type 1 diabetes. *Alternative therapies in health and medicine*, 28(1), 107-113.

Danne, T., Phillip, M., Buckingham, B. A., Jarosz-Chobot, P., Saboo, B., Urakami, T., ... & Codner, E. (2018). ISPAD Clinical Practice Consensus Guidelines 2018: Insulin treatment in children and adolescents with diabetes. *Pediatric diabetes*, 19, 115-135. DOI: 10.1111/pedi.12718

Dash, K., Goyder, E. C., & Quirk, H. (2020). A qualitative synthesis of the perceived factors that affect participation in physical activity among children and adolescents with type 1 diabetes. *Diabetic Medicine*, 37(6), 934-944. https://doi.org/10.1111/dme.14299

D'Souza, R. S., Ryan, M., Hawkes, E., Baker, C., Davies, Y., Judith, R., ... & D'Souza, N. A. (2021). Questionnaire-based service evaluation of the efficacy and usefulness of SEREN: a structured education programme for children and young people diagnosed with type 1 diabetes mellitus. *BMJ Open Quality*, 10(3), e001337. https://doi.org/10.1136/bmjoq-2021-001337

Demir, G., Çubukcu, E. & Akcay, N. (2022). Tip 1 diyabetli çocuk ve adölesanların insülin pompa yönetiminde sorunlar ve çözüm önerileri. *Türkiye Diyabet ve Obezite Dergisi*, 6 (2), 187-194. https://doi.org/10.25048/tudod.1105407

Demirdağ, S. N. (2022). Pender'in Sağlığı Geliştirme Modeline göre tip 1 diyabet tanılı çocuk ve ailenin değerlendirilmesi: kavram haritası. *Güncel Hemşirelik Araştırmaları Dergisi,* 2 (2), 95-103.

ElSayed, N. A., Aleppo, G., Aroda, V. R., Bannuru, R. R., Brown, F. M., Bruemmer, D., ... & Gabbay, R. A. (2023). 14. Children and adolescents: standards of care in diabetes—2023. *Diabetes Care*, 46(1), S230-S253. https://doi.org/10.2337/dc23-S014

Giwa, A. M., Ahmed, R., Omidian, Z., Majety, N., Karakus, K. E., Omer, S. M., ... & Hamad, A. R. A. (2020). Current understandings of the pathogenesis of type 1 diabetes: genetics to environment. *World journal of diabetes*, 11(1), 13-25. doi: 10.4239/wjd.v11.i1.13

Gülen, A. H., Arı Korkusuz, N., & Korkusuz, E. (2023). Diyabet teknolojilerinin diyabetli bireyler üzerindeki etkisi ve diyabet kabul durumları arasındaki ilişkinin incelenmesi. *Sağlık Akademisyenleri Dergisi*, 10(3), 348-355. https://doi.org/10.52880/sagakaderg.1230648.

Güzel, E. Ç., & Gülşen, H. B. (2023). Aile Sağlığı Merkezinde tanı konan Tip 1 Diyabetes Mellitus vakası. *The Journal of Turkish Family Physician*, 14(1), 42-48. doi: 10.15511/tjtfp.23.00142

Halili, X., Välimäki, M., Li, Z., Tang, S., Wang, H., & Chen, Q. (2022). Protocol: Academic-practice partnerships in evidence-based nursing practice: a scoping review protocol. *BMJ open*, 12(9). doi:10.1136/bmjopen-2022-065049

International Diabetes Federation. IDF Diabetes Atlas-10th Edition. Erişim Tarihi: 19. 12.2023, https://idf.org/about-diabetes/type-1-diabetes/.

Kardaş, G. N., & Gürol, A. (2022). İnsülin Kalemi ve pompası kullanan tip 1 diyabet hastası çocuklarda metabolik kontrol ve yaşam kalitesi düzeyleri. Kocaeli Üniversitesi *Sağlık Bilimleri Dergisi*, 8(1), 65-71. https://doi.org/10.30934/kusbed.988288

Karakoç Kumsar, A., Polat, Ş., & Afşar-Doğrusöz, L. (2020). Determining attitudes of nurses toward evidence-based nursing in a university hospital sample. *Florence Nightingale journal of nursing*, 28(3), 268. doi: 10.5152/FNJN.2020.19022

Kenger, E. B., & Ergün, C. (2019). Tip 1 Diyabet, egzersiz ve beslenme. *Turkiye Klinikleri Journal of Sports Sciences*, 11(3), 164-170. DOI: 10.5336/sportsci.2019-70286

Koç, B., Baş, M., Eliuz Tipici, B., & Bundak, R. (2018). Tip 1 diyabetli çocuk ve adölesanların beslenme durumlarının belirlenmesi ve beslenme örüntülerinin metabolik profilleri ile ilişkisinin saptanması. *Turkiye Klinikleri Journal of Pediatrics*, 27(2), 59-69. DOI: 10.5336/pediatr.2018-60826

Nevo-Shenker, M., Phillip, M., Nimri, R., & Shalitin, S. (2020). Type 1 diabetes mellitus management in young children: implementation of current technologies. *Pediatric research*, 87(4), 624-629. https://doi.org/10.1038/s41390-019-0665-4

Pedrosa, I., Cardoso, F., Martins, V., & Gama, E. (2023). Integrated care process in type 1 diabetes mellitus in children and adolescents: A quality improvement initiative. *Journal of Healthcare Quality Research*, 38(4), 245-249. https://doi.org/10.1016/j.jhqr.2022.09.005

Phelan, H., Lange, K., Cengiz, E., Gallego, P., Majaliwa, E., Pelicand, J., ... & Hofer, S. E. (2018). ISPAD Clinical Practice Consensus Guidelines 2018: Diabetes education in children and adolescents. *Pediatric diabetes,* 19, 75-83. DOI: 10.1111/pedi.12762

Pulungan, A. B., Fadiana, G., & Annisa, D. (2021). Type 1 diabetes mellitus in children: experience in Indonesia. *Clinical Pediatric Endocrinology*, 30(1), 11-18. https://doi.org/10.1297/cpe.30.11

Rahmayanti, E. I., Kadar, K. S., & Saleh, A. (2020). Readiness, barriers and potential strenght of nursing in implementing evidence-based practice. *International Journal of Caring Sciences*, 13(2), 1203-1211.

Shorey, S., Ng, E. D., Law, E. C., Wong, J., Loke, K. Y., & Tam, W. W. (2022). Physical activity and nutrition interventions for type 1 diabetes: a meta-analysis. *Pediatrics*, 150(3):e2022056540. https://doi.org/10.1542/peds.2022-056540

Skinner, T. C., Lange, K. S., Hoey, H., Mortensen, H. B., Aanstoot, H. J., Castaño, L., ... & Hvidoere Study Group. (2018). Targets and teamwork: understanding differences in pediatric diabetes centers treatment outcomes. *Pediatric diabetes*, 19(3), 559-565. https://doi.org/10.1111/pedi.12606

Syed, F. Z. (2022). Type 1 diabetes mellitus. *Annals of internal medicine*, 175(3), ITC33-ITC48. https://doi.org/10.7326/AITC20220315

Tauschmann, M., & Hovorka, R. (2018). Technology in the management of type 1 diabetes mellitus—current status and future prospects. *Nature Reviews Endocrinology*, 14(8), 464-475.

Olinder, A. L., DeAbreu, M., Greene, S., Haugstvedt, A., Lange, K., Majaliwa, E. S., ... & Mahmud, F. H. (2022). ISPAD Clinical Practice Consensus Guidelines 2022: Diabetes education in children and adolescents. *Pediatric Diabetes,* 23(8), 1229. doi: 10.1111/pedi.13418

Özgül, E, Ünsar, S., & Yacan, L. (2022). Diabetes Mellituslu bireylerin fiziksel aktivite davranışları ve iyilik hallerinin belirlenmesi. *Türkiye Diyabet ve Obezite Dergisi*, 6(1). DOI: 10.25048/tudod.1053313

Yaz, Ş. B., & Çinar, D. (2023). Parent Quality of Life scale in Type 1 Diabetes: a scale development and validation study. *European journal of pediatrics*, 182(8), 3491-3499. https://doi.org/10.1007/s00431-023-05023-y

Yılmaz, F. T. (2015). Diyabetin tedavisinde ve kontrolünde kanıta dayalı hemşirelik uygulamaları. *Turkiye Klinikleri J Intern Med Nurs-Special Topics*, 1(3), 13-9.

Yılmaz, H. Ö. (2017). Tip 1 diyabette tıbbi beslenme tedavisi. *Türkiye Klinikleri J Nutr Diet-Special Topics*, 3(3), 164-72.

Yoo, J. H., Kim, G., Lee, H. J., Sim, K. H., Jin, S. M., & Kim, J. H. (2022). Effect of structured individualized education on continuous glucose monitoring use in poorly controlled patients with type 1 diabetes: a randomized controlled trial. *Diabetes Research and Clinical Practice*, 184, 109209. https://doi.org/10.1016/j.diabres.2022.109209

Zhao, X., Huang, H., & Zheng, S. (2021). Effectiveness of Internet and Phone-Based Interventions on Diabetes Management of Children and Adolescents With Type 1 Diabetes: A Systematic Review. *Worldviews on Evidence-Based Nursing*, 18(3), 217-225. https://doi.org/10.1111/wvn.12511

Chapter 13

Evidence-Based Nursing Practices in Epilepsy Management

Zeynep Erkut[1*], PhD
and Zeynep Aközlü[2], MSc

[1]Department of Nursing, School of Nursing, Maltepe University, Istanbul, Türkiye
[2]Department of Medical Services and Techniques, Vocational School, Maltepe University, Istanbul, Türkiye

Abstract

Epilepsy is one of the most common chronic neurological diseases in childhood. It is characterized by recurrent unprovoked seizures, requires long-term medication use, and can cause various complications. Structural, genetic, infectious, metabolic, and immune factors play a role in the etiology of epilepsy and its treatment and care continue throughout life. Epilepsy negatively affects the quality of life of children and their families in physical, social, economic, and psychological aspects. Epilepsy management includes regular use of medications, minimization of medication side effects, control of seizures, reduction of the dangers associated with recurrent seizures, maintenance of healthy growth and development of the child, epilepsy management at school, and family education. The current treatment of pediatric epilepsy aims to improve health outcomes as well as to manage issues related to the quality of life of pediatric patients and their parents. Pediatric nurses have important functions to improve the quality of life of children with epilepsy and their families. In this regard, pediatric nurses should provide education to children with epilepsy and their families on issues such as drug use in epilepsy, seizure management, and prevention of seizure-related trauma. Furthermore, recognizing the psychosocial problems that can develop in the child and the family at an early stage and initiating the necessary interventions is one of the important functions of pediatric nurses in epilepsy management. Evidence-based nursing practices in pediatric epilepsy care are important in terms of integrating reliable information obtained from scientific research into clinical practice. Nurses should optimize the evidence obtained from current research in treatment and care plans by addressing the individual needs of the child. In this section, evidence-based nursing practices in the management of childhood epilepsy are included.

Keywords: children, epilepsy, nursing, parents, seizure

---

* Corresponding Author's Email: erkutzeynep@hotmail.com.

In: Evidence-Based Care Practices in Pediatric Nursing
Editors: Feyza Küçük and Serap Özdemir
ISBN: 979-8-89530-304-7

Introduction

An epileptic seizure is defined by the International League Against Epilepsy (ILAE) as a brief episode of signs and/or symptoms brought on by abnormally high or coordinated brain neuronal activity. A persistent predisposition to epileptic seizures and the ensuing neurobiological, cognitive, psychological, and social ramifications are the hallmarks of epilepsy, a brain illness (Fisher et al., 2014). Recurrent seizures, which are short bursts of involuntary movement that can affect the whole body (generalized) or only a portion of it and are sometimes accompanied by loss of consciousness, are what set epilepsy apart. Excessive electrical discharges in a cluster of brain cells are the cause of seizures. These discharges have the potential to impact different parts of the brain. Muscle jerks and short spells of inattention to severe and protracted convulsions are all possible types of seizures. Less than once a year or more than once a day can have seizures. At least one seizure will occur in the lifespan of 10% of the global population, yet not all seizures are epileptic (World Health Organization, 2024). The clinical diagnosis of epilepsy is based on the presence of at least two unprovoked seizures occurring more than 24 hours apart, an unprovoked seizure and a greater than 60% probability of recurrent seizures within the next 10 years, or the presence of one of the criteria for the diagnosis of epilepsy syndrome (Fisher et al., 2014).

Epidemiological estimates place the global prevalence of epilepsy at 50 million, with 5 million new cases reported annually. Eighty percent of people with epilepsy reside in low- and middle-income nations (World Health Organization, 2024). In the first ten years of life, one in every 150 children develops epilepsy, and between 0.5 and 1% of children worldwide are diagnosed with the condition (Aaberg et al., 2017). By the age of ten, children's incidence of epilepsy drops to adult levels, peaking in the first year of life (Beghi, 2020; P. Camfield & Camfield, 2015).

The etiology and clinical course of epilepsy are quite heterogeneous. A patient may have more than one etiologic cause or similar clinical pictures due to different etiologic causes (Günbey & Turanli, 2022). Epilepsy has multiple etiologies, including genetic, structural, infectious, metabolic, immunological, and unknown causes. A structural etiology can be hereditary, like different abnormalities of cortical development, or acquired, like stroke, trauma, infection, etc. When a confirmed or suspected genetic mutation directly causes seizures, the condition is described as epilepsy with genetic etiology. Numerous underlying genes remain unknown in the vast majority of epilepsies having a genetic origin. The direct occurrence of seizures brought on by several infectious agents, such as the Zika virus, cytomegalovirus, cerebral toxoplasmosis, tuberculosis, and human immunodeficiency virus, is known as infectious etiology (Scheffer et al., 2017). Epilepsy due to metabolic etiologies is when seizures occur as a result of a known or presumed metabolic disorder (porphyria, uremia, aminoacidopathy, or pyridoxine-induced). Immune etiology occurs as a result of autoimmune-mediated central nervous system inflammation (Falco-Walter et al., 2018).

Some epilepsy classifications have been made by ILAE for the correct diagnosis, prognosis, and treatment of epilepsy (Günbey & Turanli, 2022). The first step in the classification of epilepsy is to determine the epileptic seizure type. With the most recent update of the ILAE in 2017, epileptic seizure types are divided into four according to their onset patterns focal, generalized, unknown onset, and unclassifiable seizures (Figure 1) (Fisher et al., 2017). Finding the type of epilepsy is the second stage of the classification process. Once again, epilepsy types were categorized as "focal, generalized, combined generalized & focal, and unknown epilepsy" according to the 2017 ILAE classification. Additionally, it has been suggested to assess the etiology at every stage of the classification of epilepsy (Figure 2) (Scheffer et al., 2017). These classifications are recommended for use by general practitioners, pediatricians, neurologists, nurses, and other health care professionals (Falco-Walter et al., 2018).

In diagnosis, it is important to understand whether the child has a real seizure, to classify the type of seizure, and to determine the cause of the seizure. Nurses should guide the child and the family in these processes (Köse & Geçkil, 2023). The diagnosis of epilepsy is made primarily clinically and supported by investigations. The history of the child should be taken very carefully. After obtaining information from people who witnessed the child's seizure, the history should be elaborated by asking more detailed questions (onset, before, during, and after the attack). The presence of any trigger factor and/or aura before the attack should be questioned (Kutlu & Baklan, 2021).

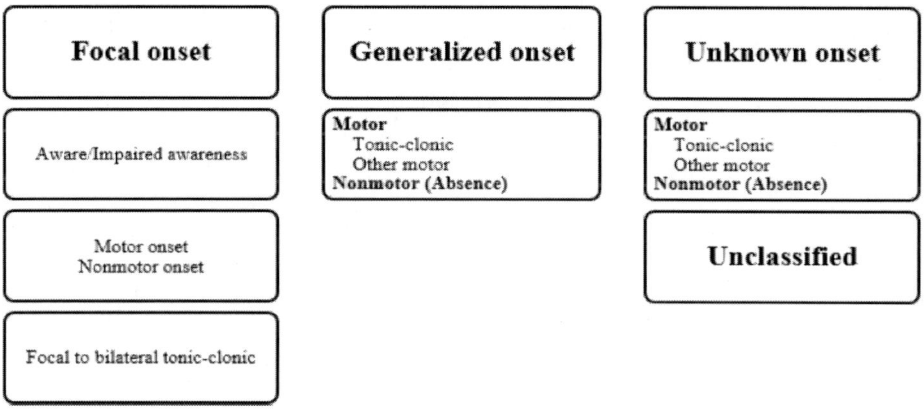

Figure 1. ILAE 2017 Classification of Seizure Types Basic Version.

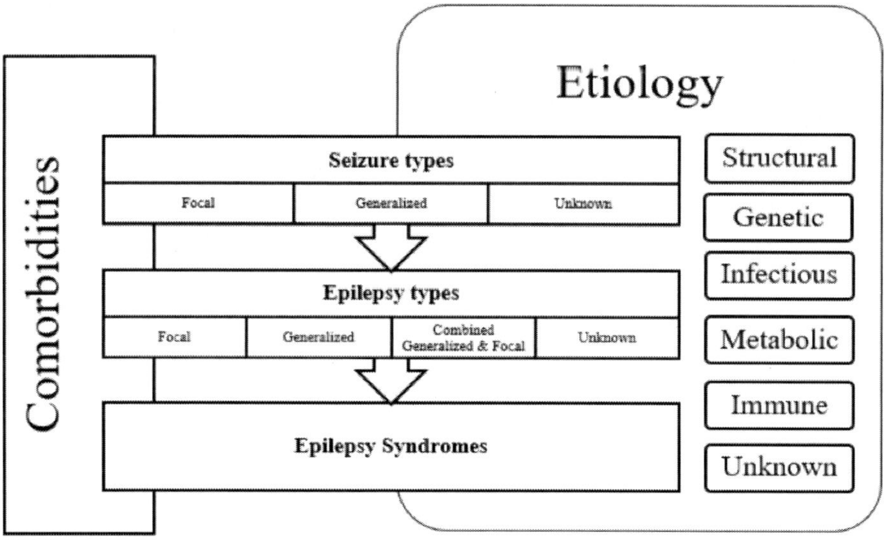

Figure 2. ILAE 2017 Classification of Epilepsies.

A complete history should be taken, including a birth and developmental history, major illnesses and injuries, a family history, a history of febrile seizures, and a thorough neurological evaluation. If necessary, the family may be asked for a video recording of the seizure. Second, a physical and neurological examination should be performed. Anthropometric measurements should be taken and laboratory tests should be ordered (Köse & Geçkil, 2023). Routine biochemical examination should be performed to exclude various secondary causes such as infectious, metabolic, and endocrine causes. Chromosome analysis can be performed if genetic predisposition is thought to be present (Kutlu & Baklan, 2021). If meningitis is suspected, a lumbar puncture (LP) may be performed to confirm the diagnosis, and structural abnormalities may be detected by radiological imaging such as computed tomography (CT), positron emission tomography (PET), or magnetic resonance imaging (MRI) (Köse & Geçkil, 2023). Electroencephalography (EEG) is an important diagnostic tool in childhood epileptic seizures. This test should be performed in every case of a presumed seizure. EEG is performed during sleep or wakefulness by giving stimuli that can trigger a seizure. These stimuli trigger abnormal electrical activity, and these discharges are seen in the EEG trace. Especially in children, an EEG should be performed in the first 24 hours after a seizure. In cases where the diagnosis cannot be made with standard EEG and the distinction between psychogenic and epileptic seizures cannot be made clearly, long-term video-EEG recording should be performed (İlgen Uslu, 2018; Rodgers, 2021).

The main goal of epilepsy treatment is to reduce the frequency, severity, or prevent seizures by controlling seizures without harming the child's development and to prevent side effects related to long-term treatment (Rodgers, 2021; Toklu, 2015). Treatment methods include antiepileptic drug therapy, ketogenic diet therapy, surgical treatment, and vagal nerve stimulation (Köse & Geçkil, 2023). Antiepileptic drugs are the first choice for seizure control (Vural et al., 2019). In 70-80% of children, seizures can be controlled with medication (Sillanpää et al., 2014). The prognosis of the disease can worsen when medications are not used regularly (Rodgers, 2021). Treatment starts with a single antiepileptic drug (monotherapy) that is most appropriate for the child's seizure type, is known to be effective and has the fewest side effects. If the initial drug treatment is insufficient to control seizures, polytherapy is applied. A second drug is started by gradually increasing the dose (Kayani & Sirsi, 2012). In children, the ketogenic diet is a successful treatment for drug-resistant epilepsy. It is a diet that emphasizes eating a lot of fat, enough protein, and carbohydrates. While the exact mode of action of the ketogenic diet is still unknown, it is believed that the ketone bodies (acetoacetate, acetone, and β-hydroxybutyrate) that are created from the body's primary energy source-fatty acids-cross the blood-brain barrier and exhibit anticonvulsant properties (Sourbron et al., 2020). Surgical treatment may be preferred in some children with refractory epilepsy whose seizures cannot be controlled despite the use of antiepileptic drugs. The main aim of epilepsy surgery is to prevent the child's seizure occurrence without any additional neurological deficit after surgery (Braun & Cross, 2018). A significant (>90%) reduction in seizures following epilepsy surgery (Jayalakshmi et al., 2014). Vagal nerve stimulation is a non-pharmacologic treatment for children with refractory epilepsy that cannot be treated surgically. The nerve stimulator consists of electrodes implanted under the skin covering the left vagus nerve at the cervical level. The electrodes work automatically and deliver small electrical currents to the nerve at short intervals. The use of vagal nerve stimulation has been reported to reduce the frequency and duration of seizures in refractory epilepsy in childhood by 16% to 65% (Sourbron et al., 2017).

Evidence-Based Nursing Practices in Epilepsy Management

Epilepsy is a disease that significantly affects the lives of diagnosed children and their families. Epilepsy management requires a multidisciplinary approach, and nurses are an important member of this team (Prevos-Morgant et al., 2019). Nurses help children with epilepsy and their families achieve the best possible health outcomes by providing disease and seizure management information, teaching self-management skills, and discussing treatment options (Smith et al., 2015).

Education of Children and Parents

One of the most important roles of nurses in the care of patients with epilepsy is to inform them about the disease, drug treatment, seizure management, etc. (Smith et al., 2019). Children and young people should be included in discussions about their information and support needs and provided with information appropriate to their developmental age (NICE Guideline, No. 217, 2022). In a study examining the effect of individual education and group counseling on epilepsy in adolescents with epilepsy, it was determined that adolescents' knowledge about epilepsy increased; in addition, their attitudes towards epilepsy and seizure self-efficacy improved positively (Frizzell et al., 2011). Compared to the control group, the children of the intervention group exhibited significantly improved knowledge, self-efficacy related to seizures, and quality of life in a study aimed at assessing the efficacy of the Modular Education Program for parents and children with epilepsy in disease management. Additionally, it was shown that, in comparison to the control group, the intervention group's parents' understanding of epilepsy had much increased (Turan Gürhopur & Işler Dalgiç, 2018). The primary treatment for epilepsy in children is typically medication. It is the responsibility of nurses to educate and monitor children to ensure that they take their medications on time and appropriately. A South Korean study looked into the connection between medication self-management and discharge education for parents of children with epilepsy. This study discovered a substantial relationship between medication self-management in children with epilepsy and parental discharge education (H. J. Lee et al., 2019).

Informing and empowering parents as well as children is a very important issue in the management of epilepsy in children. Nurses should provide parents with accurate information about epilepsy to help them care for their children in the best way possible (Brett, 2019). They can also educate parents on how to identify an epileptic seizure, what to do during a seizure, and develop a seizure action plan that shows what to do in the event of a sudden or prolonged seizure (Smith et al., 2019). Such educational interventions implemented by nurses have a high and beneficial effect on the knowledge of children with epilepsy and their parents about epilepsy and seizure management (Turan & Yangöz, 2023). Nashaat et al. (2022) found that the educational nursing intervention program was effective in improving the knowledge, practices, and attitudes of mothers of children with epilepsy and intellectual disabilities toward epilepsy management. In a multicenter study conducted in Europe, the effectiveness of a modular training program prepared for parents of children with epilepsy was evaluated. In this study, it was found that information transfer and the interactive approach with the modular training program were effective in increasing parents' knowledge about epilepsy, coping with their children's epilepsy, and reducing their fears about epilepsy (Hagemann et al., 2016). In a randomized controlled trial examining the effect of a structured curriculum on parents' knowledge about seizure management at home, it was found that the use of an information brochure with a structured curriculum was more effective than the use of an information brochure alone (Kumar et al., 2019).

Recent years have seen rapid advancement in technology, making it easier for people with epilepsy to obtain and update information on their condition, how to take their medications, how to control seizures, etc. (Escoffery et al., 2018). In a research study carried out to design and assess the efficacy of the web-based epilepsy education program (WEEP) for teenagers with epilepsy and their caregivers, it was discovered that the program was successful in raising the average scores of adolescents' knowledge, attitude, and e-health literacy. Furthermore, this study found that parents' levels of health literacy, self-management, and awareness of epilepsy increased while their levels of anxiety related to seizures reduced (Tutar Güven et al., 2020). In a study conducted in Malaysia, the effect of the Interactive Animated Epilepsy Education Program, an information technology-based epilepsy education program, was examined to improve the awareness, knowledge, and attitude of parents of children with epilepsy (aged 8-18 years) towards epilepsy. In the study, it was found that this information technology-based education program was effective in improving parents' awareness, knowledge, and attitude toward epilepsy (Fong et al., 2019). In another study, virtual reality technology was used to increase the knowledge, skills, and motivation of parents of children with epilepsy to manage epileptic seizures. It was determined that the "Virtual Reality-based Seizure Management Education Program for Parents (VR-ESMEPP)", which was implemented in line with a scenario in which a pediatric patient with epilepsy had a seizure, was effective in increasing the knowledge, skills, and motivation of parents to manage epileptic seizures (Turan et al., 2022). In a study examining the effect of a mobile application (EpApp) designed to educate adolescents with epilepsy and facilitate disease management, it was determined that the mobile application was effective in increasing adolescents' knowledge about epilepsy (Le Marne et al., 2018). All these evidence-based studies emphasize that it is important for nurses to use various educational methods to inform children with epilepsy and their families about epilepsy, improve epileptic seizure management skills, improve quality of life, and develop self-efficacy.

Education of School Staff

Children spend most of their lives at school. About one-third of epileptic seizures in children with epilepsy occur at school (Renzetti et al., 2020). Therefore, it is important that teachers and school staff are informed about epilepsy and raise awareness about epilepsy (Sharma et al., 2013). However, a systematic review reported that teachers lack knowledge and have negative attitudes about epilepsy (Jones et al., 2018). Therefore, especially school nurses should plan educational activities for teachers to gain knowledge and awareness about epilepsy. In a study aiming to increase teachers' knowledge about epilepsy in children, the Structured Teaching Program (STP) was found to be effective in increasing teachers' knowledge (Sharma et al., 2013). In a study conducted with primary school teachers in Egypt (n=143), it was found that the health education program was effective in improving teachers' knowledge about epilepsy and its management (Mohamed, 2017). An interactive one-day instructional workshop on epilepsy was arranged for teachers (n=230) in an Indian study to determine its impact. It was discovered that the educational intervention had a favorable effect on the attitudes, practices, and knowledge of the instructors on epilepsy. However, the researchers proposed that ongoing national and international efforts should be made to build the concept of "Epilepsy Smart Schools," as a single workshop would not be adequate to deliver the correct information about epilepsy (Sulena et al., 2023). In a study involving 740 school staff in Italy, school staff received information and awareness training on epilepsy and the proper management of epileptic seizures. As a result of this study, it was found that the participants' knowledge about epilepsy and seizure management increased, their anxiety toward epileptic seizure management decreased and their willingness to administer rescue medications increased (Renzetti et al., 2020).

Psychosocial Support

Epilepsy can negatively affect children's emotional and social well-being. Emotional, psychosocial, and behavioral problems, cognitive disorders, and academic difficulties are more common in children with epilepsy than in their healthy peers (Alam et al., 2020; Corrigan et al., 2016). Therefore, not only the physical but also the psychological and social needs of pediatric epilepsy patients should be taken into consideration; guidance should be provided to manage their relationships with family, friends, and school (NICE Guideline, No. 217, 2022). By providing psychosocial support to children and their families, nurses can help them develop coping skills and improve their quality of life. In a study, the effect of comprehensive nursing care for children with epilepsy and their families on children's psychological outcomes was examined. Children with epilepsy and their families who were hospitalized were informed about epilepsy by a specialist psychiatric nurse, as well as interventions such as family communication, practices that help the child express his/her emotions (playing games), distraction, and post-discharge counseling were provided. It was found that the anxiety and depression scores of the children who received comprehensive nursing care were significantly lower in the first and third months of care compared to the children who received only information (Wang et al., 2023). Cognitive behavioral therapy has been shown to be beneficial in lowering social anxiety and enhancing self-concept in children with epilepsy, according to a study done to assess the impact of nursing intervention based on this approach on these two areas (Alam et al., 2020). In the UK, a study was carried out to investigate the effects of a psychosocial intervention designed to enhance the quality of life, understanding, and self-management abilities of young individuals with epilepsy, ages 12 to 17. Six weekly 2-hour sessions utilizing role plays, group activities, and guided discussion led by a clinical psychologist and epilepsy nurse comprised the psychosocial intervention. It was discovered that while quality of life was not affected, this brief psychosocial intervention was successful in raising participants' awareness about epilepsy and boosting their self-assurance when talking to others about their condition (Dorris et al., 2017).

The long duration of epilepsy, unpredictable seizures, and problems in the child's social life negatively affect the family and put the family in crisis. If psychosocial support is provided to the family along with education about the disease, family members can develop the ability to control their negative emotions and feel better about themselves (Wo et al.,

2018). In a study including parents of epileptic children aged 6 to 18, the impact of a psychoeducational program on the care burden on families was investigated. It was found that both immediately following the psychoeducational program and one month later, the intervention group's mean care burden scale score was significantly lower than that of the control group (Balouchi et al., 2021). In another study, the effect of a family education program including drug treatment, seizure management, and home care of the child on the quality of life of families of children aged 0-6 years with newly diagnosed epilepsy was examined. It was found that the quality of life of families who received family education programs in addition to routine care was higher in the 6th and 12th months of discharge compared to families who received only routine care (Liu et al., 2020).

Safety Precautions

11% of children with epilepsy are more likely to sustain injuries from falls, burns, drownings, and auto accidents during an epileptic episode (C. Camfield & Camfield, 2015). Therefore, safety measures are critical in disease management in children with epilepsy. Nurses should teach children and their families to take the necessary precautions to ensure safety at home, school, and other outdoor settings. This can help minimize injuries and risks during seizures. In addition to organizing trainings for patients and their relatives on seizure-related safety precautions, nurses can support the trainings with written educational materials (Freedman & Albert, 2021). Children with epilepsy should not be allowed to swim unsupervised, should take showers rather than baths, should wear helmets when bicycling, skating, or rollerblading, should not engage in activities that involve climbing and should not cook or be near an open fire without adult supervision. This information should be shared with both the children and their families (American Academy of Pediatrics, 2020). In a study, a remedial standardized seizure action plan for epileptic seizures was applied to families with children with epilepsy. In this study, it was found that families who received standardization of the seizure action plan (SAP) increased their knowledge about emergency seizure intervention (Neville et al., 2020).

Training and Empowering Nurses

In the clinical context, nurses are essential to the care of children with epilepsy. Consequently, pediatric nurses ought to be well-versed in epilepsy and seizure treatment and equipped with the necessary tools (Alam et al., 2020). In a study conducted in Korea, an algorithm-based training program was used to improve the knowledge and self-efficacy of 27 nurses working in pediatric neurology and pediatric emergency services with regard to caring for children with epilepsy. According to this study, the knowledge and self-efficacy of nurses who participated in the training program on nursing care of children with epilepsy improved statistically considerably (J. H. Lee et al., 2019).

To support students with epilepsy in the classroom, school nurses play a crucial role. To oversee the care of students with epilepsy in a school setting, nurses must have the necessary knowledge and abilities. They also need to feel confident in their abilities. As a result, it is critical to empower and inform school nurses about epilepsy. School nurses received management and intervention training for children with epilepsy as part of a project carried out in the United States of America. It was discovered that school nurses who participated in the experiment had more confidence in their ability to control seizures, used seizure action plans more frequently, and finished recording 88% of the children who had received a new seizure diagnosis. Additionally, the training program was rated as "very useful" by the majority of school nurses (Brook et al., 2015).

Conclusion

The treatment of epilepsy in children is a complicated process that calls for customized attention. Optimizing treatment outcomes and enhancing the quality of life for children and their families with pediatric epilepsy can be achieved through the implementation of evidence-based nursing practices. As a result, pediatric nurses should treat children with epilepsy and their families in addition to performing their fundamental duties, which include counseling and education, using evidence-based nursing practices that they will design according to the most recent recommendations and research findings. On the other hand, educating professionals in the school environment where children spend most of their time and raising awareness should be among the important duties of school nurses.

Disclaimer

None.

References

Aaberg, K. M., Gunnes, N., Bakken, I. J., Lund Søraas, C., Berntsen, A., Magnus, P., Lossius, M. I., Stoltenberg, C., Chin, R., & Surén, P. (2017). Incidence and prevalence of childhood epilepsy: A nationwide cohort study. *Pediatrics*, *139*(5), e20163908. https://doi.org/10.1542/peds.2016-3908.

Alam, F. H., Shehata, H. S., & Hassan, G. A. (2020). Effect of implementing nursing nntervention based on cognitive behavioral therapy on social anxiety and self-concept of children with epilepsy. *International Journal of Novel Research in Healthcare and Nursing*, *7*(2), 318–330. https://doi.org/10.13140/RG.2.2.28573.03044.

American Academy of Pediatrics. (2020). *Seizure Safety: Tips for Parents—HealthyChildren.org*. https://www.healthychildren.org/English/health-issues/conditions/seizures/Pages/Seizure-Safety-Tips-for-Parents.aspx?_gl=1*o7mbe9*_ga*NjUyNzA4MTIzLjE3MDc3Mjg0Mjk.*_ga_FD9D3XZVQQ*MTcwODQxMTYwOC4yLjAuMTcwODQxMTYwOC4wLjAuMA. Accessed Date:

Balouchi, Z., Pahlavanzadeh, S., & Alimohammadi, N. (2021). Efficacy of psycho-educational program on burden of caregivers of children with epilepsy: A clinical trial. *Medical - Surgical Nursing Journal*, *10*(2), Article 2. https://doi.org/10.5812/msnj.119961.

Beghi, E. (2020). The epidemiology of epilepsy. *Neuroepidemiology*, *54*(2), 185–191. https://doi.org/10.1159/000503831.

Braun, K. P. J., & Cross, J. H. (2018). Pediatric epilepsy surgery: The earlier the better. *Expert Review of Neurotherapeutics*, *18*(4), 261–263. https://doi.org/10.1080/14737175.2018.1455503.

Brett, S. (2019). Chapter 19—Nursing Issues in Managing Comorbidities of Epilepsy. In M. Mula (Ed.), *The Comorbidities of Epilepsy* (pp. 367–387). Academic Press. https://doi.org/10.1016/B978-0-12-814877-8.00019-2.

Brook, H. A., Hiltz, C. M., Kopplin, V. L., & Lindeke, L. L. (2015). Increasing epilepsy awareness in schools: A seizure smart schools project. *The Journal of School Nursing*, *31*(4), 246–252. https://doi.org/10.1177/1059840514563761.

Camfield, C., & Camfield, P. (2015). Injuries from seizures are a serious, persistent problem in childhood onset epilepsy: A population-based study. *Seizure*, *27*, 80–83. https://doi.org/10.1016/j.seizure.2015.02.031.

Camfield, P., & Camfield, C. (2015). Incidence, prevalence and aetiology of seizures and epilepsy in children. *Epileptic Disorders: International Epilepsy Journal with Videotape*, *17*(2), 117–123. https://doi.org/
10.1684/epd.2015.0736.

Corrigan, F. M., Broome, H., & Dorris, L. (2016). A systematic review of psychosocial interventions for children and young people with epilepsy. *Epilepsy & Behavior*, *56*, 99–112. https://doi.org/10.1016/j.yebeh.2016.01.005.

Dorris, L., Broome, H., Wilson, M., Grant, C., Young, D., Baker, G., Balloo, S., Bruce, S., Campbell, J., Concannon, B., Conway, N., Cook, L., Davis, C., Downey, B., Evans, J., Flower, D., Garlovsky, J., Kearney, S., Lewis, S., … Wright, I. (2017). A randomized controlled trial of a manual-based psychosocial group intervention for young people with epilepsy [PIE]. *Epilepsy & Behavior*, *72*, 89–98. https://doi.org/10.1016/j.yebeh.2017.04.007.

Escoffery, C., McGee, R., Bidwell, J., Sims, C., Thropp, E. K., Frazier, C., & Mynatt, E. D. (2018). A review of mobile apps for epilepsy self-management. *Epilepsy & Behavior*, *81*, 62–69. https://doi.org/10.1016/j.yebeh.2017.12.010.

Falco-Walter, J. J., Scheffer, I. E., & Fisher, R. S. (2018). The new definition and classification of seizures and epilepsy. *Epilepsy Research*, *139*, 73–79. https://doi.org/10.1016/j.eplepsyres.2017.11.015.

Fisher, R. S., Acevedo, C., Arzimanoglou, A., Bogacz, A., Cross, J. H., Elger, C. E., Engel Jr, J., Forsgren, L., French, J. A., Glynn, M., Hesdorffer, D. C., Lee, B. i., Mathern, G. W., Moshé, S. L., Perucca, E., Scheffer, I. E., Tomson, T., Watanabe, M., & Wiebe, S. (2014). ILAE Official Report: A practical clinical definition of epilepsy. *Epilepsia*, *55*(4), 475–482. https://doi.org/10.1111/epi.12550.

Fisher, R. S., Cross, J. H., French, J. A., Higurashi, N., Hirsch, E., Jansen, F. E., Lagae, L., Moshé, S. L., Peltola, J., Roulet Perez, E., Scheffer, I. E., & Zuberi, S. M. (2017). Operational classification of seizure types by the International League Against Epilepsy: Position paper of the ILAE Commission for classification and terminology. *Epilepsia*, *58*(4), 522–530. https://doi.org/10.1111/epi.13670.

Fong, C. Y., Seet, Y. H., Ong, L. C., Lim, W. K., & Lua, P. L. (2019). Improving awareness, knowledge, and attitude among Malaysian parents of children with epilepsy using an Interactive Animated Epilepsy Education Programme (IAEEP). *Epilepsy & Behavior*, *94*, 52–58. https://doi.org/10.1016/j.yebeh.2019.02.008.

Freedman, D. A., & Albert, D. V. F. (2021). Seizure safety education should be provided to pediatric patients With suspected seizures. *Pediatric Neurology*, *114*, 53–54. https://doi.org/10.1016/j.pediatrneurol.2020.08.018.

Frizzell, C. K., Connolly, A. M., Beavis, E., Lawson, J. A., & Bye, A. M. (2011). Personalised epilepsy education intervention for adolescents and impact on knowledge acquisition and psychosocial function. *Journal of Paediatrics and Child Health*, *47*(5), 271–275. https://doi.org/10.1111/j.1440-1754.2010.01952.x.

Günbey, C., & Turanli, G. (2022). Epilepsi ve pediatrik epilepsi sendromları. *Türkiye Çocuk Hastalıkları Dergisi*, *16*(3), 249–257. https://doi.org/10.12956/tchd.888121.

Hagemann, A., Pfäfflin, M., Nussbeck, F. W., & May, T. W. (2016). The efficacy of an educational program for parents of children with epilepsy (FAMOSES): Results of a controlled multicenter evaluation study. *Epilepsy & Behavior*, *64*, 143–151. https://doi.org/10.1016/j.yebeh.2016.09.027.

İlgen Uslu, F. (2018). Epileptik nöbet ve epilepsi. In G. Babacan Yıldız & E. Gökçal (Eds.), *Nöroloji'nin ABC'si* (pp. 117–127). İstanbul Tıp Kitabevleri.

Jayalakshmi, S., Panigrahi, M., Nanda, S. K., & Vadapalli, R. (2014). Surgery for childhood epilepsy. *Annals of Indian Academy of Neurology*, *17*(Suppl 1), S69–S79. https://doi.org/10.4103/0972-2327.128665.

Jones, C., Atkinson, P., Helen Cross, J., & Reilly, C. (2018). Knowledge of and attitudes towards epilepsy among teachers: A systematic review. *Epilepsy & Behavior*, *87*, 59–68. https://doi.org/10.1016/j.yebeh.2018.06.044.

Kayani, S., & Sirsi, D. (2012). The safety and tolerability of newer antiepileptic drugs in children and adolescents. *Journal of Central Nervous System Disease*, *4*, 51–63. https://doi.org/10.4137/JCNSD.S5097.

Köse, S., & Geçkil, E. (2023). Nörolojik Sorunu Olan Çocuk. In S. Arslan (Ed.), *Pediatri Hemşireliğinin Temelleri* (pp. 473–492). Nobel Akademik Yayıncılık.

Kumar, R., Khakha, D. C., Gulati, S., & Kaushik, J. S. (2019). Impact of structured teaching program on the parent's knowledge of domiciliary management of seizure—A randomized controlled trial. *Epilepsy & Behavior*, *92*, 191–194. https://doi.org/10.1016/j.yebeh.2018.11.038.

Kutlu, A., & Baklan, B. (2021). *Epilepside Tanı ve Ayırıcı Tanı* (İ. Öztura, G. Kutlu, İ. Tezer, K. Ağan, & Ö. Çokar, Eds.; pp. 24–34). Galenos Yayınevi.

Le Marne, F. A., Butler, S., Beavis, E., Gill, D., & Bye, A. M. E. (2018). EpApp: Development and evaluation of a smartphone/tablet app for adolescents with epilepsy. *Journal of Clinical Neuroscience*, *50*, 214–220. https://doi.org/10.1016/j.jocn.2018.01.065.

Lee, H. J., Choi, E. K., Kim, H. S., & Kang, H. C. (2019). Medication self-management and the quality of discharge education among parents of children with epilepsy. *Epilepsy & Behavior*, *94*, 14–19. https://doi.org/10.1016/j.yebeh.2018.12.030.

Lee, J. H., Ju, H. O., Lee, Y. J., Lee, J. H., Ju, H. O., & Lee, Y. J. (2019). Effects of an algorithm-based education program on nursing care for children with epilepsy by hospital nurses. *Child Health Nursing Research*, *25*(3), 324–332. https://doi.org/10.4094/chnr.2019.25.3.324.

Liu, H., Song, Q., Zhu, L., Chen, D., Xie, J., Hu, S., Zeng, S., & Tan, L. (2020). Family management style improves family quality of life in children with epilepsy: A randomized controlled trial. *Journal of Neuroscience Nursing*, *52*(2), 84. https://doi.org/10.1097/JNN.0000000000000497.

Mohamed, M. A. (2017). Effect of health educational program on knowledge about epilepsy and its management among primary schools' teachers. *Port Said Scientific Journal of Nursing*, *4*(1), 76–87. https://doi.org/10.21608/PSSJN.2017.33089.

Nashaat, N., Abd El-Ghany, G., Mahmoud, S., El Sebaie, S., AbdelrhmanAlhanafy, S., & Mohamed, E. S. H. (2022). Effect of nursing intervention program on mothers' knowledge, practice and attitudes toward management of their children with epilepsy and intellectual disability. *Tanta Scientific Nursing Journal*, *25*(2), 198–216. https://doi.org/10.21608/TSNJ.2022.243362.

Neville, K. L., McCaffery, H., Baxter, Z., Shellhaas, R. A., & Fedak Romanowski, E. M. (2020). Implementation of a standardized seizure action plan to improve communication and parental education. *Pediatric Neurology*, *112*, 56–63. https://doi.org/10.1016/j.pediatrneurol.2020.04.005.

NICE Guideline, No. 217. (2022). *Epilepsies in children, young people and adults*. National Institute for Health and Care Excellence (NICE). http://www.ncbi.nlm.nih.gov/books/NBK581165/.

Prevos-Morgant, M., Leavy, Y., Chartrand, D., Jurasek, L., Osborne Shafer, P., Shinnar, R., & Goodwin, M. (2019). Benefits of the epilepsy specialist nurses (ESN) role, standardized practices and education around the world. *Revue Neurologique*, *175*(3), 189–193. https://doi.org/10.1016/j.neurol.2018.10.003.

Renzetti, T., Calabrese, C., Pietrafusa, N., Pannacci, I., Rainò, R., Giuffrida, A., Specchio, N., & Vigevano, F. (2020). Management of epileptic seizures in school-age children: Educational project dedicated to school staff. *Epilepsy & Behavior*, *105*, 106951. https://doi.org/10.1016/j.yebeh.2020.106951.

Rodgers, C. C. (2021). The Child with Cerebral Dysfunction. In M. J. Hockenberry, D. Wilson, & C. C. Rodgers (Eds.), *Wong's Essentials of Pediatric Nursing* (pp. 872–910). Elsevier Health Sciences.

Scheffer, I. E., Berkovic, S., Capovilla, G., Connolly, M. B., French, J., Guilhoto, L., Hirsch, E., Jain, S., Mathern, G. W., Moshé, S. L., Nordli, D. R., Perucca, E., Tomson, T., Wiebe, S., Zhang, Y.-H., & Zuberi, S. M. (2017). ILAE classification of the epilepsies: Position paper of the ILAE Commission for Classification and Terminology. *Epilepsia*, *58*(4), 512–521. https://doi.org/10.1111/epi.13709.

Sharma, N. K., Prasanna, K. L., & Kumar, A. (2013). Effectiveness of structured teaching program on knowledge regarding epilepsy in children among school teachers. *IOSR Journal of Nursing and Health Science*, *2*(6), 07–13. https://doi.org/10.9790/1959-0260713.

Sillanpää, M., Saarinen, M., & Schmidt, D. (2014). Clinical conditions of long-term cure in childhood-onset epilepsy: A 45-year follow-up study. *Epilepsy & Behavior*, *37*, 49–53. https://doi.org/10.1016/j.yebeh.2014.05.029.

Smith, G., Plueger, M., & Wagner, J. L. (2019). Evidence-based epilepsy care: Assessment, treatment, and self-management. *American Nurse Today*, *14*(7), 6–12.

Smith, G., Wagner, J. L., & Edwards, J. C. (2015). CE: Epilepsy Update, Part 2: Nursing Care and Evidence-Based Treatment. *AJN The American Journal of Nursing*, *115*(6), 34–44. https://doi.org/10.1097/01.NAJ.0000466314.46508.00.

Sourbron, J., Klinkenberg, S., Kessels, A., Schelhaas, H. J., Lagae, L., & Majoie, M. (2017). Vagus nerve stimulation in children: A focus on intellectual disability. *European Journal of Paediatric Neurology: EJPN: Official Journal of the European Paediatric Neurology Society*, *21*(3), 427–440. https://doi.org/10.1016/j.ejpn.2017.01.011.

Sourbron, J., Klinkenberg, S., van Kuijk, S. M. J., Lagae, L., Lambrechts, D., Braakman, H. M. H., & Majoie, M. (2020). Ketogenic diet for the treatment of pediatric epilepsy: Review and meta-analysis. *Child's Nervous System: ChNS: Official Journal of the International Society for Pediatric Neurosurgery*, *36*(6), 1099–1109. https://doi.org/10.1007/s00381-020-04578-7.

Sulena, S., Singh, G., Tyagi, D., Bansal, N., Padda, P., Garg, R., Kumar, R., Kaur, K., Kaur, H., & Kumar, N. (2023). Epilepsy smart schools: Educational intervention improves knowledge, attitude, and practices regarding epilepsy among school teachers. *Epilepsy & Behavior*, *141*, 109138. https://doi.org/10.1016/j.yebeh.2023.109138.

Toklu, Z. (2015). Epilepside tedavi stratejileri. *Kocatepe Tıp Dergisi*, *16*(2), Article 2. https://doi.org/10.18229/ktd.55178.

Turan, F. D., Dalgıç, A. İ., & Duman, Ö. (2022). Development of a conceptual framework for a Virtual Reality-based Seizure Management Education Program for Parents (VR-ESMEPP). *Epilepsy & Behavior*, *135*, 108875. https://doi.org/10.1016/j.yebeh.2022.108875.

Turan, F. D., & Yangöz, Ş. T. (2023). Effect of educational interventions on level of epilepsy knowledge in children with epilepsy and parents: Systematic review and meta-analysis. *Journal of Clinical Nursing*, *32*(7–8), 1381–1397. https://doi.org/10.1111/jocn.16346.

Turan Gürhopur, F. D., & Işler Dalgiç, A. (2018). The effect of a modular education program for children with epilepsy and their parents on disease management. *Epilepsy & Behavior*, *78*, 210–218. https://doi.org/
10.1016/j.yebeh.2017.07.048.

Tutar Güven, Ş., İşler Dalgiç, A., & Duman, Ö. (2020). Evaluation of the efficiency of the web-based epilepsy education program (WEEP) for youth with epilepsy and parents: A randomized controlled trial. *Epilepsy & Behavior*, *111*, 107142. https://doi.org/10.1016/j.yebeh.2020.107142.

Vural, Ö., Serdaroglu, A., Citak Kurt, A. N., Hirfanoğlu, T., & Kurt, G. (2019). The efficacy of nonpharmacologic treatment in children with pharmacoresistant epilepsy. *Güncel Pediatri*, *17*(2), 243–252. https://doi.org/10.4274/jcp.2019.0022.

Wang, J., Chen, W., & Lai, Y. (2023). Comprehensive nursing program for children with epilepsy: A randomized controlled trial. *Nigerian Journal of Clinical Practice*, *26*(10), 1498. https://doi.org/10.4103/
njcp.njcp_93_23.

Wo, S. W., Ong, L. C., Low, W. Y., & Lai, P. S. M. (2018). Exploring the needs and challenges of parents and their children in childhood epilepsy care: A qualitative study. *Epilepsy & Behavior*, *88*, 268–276. https://doi.org/10.1016/j.yebeh.2018.09.018.

World Health Organization. (2024). *Epilepsy*. https://www.who.int/news-room/fact-sheets/detail/epilepsy.

Chapter 14

Evidence-Based Multidisciplinary Approaches in Childhood Obesity

Meltem Catalbas*, PhD
Department of Nursing, Faculty of Health Sciences, Kutahya Health Sciences University, Kutahya, Türkiye

Abstract

The prevalence of childhood obesity has reached an epidemic across the world, constituting a vital public health concern. The increasing prevalence of obesity among children highlights the related health consequences and stresses the significance of using evidence-based strategies for prevention and treatment. Considering the multifaceted nature of childhood obesity encompassing, physical, psychological, and social dimensions. Intervention programs must extend beyond physical weight loss, targeting behavioral, and psychosocial changes. Recognizing obesity as a psychosocial condition, a multidisciplinary professional team comprising health promoters, nurses, physicians, physiotherapists, and psychologists is essential. Treatment modalities encompass diet, physical exercise, behavioral modification, and psychosocial support. For those already tackling childhood obesity, HCPs play a crucial role in implementing evidence-based strategies. A comprehensive understanding of the issue is essential for health professionals to effectively comprehend and mitigate its impact. The initial step toward resolving challenges involves establishing a constructive relationship marked by non-stigmatization and attentive listening, ensuring children's voices are heard in interventions exploring their agency in everyday life. Family-based interventions and support play a crucial role in promoting healthy behaviors and successful weight management among children, with parental involvement being a key factor in the long-term success of treatment. However, challenges such as inconsistent parental involvement and negative interactions with HCPs can hinder treatment effectiveness. Therefore, a collaborative approach involving HCPs, families, and children is essential to comprehensively address childhood obesity and ensure positive health outcomes.

This chapter highlights the importance of an evidence-based, multidisciplinary approach to childhood obesity. Advocating for a personalized intervention, it prioritizes children's needs in a multidisciplinary approach to minimize their physical and psychosocial problems.

* Corresponding Author's Email: meltem.catalbas@ksbu.edu.tr.

In: Evidence-Based Care Practices in Pediatric Nursing
Editors: Feyza Küçük and Serap Özdemir
ISBN: 979-8-89530-304-7

Keywords: childhood obesity, multidisciplinary approach, obsesity treatment

Introduction

The prevalence of childhood obesity has become a global concern. By 2022, more than 1 billion people worldwide were impacted by obesity, resulting in at least 2.8 million deaths annually from related health complications. This epidemic has doubled obesity rates in adults since 1990 and tripled them in children, with projections suggesting a future prevalence exceeding 70%. While historically linked to affluent nations, obesity now affects low- and middle-income countries significantly, necessitating evidence-based strategies and comprehensive interventions involving healthcare professionals and families. Addressing childhood obesity requires a multifaceted approach, encompassing not only physical health but also psychosocial well-being, with family-based interventions playing a crucial role in promoting healthy behaviors, and sustainable weight management among children. Collaborative efforts are essential to effectively combat this global health challenge.

Global Assessment of Childhood Obesity: Prevalence, Estimates and Trends

The World Health Organization (WHO) (2024) defines obesity as a physical condition characterized by excessive fat accumulation stored in the body. According to the WHO's most recent assessment in 2022, obesity has emerged as a worldwide public health issue and has reached epidemic levels, impacting more than 1 billion individuals worldwide and resulting in a minimum of 2.8 million people dying annually due to being overweight or obese (WHO, 2021, 2024). Obesity rates in adults have doubled since 1990, while in children they have increased more than tripled in the same period (WHO, 2024). By 2022, 37 million children under the age of five spotted overweight, and children and adolescents over 390 million aged 5 to 19 years are overweight, with 160 million living with obesity (WHO, 2024).

Obesity was formerly associated mainly with affluent countries; however, it is now increasingly prevalent in low- and middle-income countries as well (WHO, 2021). Accordingly, childhood obesity is growing more prevalent in all countries, with low- and middle-income countries experiencing the highest growth. The vast majority of children living with overweight or obesity reside in developing countries, where the rate of increase is more than 30% higher than in developed countries (WHO, 2016). Considering population growth and age distribution changes, and assuming that obesity prevalence trends continue, the World Obesity Federation (2022) predicts that by 2060, the vast majority of countries will have overweight and obesity prevalence rates greater than 70% of the total population, including children. According to this estimate, the majority of high obesity prevalence levels will come from middle-income nations.

Why Childhood Obesity Treatment Matters: Understanding Its Significance and Impact

As concerns about the rising rates of obesity increase, the associated health impacts also escalate (Tiwari & Balasundaram, 2021). Obesity in children can underpin and contribute to the development of potentially fatal health problems and preventable diseases such as cardiovascular disease, hyperlipidemia, type 2 diabetes mellitus, hypertension, stroke, asthma, sleep apnea, orthopedic, and fatty liver disease (Dietz, 1998; Reilly et al., 2003). In addition to the physical health effects associated with childhood obesity, psychosocial challenges have been linked as a negative consequence of childhood obesity and overweight (Kansra et al., 2021; Reilly et al., 2003), which have a significant impact on children's overall well-being and the quality of life (Sagar & Gupta, 2018). The psychological health concers of children living with obesity worsen with age (Reilly et al., 2003). The literature reports on the psychosocial problems associated with childhood obesity that impair children's quality of life in several dimensions such as low self-esteem, body discomfort, and psychosocial distress (depression, anxiety, stigmatization, and stress) (Kaufman et al., 2020; Marten et al., 2023; Rankin et al., 2016; Russell-Mayhew et al., 2012). An increasing amount of evidence indicates that children with psychosocial (dys)function are more likely to have the same issue in adulthood (Blanco et al., 2020; Reilly et al., 2003; Sanderson et al., 2011).

Childhood obesity is a crucial aim as part of a strategy to ensure a healthy life expectancy (WHO, 2016). Obesity has serious health consequences, beginning in childhood period and progressing into adulthood; hence, childhood obesity is the strongest predictor of adulthood obesity and its accompanying physical health and psychosocial implications (Dietz, 1998; Faienza et al., 2020; Reilly et al., 2003) with increased mortality and morbidity (Sutin et al., 2015), which is a worldwide health problem that cannot be ignored. Therefore, given the widespread prevalence of obesity and its associated health-related problems in children globally, it is crucial to address this critically and with evidence-based strategies, especially considering the growing need to protect future public health interventions (Reilly et al., 2003; World Obesity Federation, 2022).

Childhood Obesity Prevention and Treatment

Obesity and overweight in clinical contexts relate to an excess of body fat as measured by Body Mass Index (BMI) anthropometrics, which are calculated by dividing one's weight in kilograms by the square of their height in meters (kg/m2). Due to the growth process in children and adolescents, the height, weight, and BMI ranges differ based on age and gender. Consequently, Children's BMI is assessed in percentiles on children's growth charts considering sex and age for an accurate assessment. If the BMI is between the 85th and the 95th percentiles for a child's age and gender, they are defined as overweight (Hampl et al., 2023). Obesity is defined as being at the 95th percentile and above (Hampl et al., 2023). This criterion fulfills the standard for diagnosing weight conditions in young individuals.

Obesity is difficult to cure and can lead to long-term health problems in children, hence prevention and treatment initiatives should be prioritized within public health services. Also, managing childhood obesity is recognized as a challenging and costly endeavor (Ells et al.,

2005; World Obesity Federation., 2022). However, the emphasis has primarily been on prevention, with inadequate attention given to treatment services for children living with obesity and overweight (Viner et al., 2018; World Obesity Federation., 2022). Addressing childhood obesity has a strong rationale, and science provides several opportunities for intervention. However, there is presently no clear consensus on which interventions and combinations are likely to be most beneficial in various situations throughout the world, and there is no global accountability framework in place for stakeholders (World Obesity Federation., 2022). Also, obesity management is difficult since it focuses on diet, physical activity, and behavior modification, all of which take a large amount of time from the patient, the patient's family, and the providers (Marten et al., 2023). Therefore, the most evident and efficient methods to prevent and address current obesity are long-term preventive and intervention strategies.

Evidence-based clinical guidelines (Hampl et al., 2023; NICE, 2006, 2015; Stewart et al., 2009; WHO, 2016) agree that obesity treatment regimens should be multifaceted, with a focus on behavioral change in children with obesity or overweight to increase physical activity, decrease sedentary behaviors, improve eating habits, self-esteem, mental wellbeing and reduce energy intake. To achieve this, it is recommended that obesity intervention programs be developed using a multidisciplinary approach such as dietitians, psychologists, nurses, and pediatricians that consider the viewpoints of both children and families (Lanigan & Sauven, 2020; NICE, 2017).

The Importance of a Multidisciplinary Approach

HCPs play an important role in the evidence-based treatment of childhood obesity since they are at the forefront of diagnosis, prevention, treatment, and management of childhood obesity. To achieve effective results in the treatment of childhood obesity, complete collaboration with the child and family is essential. Childhood obesity is a long-term problem that affects children with complex needs both physically and psychologically. HCPs should enhance their understanding of childhood obesity to properly tackle it and mitigate its implications.

The first stage in addressing the issue is to develop a constructive and non-stigmatizing relationship with children and their families (Jones et al., 2019; Kirk et al., 2020; Lowenstein et al., 2013; Pont et al., 2017). One of the most negative behaviors that children with obesity are exposed to is weight stigma, with its immediate and long-term effects (Phelan et al., 2015). Phelan et al. (2015) objectively evaluated empirical data and discussed obesity stigma across all relevant areas, and they found that the HCPs' attitudes regarding obesity-centered care may lower the quality of the individuals' interaction with treatments, have a detrimental influence on patients' results, and impair patient satisfaction. Similarly, in the systematic reviews conducted by Jones et al. (2019), they found that negative feedback from professionals resulted in adolescents experiencing heightened levels of dissatisfaction and reduced compliance with obesity treatment protocols. Again, these findings are consistent with the scoping review conducted by Roberts et al. (2021), which highlighted that unfavorable encounters with HCPs, resulting in dissatisfaction among children and families, are identified as noteworthy barriers.

According to evidence-based research, children receiving obesity treatment prefer to have continual connections with regular HCPs with whom they have developed a trusting relationship (Jones et al., 2019). Similarly, the findings from children's accounts illustrate that children's trust in providers has a positive influence on their adherence to treatment programs, whereas meeting with different professional teams each time results in emotions of neglect and disappointment (Morinder et al., 2011).

Children with obesity experience not only physical health concerns but also severe psychological (dsy)function (Lanigan & Sauven, 2020). In the context of obesity, while physical transformation may manifest rapidly or visibly, the improvement of children's psychological well-being and overall quality of life ascribed to weight-related issues may take a longer length of time to observe (Smith et al., 2020). An evidence-based study highlighted that while adolescents with obesity desire to lose weight, they also value receiving support that encompasses aspects beyond weight loss alone, including interventions that address self-esteem and overall well-being, indicating a holistic approach to their healthcare needs (Jones et al., 2019). Likewise, study of Morinder et al. (2011) on children living with obesity discovered that weight management programs should focus not only on weight loss, but also on meeting other needs such as feeling content and accepting oneself, being healthy and physically well, having more self-esteem, and not worrying about weight-related management. Furthermore, the literature highlighted that when children experience stress or encounter adverse events such as trauma, bullying, or exposure to stereotypes, these situations trigger their emotional eating behavior as a coping mechanism (Howie et al., 2016; Milaneschi et al., 2019). This behavior not only leads to relapses but also contributes significantly to the cycles of obesity and depression (Howie et al., 2016; Milaneschi et al., 2019). In alignment with clinical guidelines, it is recommended that treatment goals for childhood obesity extend beyond simply reducing or stabilizing BMI (Hampl et al., 2023; Kirk et al., 2020; WHO, 2016). Instead, treatment goals should encompass a broader perspective, including aspects such as improving or resolving comorbidities, health-related quality of life, self-perception, psychosocial distress (self-confidence, low self-esteem, teasing, bullying), and other aspects associated with a holistic approach (Hampl et al., 2023; Kirk et al., 2020; NICE, 2014; Rankin et al., 2016; WHO, 2016). This approach emphasizes the importance of addressing the overall well-being and psychological health of children with obesity, alongside physical health considerations, to ensure comprehensive and effective treatment outcomes.

Family-Based Intervention Programs

Children are mostly dependent on their families until they mature physically, intellectually, and gain independence. As a result, families are usually responsible for preparing food, selecting appropriate foods as needed, and providing a social environment that meets the child's requirements. Pamungkas and Chamroonsawasdi's (2019) systematic review highlighted that incorporating families to combat childhood obesity offers favorable results in treating and preventing obesity. Their research revealed that involving parents enhances their skills in childcare and child rearing, particularly in terms of problem-solving ability to address weight-related challenges faced by children. These challenges include emotional support, setting goals, availability, and accessibility of nutritious meals at home to build a healthy eating pattern, and managing healthy behaviors by monitoring their child's activities. They highlighted the necessity of involving parents as a part of the childhood obesity intervention program. Therefore, in addition to children's weight-lost, family involvement in weight-management programs helps them better handle their emotional and social difficulties.

The key finding of the evidence-based studies presented at the conference supported by the Agency for Healthcare Research and Quality, the American Academy of Paediatrics Institute for Healthy Childhood Weight, and The Obesity Society, indicated that despite the rising prevalence of childhood obesity, a family-centered therapeutic approach has shown promising outcomes over a period of 30 years (Wilfley et al., 2017). Likewise, evidence-based research indicates that family/caregiver support and dynamics have a significant impact on children's behavioral and emotional status when treating obesity by implementing strategies such as monitoring their children, setting limits, overcoming obstacles, managing conflicts, and adjusting the home climate (Andersson et al., 2016; Campbell-Voytal et al., 2018; Hampl et al., 2023; Schalkwijk et al., 2015). A recent umbrella review found that involving parents in both preventative and treatment interventions improved child BMI outcomes, particularly the effectiveness of diet and physical activity-focused programs to prevent and treat children living with overweight and obesity aged 3 to 12 years (Tomayko et al., 2021). They stated that a positive interaction between parental involvement in any setting (home, preschool, school, and hospital) and weight control in children under 18 years of age, particularly in interventions focused on parents-centered or parent-child treatments. This effectiveness was achieved by providing flexibility and intensity in the level of parents' participation in the intervention program such as parent-child interventions, family-based approaches, and solitary parental interventions (Tomayko et al., 2021). Similarly, Kruk et al. (2013) underline in their systematic study that the level of parenteral involvement in children's long-term participation in the weight management program has a beneficial influence on weight-related measures of obesity treatment success.

Additionally, family support is highly valued by adolescents, Jones et al.'s (2019) qualitative systematic study examined the perspectives of adolescents with overweight and obesity attending lifestyle obesity treatment interventions. The study places a strong emphasize on how supportive families can be to children throughout their weight-loss journeys by offering a positive environment for behavior change and making healthier choices. However, according to a recent different viewpoint (Bean et al., 2020), families have increasing difficulty in being consistent in treating and preventing childhood obesity as their children become older and their control over their weight-loss journey decreases. Since adolescents tend to seek more independence and autonomy, parent involvement in treating adolescent obesity varies and is inconsistent. There are differing opinions on the most effective level of parental involvement and the specific strategies that can improve obesity intervention outcomes. As highlighted in Hampl et al. (2023) and Bean et al. (2020) to optimize and effectiveness of the involvement of parents in treating adolescent obesity, clinical guidelines requiring further research and thorough reporting are required. Hence, it is clear that healthy lifestyle changes require assistance, and families play a crucial role in this regard. Without such support, there may be a risk of reverting to old habits and patterns, leading to a relapse into unhealthy behaviors.

Conclusion

Childhood obesity treatment is of essential importance due to its considerable health consequences and the possible development of fatal health conditions. Addressing childhood obesity is crucial for ensuring a healthy life expectancy, as it strongly predicts obesity in adulthood and its associated health and psychosocial implications.

HCPs are crucial in the diagnosis, prevention, treatment, and management of childhood obesity, requiring collaboration with the child and the family for effective results. Establishing a supportive relationship without stigmatization is essential, as weight stigma can negatively impact treatment outcomes and patient satisfaction. Continual connection with regular HCPs builds trust and enhances adherence to treatment programs. Childhood obesity not only involves physical health concerns but also severe psychological dysfunction, highlighting the need for a holistic approach that addresses self-esteem, overall well-being, and psychological distress. Treatment goals should extend beyond BMI reduction, focusing on improving overall quality of life and addressing psychosocial aspects for comprehensive and effective outcomes in the management of childhood obesity.

Additionally, research on childhood obesity highlighted the critical role of family-based intervention programs and family support in promoting healthy behaviors and successful weight management among children. Studies have identified key components such as monitoring, setting limits, overcoming obstacles, managing conflicts, and creating a supportive home environment as crucial for improving behavioral and emotional outcomes during obesity treatment. Including a parent component in interventions has shown positive effects on child weight outcomes, with parental involvement across various intervention types leading to better long-term participation and success in weight management programs. Additionally, involving families in obesity interventions enhances parents' skills in childcare and problem-solving, contributing to better management of the emotional and social difficulties faced by children with obesity. Adolescents value family support, but challenges arise with increasing independence, leading to inconsistent parental involvement in treatment. HCPs play a critical role, yet negative interactions can hinder the effectiveness of treatment. Therefore, establishing a constructive relationship with children and their families is essential to address childhood obesity comprehensively, focusing not only on weight loss but also on emotional well-being and supportive environments.

Despite the challenges in obesity management, evidence-based strategies and a multidisciplinary approach involving healthcare professionals and families are essential for effective prevention and treatment outcomes, emphasizing the need for long-term strategies and holistic interventions to address this global health concern.

References

Andersson, K., Shadloo, M., & Rudolfsson, G. (2016). Growing as a Human Being-Obese Adolescents' Experiences of the Changing Body. *Journal of Pediatric Nursing*, *31*(1), e53–e62. https://doi.org/10.1016/j.pedn.2015.07.007.

Bean, M., Caccavale, L., Adams, E., Burnette, C., Larose, G., Raynor, H. A., Wickham, E. P., & Mazzeo, S. E. (2020). Parent Involvement in Adolescent Obesity Treatment: A Systematic Review. *Pediatrics*, *146*(3). https://doi.org/10.1542/peds.2019-3315.

Blanco, M., Solano, S., Alcántara, A. I., Parks, M., Román, F. J., & Sepúlveda, A. R. (2020). Psychological well-being and weight-related teasing in childhood obesity: a case–control study. *Eating and Weight Disorders*, *25*(3), 751–759. https://doi.org/10.1007/s40519-019-00683-y.

Campbell-Voytal, K. D., Brogan Hartlieb, K., Cunningham, P. B., Jacques-Tiura, A. J., Ellis, D. A., Jen, K. L. C., & Naar-King, S. (2018). African American Adolescent-Caregiver Relationships in a Weight Loss Trial. *Journal of Child and Family Studies*, *27*(3), 835–842. https://doi.org/10.1007/s10826-017-0920-4.

Dietz, W. H. (1998). Health consequences of obesity in youth: childhood predictors of adult disease. *Pediatrics*, *101 (3 Pt*, 518–525.

Ells, L. J., Campbell, K., Lidstone, J., Kelly, S., Lang, R., & Summerbell, C. (2005). Prevention of childhood obesity. *Best Practice and Research: Clinical Endocrinology and Metabolism*, *19*(3 SPEC. ISS.), 441–454. https://doi.org/10.1016/j.beem.2005.04.008.

Faienza, M. F., Chiarito, M., Molina-Molina, E., Shanmugam, H., Lammert, F., Krawczyk, M., D'Amato, G., & Portincasa, P. (2020). Childhood obesity, cardiovascular and liver health: a growing epidemic with age. *World Journal of Pediatrics*, *16*(5), 438–445. https://doi.org/10.1007/s12519-020-00341-9.

Hampl, S. E., Hassink, S. G., Skinner, A. C., Armstrong, S. C., Barlow, S. E., Bolling, C. F., Edwards, C. A., Eneli, I., Hamre, R., Joseph, M. M., Lunsford, D., Mendonca, E., Michalsky, M. P., & Mirza, N. (2023). *Clinical Practice Guideline for the Evaluation and Treatment of Children and Adolescents With Obesity*. *151*(2).

Howie, E. K., McManus, A., Smith, K. L., Fenner, A. A., & Straker, L. M. (2016). Practical Lessons Learned from Adolescent and Parent Experiences Immediately and 12 Months following a Family-Based Healthy Lifestyle Intervention. *Childhood Obesity*, *12*(5), 401–409. https://doi.org/10.1089/chi.2016.0091.

Jones, H. M., Al-Khudairy, L., Melendez-Torres, G. J., & Oyebode, O. (2019). Viewpoints of adolescents with overweight and obesity attending lifestyle obesity treatment interventions: a qualitative systematic review. *Obesity Reviews*, *20*(1), 156–169. https://doi.org/10.1111/obr.12771.

Kansra, A. R., Lakkunarajah, S., & Jay, M. S. (2021). Childhood and Adolescent Obesity: A Review. *Frontiers in Pediatrics*, *8*(January), 1–16. https://doi.org/10.3389/fped.2020.581461.

Kaufman, T. K., Lynch, B. A., & Wilkinson, J. M. (2020). *Childhood Obesity : An Evidence-Based Approach to Family-Centered Advice and Support*. https://doi.org/10.1177/2150132720926279.

Kirk, S., Ramos Salas, X., Alberga, A., & Russell-Mayhew, S. (2020). *Canadian Adult Obesity Clinical Practice Guidelines: Reducing Weight Bias, Stigma and Discrimination in Obesity Management, Practice and Policy*. https://obesitycanada.ca/guidelines/weightbias.

Kruk, J. J. Van Der, Kortekaas, F., & Lucas, C. (2013). Obesity: a systematic review on parental involvement in long-term European childhood weight control interventions with a nutritional focus. *Obesity Reviews*, *5*, 745–760. https://doi.org/10.1111/obr.12046.

Lanigan, J., & Sauven, N. (2020). Treatment of childhood obesity : a multidisciplinary approach Key points. *Clinics in Integrated Care*, *3*, 100026.

Lowenstein, L. M., Perrin, E. M., Berry, D., Vu, M. B., Davis, L. P., Cai, J., Tzeng, J. P., & Ammerman, A. S. (2013). Childhood Obesity Prevention: Fathers' Reflections with Healthcare Providers. *Childhood Obesity*, *9*(2), 137–143. https://doi.org/10.1089/chi.2012.0111.

Marten, K. A., Allen, D. B., Rehm, J., Vanderwall, C., Peterson, A. L., & Carrel, A. L. (2023). A Multidisciplinary Approach to Pediatric Obesity Shows Improvement Postintervention. *Academic Pediatrics*, *23*(5), 947–951. https://doi.org/10.1016/j.acap.2022.10.019.

Milaneschi, Y., Simmons, W. K., Rossum, E. F. C. Van, & Pennix, B. W. (2019). Depression and obesity : evidence of shared biological mechanisms. *Molecular Psychiatry*, *24*, 18–33. https://doi.org/10.1038/s41380-018-0017-5.

Morinder, G., Biguet, G., Mattsson, E. V. A., Marcus, C., & Larsson, U. E. (2011). Adolescents ' perceptions of obesity treatment – an interview study. *Disability and Rehabilitation*, *33*(12), 999–1009. https://doi.org/
10.3109/09638288.2010.520800.

NICE. (2006). *NICE Clinical Guidelines, No. 43; Obesity: the prevention, identification, assessment and management of overweight and obesity in adults and children (CG 43)*. https://www.nice.org.uk/guidance/cg43/evidence/cg43-obesity-full-guideline-section-1-introduction-methods-and-recommendations2.

NICE. (2014). NICE Obesity: Identification, assessment and management. In *Nice* (Issue November 2014). https://www.nice.org.uk/guidance/cg189/resources/obesity-identification-assessment-and-management.

NICE. (2015). Obesity in children and young people: prevention and lifestyle weight management programmes (QS94). In *NICE National Institute for Health and Care Excellence* (Issue July 2015). Quality Standard 94.

NICE. (2017). NICE Pathways: Lifestyle weight management services for overweight or obese children and young people overview. In *NICE National Institute for Health and Care Excellence* (02.01.2017). https://pathways.nice.org.uk/pathways/lifestyle-weight-management-services-for-overweight-or-obese-children-and-young-people.

Pamungkas, R. A., & Chamroonsawasdi, K. (2019). Home-Based Interventions to Treat and Prevent Childhood Obesity: A Systematic Review and Meta-Analysis. *Behavioral Sciences*, *9*(38).

Phelan, S. M., Burgess, D. J., Yeazel, M. W., Hellerstedt, W. L., Griffin, J. M., & Ryn, M. Van. (2015). Impact of weight bias and stigma on quality of care and outcomes for patients with obesity. *Obesity Reviews*, *16*, 319–326. https://doi.org/10.1111/obr.12266.

Pont, S., R, P., SR, C., & Al., E. (2017). AAP SECTION ON OBESITY, THE OBESITY SOCIETY. Stigma Experienced by Children and Adolescents With Obesity. *Pediatrics*, *140*(6), e20173034.

Rankin, J., Matthews, L., Cobley, S., Han, A., Sanders, R., Wiltshire, H. D., & Baker, J. S. (2016). Psychological consequences of childhood obesity: psychiatric comorbidity and prevention. *Adolescent Health, Medicine and Therapeutics*, *7*, 125–146.

Reilly, J. J., Methven, E., Mcdowell, Z. C., Hacking, B., Alexander, D., Stewart, L., & Kelnar, C. J. H. (2003). Health consequences of obesity. *Archives of Disease in Childhood*, *88*, 748–752. https://doi.org/10.1136/adc.88.9.748.

Roberts, K. J., Binns, H. J., Vincent, C., & Koenig, M. D. (2021). A Scoping Review : Family and Child Perspectives of Clinic-Based Obesity Treatment. *Journal of Pediatric Nursing*, *57*, 56–72. https://doi.org/
10.1016/j.pedn.2020.10.025.

Russell-Mayhew, S., Mcvey, G., Bardick, A., & Ireland, A. (2012). Mental Health , Wellness , and Childhood Overweight / Obesity. *Journal OfObesity*. https://doi.org/10.1155/2012/281801.

Sagar, R., & Gupta, T. (2018). Psychological Aspects of Obesity in Children and Adolescents. *Indian Journal of Pediatrics*, *85*(7), 554–559. https://doi.org/10.1007/s12098-017-2539-2.

Sanderson, K., Patton, G. C., McKercher, C., Dwyer, T., & Venn, A. J. (2011). Overweight and obesity in childhood and risk of mental disorder: A 20-year cohort study. *Australian and New Zealand Journal of Psychiatry*, *45*(5), 384–392. https://doi.org/10.3109/00048674.2011.570309.

Schalkwijk, A. A. H., Bot, S. D. M., de Vries, L., Westerman, M. J., Nijpels, G., & Elders, P. J. M. (2015). Perspectives of obese children and their parents on lifestyle behavior change: A qualitative study. *International Journal of Behavioral Nutrition and Physical Activity*, *12*(102). https://doi.org/10.1186/s12966-015-0263-8.

Smith, J. D., Fu, E., Kobayashi, M. A., Yerges, A. L., Snethen, J. A., Carrel, A. L., Pan, H. J., Hung, L. J., Chen, C. Y., Li, J. C., Welsh, J. A., DiNallo, J. M., & Nix, R. L. (2020). Prevention and Management of Childhood Obesity and Its Psychological and Health Comorbidities and health comorbidities. *SAGE Open Nursing*, *58*(2), 1–11. https://doi.org/10.1146/annurev-clinpsy-100219-060201.

Stewart, L., Reilly, J. J., & Hughes, A. R. (2009). Evidence-based behavioral treatment of obesity in children and adolescents. *Child and Adolescent Psychiatric Clinics of North America*, *18*(1), 189–198.

Sutin, A. R., Stephan, Y., & Terracciano, A. (2015). Weight Discrimination and Risk of Mortality. *Psychological Science*, *26*(11), 1803–1811. https://doi.org/10.1177/0956797615601103.

Tiwari, A., & Balasundaram, P. (2021). Public Health Considerations Regarding Obesity. *StatPearls [Internet]*. https://www.ncbi.nlm.nih.gov/books/NBK572122/.

Tomayko, E. J., Tovar, A., Fitzgerald, N., Howe, C. L., Hingle, M. D., Murphy, M. P., Muzaffar, H., Going, S. B., & Hubbs-tait, L. (2021). Parent Involvement in Diet or Physical Activity Interventions to Treat or Prevent Childhood Obesity : An Umbrella Review. *Nutriens*, *13*, 1–26.

Viner, R. M., Kinra, S., Nicholls, D., Cole, T., Kessel, A., Christie, D., White, B., Croker, H., Wong, I. C. K., & Saxena, S. (2018). Burden of child and adolescent obesity on health services in England. *Archives of Disease in Childhood*, *103*(3), 247–254. https://doi.org/10.1136/archdischild-2017-313009.

WHO. (2016). Consideration of the evidence on childhood obesity for the Commission on Ending Childhood Obesity: report of the ad hoc working group on science and evidence for ending childhood obesity. In *Geneva, Switzerland.*

WHO. (2021). *Obesity*. https://www.who.int/news-room/facts-in-pictures/detail/6-facts-on-obesity.

WHO. (2024). *Obesity and overweight*. https://www.who.int/news-room/fact-sheets/detail/obesity-and-overweight#:~:text=Worldwide adult obesity has more,16%25 were living with obesity.

Wilfley, D. E., Staiano, A. E., Altman, M., Lindros, J., Lima, A., Hassink, S. G., & Dietz, W. H. (2017). Improving Access and Systems of Care for Evidence-Based Childhood Obesity Treatment : Conference Key Findings and Next Steps. *Obesity*, *25*, 16–29. https://doi.org/10.1002/oby.21712.

World Obesity Federation. (2022). *The Economic Impact of Overweight & Obesity in 2020 and 2060: 2nd Edition with Estimates for 161 Countries*.

Chapter 15

Evidence-Based Nursing Practices in Oncological Pediatric Palliative Care

Sümeyye Yıldız*, PhD
Department of Nursing, Nursing Faculty, Gazi University, Ankara, Türkiye

Abstract

Although childhood cancers have a lower prevalence than adult cancers, the number of children diagnosed with new cancers increases every year. Palliative care is a care approach that aims to reduce the suffering of infants, children, adolescents, and their families in case of life-threatening illness, alleviating pain and other symptoms, and improve the quality of life by treating psychological, social, and spiritual problems. Pediatric palliative care (PPC) aims to improve the quality of life for children and their families through the prevention and reduction of physical and psychosocial symptoms. Children with oncological problems and in the palliative care period may have physical and emotional symptoms due to their diseases. In this period, especially pain, nausea-vomiting, fatigue, anorexia, diarrhea, anemia, constipation, dyspnea, death anxiety, stomatitis, and spiritual distress symptoms appear intensely. Prevention and reduction of symptoms experienced by children and their families are very important in terms of improving their quality of life. It is very important to prefer evidence-based practices while providing symptom control. In palliative care, which requires a multidisciplinary team approach, it is also necessary to include evidence-based and a high level of evidence-based practices in the care process of the child and the family and to provide patient-centered care. Today, the importance of evidence-based practices is gradually increasing to reduce differences in practices and medical errors, to standardize care, and to improve the quality of health care. In this section, evidence-based nursing practices for physical and psychosocial symptoms experienced by children with oncological problems during the palliative care period are discussed. In the palliative care period, studies are needed to establish evidence-based practices in the care of patients by nurses.

Keywords: nausea and vomiting, pain, palliative care, psychosocial problems, oral mucositis

* Corresponding Author's Email: smyldz24@gmail.com.

In: Evidence-Based Care Practices in Pediatric Nursing
Editors: Feyza Küçük and Serap Özdemir
ISBN: 979-8-89530-304-7

Introduction

Childhood cancers are cancers seen in infants, children, and adolescents aged 0-18 years. An estimated 400 thousand infants, children, and adolescents aged 0-19 years are diagnosed with cancer each year (World Health Organization-WHO, 2021). Children and adolescents diagnosed with cancer or oncology due to symptoms die or need palliative care (National Cancer Institute, 2016). Only two-thirds of people with life-threatening diseases have access to palliative care. Only 14% of people in need of palliative care worldwide can access this care (WHO, 2020). Of the 20.4 million individuals in need of palliative care, 25% are aged 15-50 years and 6% are aged 0-14 years (Connor and Sepulveda, 2014). Palliative care is important to meet the physical, psychosocial, and spiritual needs of individuals who are at the end of life or diagnosed with life-threatening diseases and to improve their quality of life (Danış and Özhan, 2019).

Palliative care; "In patients and families who face problems arising from life-threatening diseases; pain and other problems, early diagnosis and perfect evaluation of pain and other problems, meeting physical, psychosocial, and spiritual needs, preventing and alleviating suffering, and is an approach that includes practices aimed at improving quality of life." (WHO, 2020). Palliative care is both a philosophy of care and a highly structured care-giving system. Palliative care is a care process that starts from the diagnosis of a life-threatening disease and continues during active treatment and the end of life. Various care models have been developed to express this process. In all care models, it is stated that the patient will not always lose his/her life at the end of palliative care and that the rehabilitation process of the patient comes into play in the continuity of life (Demir, 2016; Hawley, 2014). Pediatric palliative care, which has the same purpose, philosophy, and components as general palliative care, is different from adult palliative care due to the differences in children's perceptions, reactions, and communication according to age, the lack of self-expression skills of young age groups, and difficulties in adjusting drug doses (American Academy of Pediatrics-AAP, 2013; Shapiro et al., 2017).

The main aim of pediatric palliative care (PPC) is to relieve pain in the child and the family, manage the disease process well, prevent physical and psychosocial symptoms, and improve the quality of life of children and their families (Postier et al., 2014). Pediatric palliative care addresses the physical, psychosocial, and spiritual needs of the child and family from the moment of diagnosis. It includes determining and meeting the needs of the child in the diagnosis and treatment process, symptom management, end-of-life, and mourning process (Yıldız, 2022).

Children with oncological problems and in the palliative period may have physical and psychosocial symptoms due to their illness. In this period, especially pain, oral mucositis, nausea-vomiting, fatigue, anxiety, depression, and spiritual distress symptoms appear intensely (Craig et al., 2015). The main aim of all interventions in symptom management should be to reduce symptoms and improve the quality of life of the child and family (Mandac and Battista, 2014). The appropriate management of symptoms seen in children and the interventions to be made have an important place in terms of improving the quality of care and quality of life of the child (Vollenbroich et al., 2016).

Evidence-based practices ensure that the nursing care provided to children followed up with a diagnosis of cancer in the clinical setting is reliable, effective, and appropriate for the purpose, and that the development of undesirable outcomes and patient victimization is prevented. Therefore, pediatric oncology/hematology nurses should include evidence-based practices in their interventions (Çolaklar, 2017). The care needs of the children should be determined from the moment of diagnosis. It is thought that providing effective symptom management with the integration of palliative care philosophy into planned care will significantly affect the quality of life of children and increase patient satisfaction. Conducting evidence-based practices in the management of pain, oral mucositis, nausea-vomiting, psychosocial symptoms that frequently occur during the palliative care period, and alleviating symptoms are effective in improving the quality of life of children.

Research

Pain

Pain is one of the most common symptoms expressed by children with a cancer diagnosis and who are receiving palliative care (Kuhlen et al., 2016). The majority of children in the terminal period (89%) experience the most pain in the last periods of their lives (Jibb et al., 2017). Lifelong activities to relieve pain and anxiety are a fundamental aspect of palliative care (Vollenbroich et al., 2016). The important part of the pain experienced by children is to ensure that pain management is carried out appropriately (Törüner and Büyükgönenç, 2017). Effective pain management in children includes various pharmacological and non-pharmacological applications and requires cooperation between health team members.

Non-pharmacological methods are effective both alone and in combination with pharmacological methods for effective pain management and reduction of pain intensity. Between 31-84% of children and adolescents diagnosed with cancer use non-pharmacological methods to reduce pain. Non-pharmacological methods reduce the cost of treatment, the rate of analgesic use, and improve the quality of life of the child and family (Downing et al., 2015).

Many evidence-based studies are carried out to provide pain management and improve the quality of life of children and adolescents followed up with a diagnosis of cancer. Among the physical pain relief methods in children; technology-based applications, aromatherapy, massage, therapeutic touch, music, and animal therapies were included.

Technology-Based Applications

Studies have been conducted to evaluate the effectiveness of virtual reality in pain management in children and adolescents receiving cancer treatment. In studies conducted with pediatric oncology randomized controlled method, it was reported that the application of virtual reality was effective in reducing the pain of children and adolescents (Hundert et al., 2021; Semerci et al., 2021; Tennant et al., 2020). A mobile application called Pain Squad+ was developed to reduce pain and improve the quality of life in adolescents diagnosed with cancer. As a result of a 28-day study with 40 adolescents, it was reported that the application developed was moderately effective in pain management (Jibb et al., 2017). In a systematic review conducted to determine the effectiveness of distraction as a procedural pain management technique in pediatric oncology patients, it was reported that distraction was effective in reducing pain during the procedure (Bukola et al., 2017).

Aromatherapy

In a randomized controlled study conducted with adolescents receiving palliative care, it was reported that the pain of adolescents receiving the application of aromatherapy (lavender oil) decreased (Weaver et al., 2020). Mistletoe has been found to have an analgesic effect in children and to be effective in alleviating pain and other symptoms (Schutzeet al., 2016).

Massage and Therapeutic Touch

It was found that the 4-week massage practice carried out to improve the quality of life of adolescents diagnosed with cancer during the palliative care period significantly reduced the pain of children and significantly improved their quality of life (Genik et al., 2020; Weekly et al., 2019). Furthermore, it was determined that therapeutic touch reduces pain, stress, and fatigue (Won et al., 2013). In palliative care, reiki is effective in reducing anxiety, pain, heart, and respiratory rate (Thrane et al., 2017). Thrane et al. (2021) stated that two 24-minute sessions of Reiki application conducted by Thrane et al. (2021) in children aged 7-16 years receiving palliative care were effective in reducing pain of children (Thrane et al., 2021).

Other Techniques

In palliative care, animal-assisted therapies are used to improve children's coping and reduce pain and suffering. It has been found that interacting with animals increases hormones such as oxytocin, dopamine, serotonin, and prolactin while reducing stress hormone levels and creating a sense of peace (Gilmer et al., 2016). A mindfulness-based stress reduction program combined with music therapy applied to adolescents with osteosarcoma is important in reducing the pain of children (Liu et al., 2019). In 2005 and 2016, in the statistical review on pediatric palliative care and pain management, it was stated that patient and family experience, pain assessment, pharmacological pain management, and non-pharmacological pain management are important in pain management, and their use should increase (Thomas et al., 2018).

Oral Mucositis

Oral mucositis (OM) is an inflammatory reaction that occurs in the mucosa of children diagnosed with cancer, especially after chemotherapy treatment or head and neck radiation therapy. The rate of mucositis in children receiving chemotherapy varies between 20% and 80.4% (de Farias et al., 2021), and the incidence of oral mucositis in children under 12 years of age is more than 90% (Velten et al., 2017). The effective management of oral mucositis in children receiving chemotherapy is important in terms of nutrition and quality of life. Physical therapies and natural products are used for the management of oral mucositis, and many evidence-based studies have been conducted (Miranda-Silva et al., 2020).

Physical Therapies

Cryotherapy

Cryotherapy, ice cubes applied to the oral cavity lead to vasoconstriction of the superficial blood vessels, thereby reduce damage to the oral mucosa. Compared plain ice cubes and flavored (honey and basil) ice cubes in the development of oral mucositis in a group of pediatric patients, and found that flavored ice cubes were more effective in preventing the development of oral mucositis (Mishra and Nayak). The Joanna Briggs Institute (JBI) recommends ice cube application for 30 minutes during chemotherapy treatment for the prevention of oral mucositis (Marin, 2019). Due to insufficient evidence in the pediatric population, it is currently not possible to make a strong recommendation (Sung et al., 2017).

Photobiomodulation

Photobiomodulation, which applies low-level laser and light therapy to rapidly growing areas to stimulate biological responses, is used in Grade 2 and 3 (Quinn et al., 2020). It has been reported that photobiomodulation applied inside and outside the mouth is applicable to pediatric hematology-oncology patients and is perfectly tolerated by young children. It has also been reported to relieve pain associated with oral mucositis, as well as oral hygiene and analgesic treatment (Noirrit-Esclassan et al., 2019). The MASCC/ISOO guidelines for children do not clearly state the definitive evidence for the use of photobiomodulation in children (Miranda et al., 2020).

Cryoprotective Agents

Glutamine

Glutamine acts as an antioxidant in increasing cell proliferation and growth functions of gastrointestinal cells, regulating immunity and protein synthesis (Ramezani et al., 2019). Intravenous glutamine administration reduces the rate of oral mucositis in children; it is reported that Grade 3 and 4 oral mucositis is not seen and there are no side effects (Chang et al., 2017). In the MASCC/ISOO guideline for children, it was stated that oral glutamine can be effective in reducing severe oral mucositis and mucositis-related pain in children with stem cell transplantation, and parenteral glutamine administration did not have any oral mucositis effect (Miranda-Silva et al., 2020).

Vitamin E

Vitamin E, which has antioxidant properties, prevents mucositis by protecting the cell membrane. Vitamin E is reported to be effective in the improvement of all stages of oral mucositis (Khurana et al., 2013). It is stated that vitamin E is effective in reducing the severity of oral mucositis in children receiving chemotherapy and radiotherapy (Chaitanya et al., 2017). It is stated that vitamin E used in the treatment of oral mucositis is more effective than honey and chlorhexidine (Konuk et al., 2019).

Natural Products

Honey

Honey, which has antioxidant properties and anti-inflammatory effects, has a wide variety of structures is an effective factor in not reaching the final result of the studies. In honey with the same variety, low-grade mucositis, less pain, and increased quality of life are observed (Münstedt et al., 2019). In a study conducted on children followed up with a diagnosis of cancer; it was reported that the number of days of oral mucositis follow-up was less and the mucositis recovery time was shorter in children with honey application (Bulut and Tüfekçi, 2016; Singh et al., 2019).

Aloe-vera

An experimental study was conducted to evaluate the use of aloe-vera in the prevention of chemotherapy-related oral mucositis in children with acute lymphoblastic leukemia. A statistically significant difference was found between the group administered with 70% aloe-vera solution and the group administered with sodium bicarbonate solution, and oral mucositis was less observed in the experimental group. Furthermore, it was determined that the onset of oral mucositis in children treated with sodium bicarbonate was higher than in children in the aloe-vera group (Alkhouli et al., 2021).

Nausea and Vomiting

Nausea and vomiting are one of the most common symptoms experienced by children in the treatment of childhood cancers (Sherani et al., 2019). Chemotherapy-induced nausea and vomiting are one of the most common symptoms in children with a prevalence of over 60% and require a multidisciplinary approach. Nausea and vomiting seen in children followed up with a diagnosis of cancer can negatively affect the child's daily life activities and quality of life (Vol et al., 2016). Nanopharmacological methods that are frequently preferred to cope with nausea and vomiting in children followed up with a diagnosis of cancer include acupuncture/acupressure, aromatherapy, massage, muscle relaxation, music, and additional methods.

Acupuncture/Acupressure

Traditional Chinese medicine techniques that aim to improve health by regulating the basal energy by stimulating the acupuncture point. In the systematic review, it was reported that the use of acupuncture/acupressure methods in combination with antiemetics decreased the severity of nausea and vomiting in children (Mckeon et al., 2013). Children's Oncology Group- COG supportive care guidelines state that "acupuncture and acupressure can be effective in children receiving antineoplastic agents" to reduce chemotherapy-induced nausea/vomiting and the quality of evidence is classified as "very low" (Children's Oncology Group, 2020).

Massage

Massage, which is applied as a kind of complementary/alternative medicine, can be applied to different areas with various techniques such as Swedish massage with olive oil, effleurage, petrissage, and friction. Body massage in children has been reported to be effective in reducing nausea and vomiting (Shin et al., 2016). Positive results were obtained in reducing nausea-vomiting in children receiving chemotherapy when reflexology, one of the massage therapy methods, was applied together with aromatherapy (Zorba and Özdemir, 2018).

Aromatherapy

Aromatherapy is the inhalation of essential oils or fragrances for therapeutic or medical purposes. Studies have been conducted indicating that aromatherapy is effective in reducing nausea and vomiting. In a systematic review, ginger and peppermint oils were reported to have antiemetic and antispasmodic effects on the stomach wall and colon (Evans et al, 2018; Momani and Berry, 2017).

Progressive Muscle Relaxation

Children are allowed muscle relaxation in response to triggers of nausea and vomiting, including chemotherapy. Progressive relaxation exercises applied after chemotherapy in children with leukemia diagnosis were effective in reducing nausea and vomiting (Amer et al., 2020).

Music

Music therapy for children with pediatric oncology patients can be useful in the management of nausea and vomiting by providing relaxation and distraction of attention. In studies, music played to children receiving cancer treatment before and after chemotherapy reduced nausea complaints of children (Sickel et al., 2018).

Psychosocial Symptoms

Children with cancer are trying to cope with negative situations such as repeated hospitalizations, invasive interventions, isolation, physical side effects, and as a result, they experience psychosocial problems (Garcia et al., 2017; Kupst and Patenaude, 2016). The fact that children and adolescents who are followed up with a diagnosis of cancer are in the palliative care period, the loss of function due to their disease, and the developing mourning process, the intensive and painful treatments they receive are very effective in the development of problems such as anxiety and depression. Various non-medical methods are used in the management of these problems that develop in children during the palliative care process (Çıtak and Törüner, 2018).

Psychosocial Programs

In psychosocial intervention programs applied to children with cancer diagnosis based on the family-centered care model, children's anxiety levels decrease, and their quality of life and social adaptation capacity increase (Lyon et al., 2014; Wu et al., 2014). Psychosocial programs including physical activity, relaxation, stretching, and deep breathing exercises increase the quality of life of children diagnosed with cancer (van DijkLokkart et al., 2016). At the end of the cognitive behavioral therapy-CBT-based intervention program conducted with adolescents with a cancer diagnosis, anxiety, stress, and depression levels of adolescents decreased significantly (Zhang et al., 2019). A CBT game including activities such as relaxation training, positive thought development, and recognition of emotions was applied to children with leukemia and the anxiety level of children decreased (Mehrara et al., 2019). At the end of the programs including guided imagery, deep breathing exercises, and relaxation techniques for children with a cancer diagnosis, children's anxiety levels decreased (Aney, 2020; Shockey et al., 2013).

Therapeutic play methods used in children have reduced anxiety and depression in children and strengthened their coping (Chari et al., 2013; Çıtak and Törüner, 2018). Music, instrument playing, and drawing methods used in children also alleviate the coping with disease, anxiety, and depression (Ångström-Brännström and Norberg, 2014). Painting therapies have strengthened coping, reduced symptoms, and improved the quality of life of children (Aguilar, 2017). In a systematic review conducted to determine the benefit of psychosocial interventions in pediatric oncology, it was found that psychosocial interventions were effective in reducing the problems experienced by children (Melesse et al., 2022).

Technology-Based Psychosocial Programs

The use of technology-based applications is becoming widespread in solving psychosocial problems experienced by children with a diagnosis of cancer receiving palliative care. Evidence-based interventions are needed to reduce the psychosocial effects of cancer and increase the use of technology-based interventions in children. E-health applications, virtual reality (VR), a social robot and M-health applications, music therapy, and mobile application-based psychosocial intervention programs have a significant effect on reducing children's anxiety (Alemi et al., 2016; Gerçeker et al., 2021; Hamedi et al., 2020; Wong et al., 2021; Zhang et al., 2019). Technology-based psychosocial interventions based on E-health, virtual reality, and M-health, which were carried out to alleviate the depression experienced by children, alleviated depression (Alemi et al., 2016; Hamedi et al., 2020; Zhang et al., 2019).

There are technology-based psychosocial interventions carried out for a high quality of life, which is among the most important goals of palliative care. Digital stories, video game, and interactive CD-ROM content psychosocial interventions are beneficial in improving the quality of life of children (Akard et al., 2015; Fazelniya et al., 2017). In a meta-analysis examining the effectiveness of technology-based psychosocial interventions applied to children, adolescents, and young adults receiving cancer treatment, psychosocial interventions are moderately effective in reducing anger, anxiety, and depression (Ozturk and Toruner, 2022). In a meta-analysis study investigating the effect of virtual reality interventions on relieving pain and anxiety in children and adolescents undergoing cancer treatment, virtual reality applications were moderately effective in reducing pain and anxiety in pediatric oncology (Ozturk and Toruner, 2023).

Conclusion

Pediatric palliative care is an important care approach that addresses children holistically in the presence of a life-threatening disease. Reducing the problems experienced by children and adolescents from the moment of diagnosis and improving the quality of life are very important in improving the quality of treatment and care. Many different methods are used to reduce the physical and psychosocial problems experienced by children and adolescents who are followed up with a diagnosis of cancer and receive palliative care. Experimental studies with a high level of evidence are needed to perform and maintain effective symptom management. Health professionals working with children should know the basic principles of palliative care, and their application may play a critical role in terms of quality of care. They should be able to assess and manage the complex needs of children with a chronic or life-threatening illness and their parents, symptom control, and support the family throughout the illness and grief process. Thus, they will be able to contribute to improving the quality of life of this group with special needs. Health professionals working with children and families with palliative care needs can have the chance to develop both individually and professionally by being with children and families facing death and sharing their life stories.

References

Aguilar B. A. (2017). The Efficacy of Art Therapy in Pediatric Oncology Patients: An Integrative Literature Review. *Journal of Pediatric Nursing*, *36*, 173–178. https://doi.org/10.1016/j.pedn.2017.06.015.

Akard, T. F., Dietrich, M. S., Friedman, D. L., Hinds, P. S., Given, B., Wray, S., & Gilmer, M. J. (2015). Digital storytelling: an innovative legacy-making intervention for children with cancer. *Pediatric Blood & Cancer*, *62*(4), 658–665. https://doi.org/10.1002/pbc.25337.

Alkhouli, M., Laflouf, M., & Alhaddad, M. (2021). Efficacy of Aloe-Vera Use for Prevention of Chemotherapy-Induced Oral Mucositis in Children with Acute Lymphoblastic Leukemia: A

Randomized Controlled Clinical Trial. *Comprehensive Child and Adolescent Nursing*, *44*(1), 49–62. https://doi.org/10.1080/24694193.2020.1727065.

Amer, R. S. R. M., Hamad, M. M., and El-Sayed, RESH. (2020). The effect of applying a progressive muscle relaxation technique on nausea and vomiting ınduced by chemotherapy among leukemic children. *American Journal of Nursing*, *8*(3), 331-343.

American Academy of Pediatrics (AAP) Commıttee On Bıoethıcs. Informed Consent in Decision-Making in Pediatric Practice. Pediatrics(2016). URL: https://pediatrics.aappublications.org/content/pediatrics/138/2/e20161484.full.pdf. (Erişim tarihi 21.01.2024).

Ångström-Brännström, C., & Norberg, A. (2014). Children undergoing cancer treatment describe their experiences of comfort in interviews and drawings. *Journal of Pediatric Oncology Nursing*, *31*(3), 135-146.

Bukola, I. M., & Paula, D. (2017). The Effectiveness of Distraction as Procedural Pain Management Technique in Pediatric Oncology Patients: A Meta-analysis and Systematic Review. *Journal of Pain and Symptom Management, 54*(4), 589–600.e1. https://doi.org/10.1016/j.jpainsymman.2017.07.006.

Bulut, H., & Güdücü Tüfekci, F. (2016). Honey prevents oral mocositis in children undergoing chemotherapy: A quasi-experimental study with a control group. *Complementary Therapies in Medicine, 29*, 132–140. https://doi.org/10.1016/j.ctim.2016.09.018.

Chaitanya, N. C., Muthukrishnan, A., Babu, D. B. G., Kumari, C. S., Lakshmi, M. A., Palat, G., & Alam, K. S. (2017). Role of Vitamin E and Vitamin A in Oral Mucositis Induced by Cancer Chemo/Radiotherapy-A Meta-analysis. *Journal of Clinical and Diagnostic Research, 11*(5), ZE06–ZE09. https://doi.org/10.7860/JCDR/2017/26845.9905.

Chang, Y. H., Yu, M. S., Wu, K. H., Hsu, M. C., Chiou, Y. H., Wu, H. P., Peng, C. T., & Chao, Y. H. (2017). Effectiveness of Parenteral Glutamine on Methotrexate-induced Oral Mucositis in Children with Acute Lymphoblastic Leukemia. *Nutrition and Cancer, 69*(5), 746–751. https://doi.org/10.1080/01635581.2017.1324995.

Children's Oncology Group (2020). Guidelines on Chemotherapy-induced Nausea and Vomiting in Pediatric Cancer Patients. *COG Supportive Care Endorsed Guidelines* chrome-extension://efaidnbmnnnibpcajpcglclefindmkaj/https://childrensoncologygroup.org/docs/default-source/pdf/COG_SC_CINV_Guidelines_Document.pdf.

Connor SR, Sepulveda Bermedo MC(2014). Global Atlas of Palliative Care at the End of Life. URL: https://www.who.int/nmh/Global_Atlas_of_Palliative_Care.pdf. (Erişim tarihi: 01.03.2024).

Craig, F., Henderson, E. M., & Bluebond-Langner, M. (2015). Management of respiratory symptoms in paediatric palliative care. *Current Opinion in Supportive and Palliative Care*, *9*(3), 217–226. https://doi.org/10.1097/SPC.0000000000000154.

Çolaklar, H. (2017). Evidence-based information services: An example of a literature review. *Journal of Balkan Libraries Union, 5*(1), 11-20.

Danış, M. Z., & Özhan, E.(2019). Sağlık hizmetlerinde palyatif bakım, kanser ve sosyal destek: bir vaka örneğinde güçlendirme yaklaşımının uygulanması. *Kesit Akademi Dergisi, 5(*18), 305-320.

de Farias Gabriel, A., Silveira, F. M., Curra, M., Schuch, L. F., Wagner, V. P., Martins, M. A. T., da Silveira Matte, U., Siebert, M., Botton, M. R., Brunetto, A. T., Gregianin, L. J., & Martins, M. D. (2022). Risk factors associated with the development of oral mucositis in pediatric oncology patients: Systematic review and meta-analysis. *Oral diseases, 28*(4), 1068–1084. https://doi.org/10.1111/odi.13863.

Demir M. (2016). Palliative Care Ethics. *Turkish J Med Surg Intensive Care. 151*, *7*(2):62–6.

Downing, J., Jassal, S. S., Mathews, L., Brits, H., & Friedrichsdorf, S. J. (2015). Pediatric pain management in palliative care. *Pain Management*, *5(*1), 23–35. https://doi.org/10.2217/pmt.14.45.

Evans, A., Malvar, J., Garretson, C., Pedroja Kolovos, E., & Baron Nelson, M. (2018). The Use of Aromatherapy to Reduce Chemotherapy-Induced Nausea in Children With Cancer: A Randomized, Double-Blind, Placebo-Controlled Trial. *Journal of Pediatric Oncology Nursing: Official Journal of the Association of Pediatric Oncology Nurses*, *35*(6), 392–398. https://doi.org/10.1177/1043454218782133.

Fazelniya, Z., Najafi, M., Moafi, A., & Talakoub, S. (2017). The Impact of an Interactive Computer Game on the Quality of Life of Children Undergoing Chemotherapy. *Iranian Journal of Nursing and Midwifery Research, 22*(6), 431–435. https://doi.org/10.4103/ijnmr.IJNMR_215_15.

Garcia, E., Wijesekera, K., & Lester, P. (2017). A family-centered preventive intervention within pediatric oncology: Adapting the FOCUS intervention for Latino youth and their families. *Journal of Educational and Psychological Consultation, 27*(3), 393-410.

Genik, L. M., McMurtry, C. M., Marshall, S., Rapoport, A., & Stinson, J. (2020). Massage therapy for symptom reduction and improved quality of life in children with cancer in palliative care: A pilot study. *Complementary Therapies in Medicine, 48,* 102263. https://doi.org/10.1016/j.ctim.2019.102263.

Gerçeker, G. Ö., Bektaş, M., Aydınok, Y., Ören, H., Ellidokuz, H., & Olgun, N. (2021). The effect of virtual reality on pain, fear, and anxiety during access of a port with huber needle in pediatric hematology-oncology patients: Randomized controlled trial. *European Journal of Oncology Nursing: The Official Journal of European Oncology Nursing Society, 50,* 101886. https://doi.org/10.1016/j.ejon.2020.101886.

Gilmer, M. J., Baudino, M. N., Tielsch Goddard, A., Vickers, D. C., & Akard, T. F. (2016). Animal-Assisted Therapy in Pediatric Palliative Care. *The Nursing Clinics of North America, 51*(3), 381–395. https://doi.org/10.1016/j.cnur.2016.05.007.

Hamedi, V., Hamid, N., Beshlideh, K., Marashi, S. A., & Shabani, S. E. H. S. (2020). Effectiveness of conventional cognitive-behavioral therapy and its computerized version on reduction in pain intensity, depression, anger, and anxiety in children with cancer: A randomized, controlled trial. *Iranian Journal of Psychiatry and Behavioral Sciences, 14*(4), e83110.

Hawley P. H. (2014). The bow tie model of 21st century palliative care. *Journal of Pain and Symptom Management, 47*(1), 2–5. https://doi.org/10.1016/j.jpainsymman.2013.10.009.

He, M., Zhang, B., Shen, N., Wu, N., & Sun, J. (2018). A systematic review and meta-analysis of the effect of low-level laser therapy (LLLT) on chemotherapy-induced oral mucositis in pediatric and young patients. *European Journal of Pediatrics, 177*(1), 7–17. https://doi.org/10.1007/s00431-017-3043-4.

Hundert, A. S., Birnie, K. A., Abla, O., Positano, K., Cassiani, C., Lloyd, S., Tiessen, P. H., Lalloo, C., Jibb, L. A., & Stinson, J. (2021). A Pilot Randomized Controlled Trial of Virtual Reality Distraction to Reduce Procedural Pain During Subcutaneous Port Access in Children and Adolescents With Cancer. *The Clinical Journal of Pain, 38*(3), 189–196. https://doi.org/10.1097/AJP.0000000000001017.

Jibb, L. A., Stevens, B. J., Nathan, P. C., Seto, E., Cafazzo, J. A., Johnston, D. L., Hum, V., & Stinson, J. N. (2017). Implementation and preliminary effectiveness of a real-time pain management smartphone app for adolescents with cancer: A multicenter pilot clinical study. *Pediatric Blood & Cancer, 64*(10), 10.1002/pbc.26554. https://doi.org/10.1002/pbc.26554.

Khurana, H., Pandey, R. K., Saksena, A. K., & Kumar, A. (2013). An evaluation of Vitamin E and Pycnogenol in children suffering from oral mucositis during cancer chemotherapy. *Oral Diseases, 19*(5), 456–464. https://doi.org/10.1111/odi.12024.

Konuk Sener, D., Aydin, M., Cangur, S., & Guven, E. (2019). The Effect of Oral Care with Chlorhexidine, Vitamin E and Honey on Mucositis in Pediatric Intensive Care Patients: A Randomized Controlled Trial. *Journal of Pediatric Nursing, 45*, e95–e101. https://doi.org/10.1016/j.pedn.2019.02.001.

Kupst, M. J., & Patenaude, A. F. (2016). Coping and adaptation in pediatric cancer: Current perspectives. *Pediatric Psychosocial Oncology: Textbook for Multidisciplinary Care,* 67-79.

Liu, H., Gao, X., & Hou, Y. (2019). Effects of mindfulness-based stress reduction combined with music therapy on pain, anxiety, and sleep quality in patients with osteosarcoma. *Revista brasileira de psiquiatria (Sao Paulo, Brazil: 1999), 41*(6), 540–545. https://doi.org/10.1590/1516-4446-2018-0346.

Lyon, M. E., Jacobs, S., Briggs, L., Cheng, Y. I., & Wang, J. (2014). A longitudinal, randomized, controlled trial of advance care planning for teens with cancer: anxiety, depression, quality of life, advance directives, spirituality. *The Journal of Adolescent Health: Official Publication of the Society for Adolescent Medicine, 54*(6), 710–717. https://doi.org/10.1016/j.jadohealth.2013.10.206.

Mandac, C., & Battista, V. (2014). Contributions of palliative care to pediatric patient care. *Seminars in Oncology Nursing, 30*(4), 212–226. https://doi.org/10.1016/j.soncn.2014.08.003.

Marin, T. (2019). Oral mucositis: Cryotherapy, JBI Evidence Summary, p. 1-2.

McKeon, C., Smith, C. A., Hardy, J., & Chang, E. (2013). Acupuncture and acupressure for chemotherapy-induced nausea and vomiting: a systematic review. *Australian Journal of Acupuncture and Chinese Medicine, 8*(1), 2-27.

Mehrara, M., Ghaffari, Z., Ghezelghabr, R. M., Ghavasi, F., & Fatemizadeh, M. (2018). The Effectiveness of Cognitive-Behavioral Play Therapy on Pain Tolerance and Trait-State Anxiety Among Children with leukemia cancer in Isfahan City. *International Journal of Applied Behavioral Sciences, 5*(2), 22-27.

Melesse, T. G., Chau, J. P. C., & Nan, M. A. (2022). Effectiveness of psychosocial interventions on health outcomes of children with cancer: A systematic review of randomised controlled trials. *European Journal of Cancer Care, 31*(6), e13695. https://doi.org/10.1111/ecc.13695.

Miranda-Silva, W., Gomes-Silva, W., Zadik, Y., Yarom, N., Al-Azri, A. R., Hong, C. H. L., Ariyawardana, A., Saunders, D. P., Correa, M. E., Arany, P. R., Bowen, J., Cheng, K. K. F., Tissing, W. J. E., Bossi, P., Elad, S., & Mucositis Study Group of the Multinational Association of Supportive Care in Cancer / International Society for Oral Oncology (MASCC/ISOO) (2021). MASCC/ISOO clinical practice guidelines for the management of mucositis: sub-analysis of current interventions for the management of oral mucositis in pediatric cancer patients. *Supportive Care in Cancer: Official Journal of the Multinational Association of Supportive Care in Cancer, 29*(7), 3539–3562. https://doi.org/10.1007/s00520-020-05803-4.

Mishra, L. & Nayak, G. (2017). Effect of flavoured ice chips in reduction of oral mucositis among children receiving chemotherapy. *International Journal of Pharmaceutical Sciences Review and Research, 43*(107), 25-28.

Momani, T. G., & Berry, D. L. (2017). Integrative Therapeutic Approaches for the Management and Control of Nausea in Children Undergoing Cancer Treatment: A Systematic Review of Literature. *Journal of Pediatric Oncology Nursing: Official Journal of the Association of Pediatric Oncology Nurses, 34*(3), 173–184. https://doi.org/10.1177/1043454216688638.

Noirrit-Esclassan, E., Valera, M. C., Vignes, E., Munzer, C., Bonal, S., Daries, M., Vaysse, F., Puiseux, C., Castex, M. P., Boulanger, C., & Pasquet, M. (2019). Photobiomodulation with a combination of two wavelengths in the treatment of oral mucositis in children: The PEDIALASE feasibility study. *Archives de pediatrie: organe officiel de la Societe francaise de pediatrie, 26*(5), 268–274. https://doi.org/10.1016/
j.arcped.2019.05.012.

Ozturk, C. S., & Toruner, E. K. (2022). Effectiveness of technology-based psychosocial interventions for child, adolescents and young adults undergoing cancer treatment: A meta-analysis of randomised controlled trials. *European Journal of Cancer Care, 31*(1), e13515. https://doi.org/10.1111/ecc.13515.

Ozturk, C. S., & Toruner, E. K. (2023). Effectiveness of Virtual Reality in Anxiety and Pain Management in Children and Adolescents Receiving Cancer Treatment: A Systematic Review and Meta-analysis of Randomized Controlled Trials. *Journal of Medical Systems, 47*(1), 103. https://doi.org/10.1007/s10916-023-01995-4.

Postier, A., Chrastek, J., Nugent, S., Osenga, K., & Friedrichsdorf, S. J. (2014). Exposure to home-based pediatric palliative and hospice care and its impact on hospital and emergency care charges at a single institution. *Journal of palliative medicine, 17*(2), 183–188. https://doi.org/10.1089/jpm.2013.0287.

Quinn, A., Clump, D., Holeva, K., & Heron, D. The Use of Photobiomodulation for Oral Mucositis in Patients Receiving Chemoradiotherapy for Head and Neck Cancer: A University of Pittsburgh Cancer Center Experience. *Oralhealth* (03/03/2020).

Ramezani Ahmadi, A., Rayyani, E., Bahreini, M., & Mansoori, A. (2019). The effect of glutamine supplementation on athletic performance, body composition, and immune function: A systematic review and a meta-analysis of clinical trials. *Clinical Nutrition (Edinburgh, Scotland), 38*(3), 1076–1091. https://doi.org/10.1016/j.clnu.2018.05.001.

Schütze, T., Längler, A., Zuzak, T. J., Schmidt, P., & Zernikow, B. (2016). Use of complementary and alternative medicine by pediatric oncology patients during palliative care. *Supportive Care in Cancer : Official Journal of the Multinational Association of Supportive Care in Cancer, 24*(7), 2869–2875. https://doi.org/10.1007/s00520-016-3097-2.

Semerci, R., Akgün Kostak, M., Eren, T., & Avci, G. (2021). Effects of Virtual Reality on Pain During Venous Port Access in Pediatric Oncology Patients: A Randomized Controlled Study. *Journal of Pediatric Oncology nursing: Official Journal of the Association of Pediatric Oncology Nurses, 38*(2), 142–151. https://doi.org/10.1177/1043454220975702.

Shapiro, M. C., Henderson, C. M., Hutton, N., & Boss, R. D. (2017). Defining Pediatric Chronic Critical Illness for Clinical Care, Research, and Policy. *Hospital Pediatrics, 7*(4), 236–244. https://doi.org/10.1542/hpeds.2016-0107.

Sherani, F., Boston, C., & Mba, N. (2019). Latest Update on Prevention of Acute Chemotherapy-Induced Nausea and Vomiting in Pediatric Cancer Patients. *Current Oncology Reports, 21*(10), 89. https://doi.org/10.1007/s11912-019-0840-0.

Sickel, K., Barrett, M., & Siegenthaler, A. (2018). The effect of complementary therapies on the treatment of chemotherapeutic induced nausea and vomiting: A systematic review. *Honors Research Projects*. 706.

Singh, R., Sharma, S., Kaur, S., Medhi, B., Trehan, A., & Bijarania, S. K. (2019). Effectiveness of Topical Application of Honey on Oral Mucosa of Children for the Management of Oral Mucositis Associated with Chemotherapy. *Indian Journal of Pediatrics, 86*(3), 224–228. https://doi.org/10.1007/s12098-018-2733-x.

Sung, L., Robinson, P., Treister, N., Baggott, T., Gibson, P., Tissing, W., Wiernikowski, J., Brinklow, J., & Dupuis, L. L. (2017). Guideline for the prevention of oral and oropharyngeal mucositis in children receiving treatment for cancer or undergoing haematopoietic stem cell transplantation. *BMJ Supportive & Palliative Care, 7*(1), 7–16. https://doi.org/10.1136/bmjspcare-2014-000804.

Tennant, M., Youssef, G. J., McGillivray, J., Clark, T. J., McMillan, L., & McCarthy, M. C. (2020). Exploring the use of Immersive Virtual Reality to enhance Psychological Well-Being in Pediatric Oncology: A pilot randomized controlled trial. *European Journal of Oncology Nursing : The Official Journal of European Oncology Nursing Society, 48,* 101804. https://doi.org/10.1016/j.ejon.2020.101804.

Thomas, R., Phillips, M., & Hamilton, R. J. (2018). Pain Management in the Pediatric Palliative Care Population. *Journal of Nursing Scholarship : An official Publication of Sigma Theta Tau International Honor Society of Nursing, 50*(4), 375–382. https://doi.org/10.1111/jnu.12389.

Thrane, S. E., Grossoehme, D. H., Tan, A., Shaner, V., & Friebert, S. (2021). Feasibility and Acceptability of a Reiki Intervention With Very Young Children Receiving Palliative Care. *Nursing Research, 70*(6), 469–474. https://doi.org/10.1097/NNR.0000000000000540.

Törüner EK, Büyükgönenç L. (2017). *Çocuk sağlığı: Temel hemşirelik yaklaşımları.* 1. Basım. Ankara: Nobel Tıp; 122, 732.

van Dijk-Lokkart, E. M., Braam, K. I., van Dulmen-den Broeder, E., Kaspers, G. J., Takken, T., Grootenhuis, M. A., Streng, I. C., Bierings, M., Merks, J. H., van den Heuvel-Eibrink, M. M., Veening, M. A., & Huisman, J. (2016). Effects of a combined physical and psychosocial intervention program for childhood cancer patients on quality of life and psychosocial functioning: results of the QLIM randomized clinical trial. *Psycho-oncology, 25*(7), 815–822. https://doi.org/10.1002/pon.4016.

Velten, D. B., Zandonade, E., & Monteiro de Barros Miotto, M. H. (2017). Prevalence of oral manifestations in children and adolescents with cancer submitted to chemotherapy. *BMC Oral Health, 17*(1), 49. https://doi.org/10.1186/s12903-016-0331-8.

Vol, H., Flank, J., Lavoratore, S. R., Nathan, P. C., Taylor, T., Zelunka, E., Maloney, A. M., & Lee Dupuis, L. (2016). Poor chemotherapy-induced nausea and vomiting control in children receiving intermediate or high dose methotrexate. S*upportive Care in Cancer: Official Journal of the Multinational Association of Supportive Care in Cancer, 24*(3), 1365–1371. https://doi.org/10.1007/s00520-015-2924-1.

Vollenbroich, R., Borasio, G. D., Duroux, A., Grasser, M., Brandstätter, M., & Führer, M. (2016). Listening to parents: The role of symptom perception in pediatric palliative home care. *Palliative & Supportive Care, 14*(1), 13–19. https://doi.org/10.1017/S1478951515000462.

Weaver, M. S., Robinson, J., & Wichman, C. (2020). Aromatherapy improves nausea, pain, and mood for patients receiving pediatric palliative care symptom-based consults: A pilot design trial. *Palliative & Supportive Care, 18*(2), 158–163. https://doi.org/10.1017/S1478951519000555.

Weekly, T., Riley, B., Wichman, C., Tibbits, M., & Weaver, M. (2019). Impact of a Massage Therapy Intervention for Pediatric Palliative Care Patients and Their Family Caregivers. *Journal of Palliative Care, 34*(3), 164–167. https://doi.org/10.1177/0825859718810727.

Wong, C. L., Li, C. K., Chan, C. W. H., Choi, K. C., Chen, J., Yeung, M. T., & Chan, O. N. (2021). Virtual Reality Intervention Targeting Pain and Anxiety Among Pediatric Cancer Patients Undergoing

Peripheral Intravenous Cannulation: A Randomized Controlled Trial. *Cancer Nursing, 44*(6), 435–442. https://doi.org/10.1097/NCC.0000000000000844.

World Health Organization. (2021). Palliative Care. https://www.who.int/news-room/fact-sheets/detail/palliative-care. (Date of access: 21.02.2024).

World Health Organization (2021). CureAll framework: WHO global initiative for childhood cancer: increasing access, advancing quality, saving lives. https://iris.who.int/handle/10665/347370 (Date of access: 21.02.2024).

Wu, L. M., Chiou, S. S., Sheen, J. M., Lin, P. C., Liao, Y. M., Chen, H. M., & Hsiao, C. C. (2014). Evaluating the acceptability and efficacy of a psycho-educational intervention for coping and symptom management by children with cancer: a randomized controlled study. *Journal of Advanced Nursing, 70*(7), 1653–1662. https://doi.org/10.1111/jan.12328.

Yıldız, S., (2022). Pediatrik Palyatif Bakım ve Spirtüel Bakım. *Pediatrik Hematoloji Onkoloji Hemşireliği* (pp. 521-545), Ankara: Ankara Nobel Tıp Kitabevi.

Zhang, P., Mo, L., Torres, J., & Huang, X. (2019). Effects of cognitive behavioral therapy on psychological adjustment in Chinese pediatric cancer patients receiving chemotherapy: A randomized trial. *Medicine, 98*(27), e16319.

Zorba, P., & Ozdemir, L. (2018). The Preliminary Effects of Massage and Inhalation Aromatherapy on Chemotherapy-Induced Acute Nausea and Vomiting: A Quasi-Randomized Controlled Pilot Trial. *Cancer Nursing, 41*(5), 359–366. https://doi.org/10.1097/NCC.0000000000000496.

Chapter 16

Evidence-Based Practices for Energy Therapies Used in Pain Management in Pediatric Oncology

Duygu Demir*, PhD
Pediatric Nursing, Department of Nursing, Faculty of Health Sciences, Yalova University, Yalova, Türkiye

Abstract

Every year, more than 400,000 children aged 0-19 are diagnosed with cancer in the world. Children with cancer face a wide range of undesirable symptoms as a result of the disease and its treatment. Pain is one of the most common findings in pediatric oncology patients due to treatment and invasive procedures. As the pain experienced increases, the child's coping status and quality of life are negatively affected. Pediatric nurses and physicians can use non-pharmacological complementary and alternative therapy methods with a high level of evidence together with pharmacological methods, to reduce the child's pain. One of the complementary therapies accepted by the World Health Organization and the National Center for Complementary and Alternative Medicine is energy therapies. Energy therapies include reiki, therapeutic touch, and healing touch. Energy therapies can be used as an adjunct to medical treatment because they are non-invasive, have no side effects, and are not cost-effective. Energy therapies are applied to strengthen the body's healing capacity by influencing the energy fields of the body. The use of energy therapies in international nursing studies dates back to ancient times. Nurses should know the importance of mental balance in accelerating recovery and supporting the individual with methods that do not have side effects. Therefore, the use of energy therapies that are applied without cost in the field of health is increasing. It is said in the literature that energy therapies are used in pediatric, neonatal services, and intensive care units, and it is stated that they may be useful in reducing pain.
In this section, evidence-based results regarding the effect of energy therapies, which are used to reduce the pain of pediatric oncology patients, support the independent functions of nurses, and have no cost and side effects, are examined in line with the literature.

Keywords: child, energy therapy, healing touch, reiki, therapeutic touch

---

* Corresponding Author's Email: duygu.dmr@outlook.com.

In: Evidence-Based Care Practices in Pediatric Nursing
Editors: Feyza Küçük and Serap Özdemir
ISBN: 979-8-89530-304-7

Introduction

After accidents, cancer is the second most common cause of death for children under the age of 14. Every year, around 400,000 children aged 0 to 19 are diagnosed with cancer worldwide (World Health Organization-WHO, 2021). The most prevalent types of cancer in children are leukemia, central nervous system tumors (CNS), and lymphoma (National Cancer Institute-NCI, 2022). Children with cancer experience a variety of negative symptoms, including pain, nausea, vomiting, and weariness, because of the disease and its treatment (Dommett and Morgenstern, 2018; Hackney and Welch, 2017).

Pain is one of the most common findings in pediatric oncology patients due to disease, treatment, and invasive interventions (Agrawal and Feusner, 2016; Kyle and Carman, 2013). Pain is a personal experience associated with existing or potential tissue damage and is affected by biological, psychological, and social factors at different levels (International Association for the Study of Pain, 2011). As the pain experienced increases, the coping status and quality of life of the child are negatively affected. Therefore, effective management of the child's pain is extremely important in nursing care. Nurses should use evidence-based practices with proven scientific efficacy as a supportive treatment together with pharmacological agents in the effective management of pain in children with cancer. Nurses should support the child and family by integrating a high level of evidence-based practices into care by using education and counseling roles (WHO, 2021; Rodgers, 2017; Agrawal and Feusner, 2016).

Evidence-based practice is defined as the integration of best research, clinical expertise, and patient values to make decisions about the individualized care of patients and to solve clinical problems. The aim of evidence-based practice is to synthesize the best and most up-to-date evidence published in line with patient preferences and needs in the decision-making process for medical care and to integrate these results into clinical practice (Kapucu et al., 2021; Robbins, 2017). Evidence-based nursing is the use of the best evidence from research together with clinical experience and patient preferences when making decisions about nursing practice. Evidence-based nursing creates a bridge between research and practice and eliminates the gap between research and clinical care (Kapucu et al., 2021). In the literature, evidence-based methods emphasize that they use resources more effectively, enhance patient care, reduce costs and duration of hospital stay, increase patient satisfaction, and remove unnecessary, and inefficient activities (Kapucu et al., 2021; Alqahtani et al., 2020). Pediatric nurses and doctors can use non-pharmacological complementary and alternative therapy methods with a high level of evidence together with pharmacological methods to reduce the pain of the child.

Energy therapies are one of the complementary therapies recognized by the WHO and the National Center of Complementary and Alternative Medicine (NCCAM). (NCCAM, 2018). Energy therapies include reiki, therapeutic touch, and healing touch (Shaybak et al., 2017; Natale, 2010). Energy therapies can be used as an adjunct to medical treatment because they are non-invasive, and have no side effects and cost. Energy therapies are practiced to strengthen the healing capacity of the body by affecting the energy fields of the body. The use of energy therapies in international nursing practices dates back to ancient times (Miles and True, 2003). Nurses should know the importance of mental balance in accelerating recovery and supporting the individual with methods that do not have side effects. Therefore, the use of energy therapies that are applied without cost in the field of health is increasing. In the literature, it has been reported that energy therapies are used in pediatric, neonatal units, and intensive care units and may be useful in reducing pain (Demir, 2022; Plotnikoff et al., 2017; Thrane et al., 2017; Wong et al., 2013; Hanley, 2008; Whitley and Rich, 2008).

In this section, evidence-based results regarding the effect of energy therapies, which are used to reduce the pain of pediatric oncology patients, support the autonomous functions of nurses, and have no cost and side effects, are examined in line with the literature.

Childhood Cancers

The type of cancer that occurs between birth and 19 years of age is called childhood cancer. Childhood cancers are cancers that occur in the specified age group and are caused by the uncontrolled growth and proliferation of abnormal cells and rapid spread (metastasis) throughout the body. With early diagnosis and then appropriate treatments, cancer cells are eliminated or killed. Thus, treatment is provided (WHO, 2021).

More than 400,000 children aged 0-19 are diagnosed with cancer each year (WHO, 2021). Cancer is the second most prevalent cause of death in the United States among children aged 0-14, after accidents, and the fourth leading cause of death among adolescents (15-19 years) (Siegel et al., 2022). The most common types of cancer among children (between 2001-2018) are leukemia, CNS tumors, and lymphoma, respectively (NCI, 2022). In the UK, leukemia is the leading first among childhood cancers (32%), followed by brain and spinal tumors (24%) and lymphoma (10%) (Dommett and Morgenstern, 2018). In Turkey, leukemia (33%), CNS tumors (20%), and lymphoma (13%) are the three most common childhood cancers in the 0-14 age group. When looked at by gender, in the 0-14 age group (2018 data), leukemia (Boy: 53.7%; Girl: 45.5%), CNS tumors (B: 30.5%; G: 28%) and lymphoma (B: 24%; G: 11.4%) are the top three in boys and girls, respectively. In the 15-19 age group, males by gender; while leukemia (17%), testicular cancer (16%), and Hodgkin's lymphoma (11%) are the top three most common, thyroid cancer is the most prevalent among girls with 36% (Republic of Türkiye Ministry of Health General Directorate of Public Health, 2022).

Although the etiology of childhood cancers is unknown, it is multifactorial. The interaction between genetic factors, environmental factors, viral infections, and chemicals can predispose to childhood cancers (WHO, 2021; Dommett and Morgenstern, 2018). The first symptoms may be nonspecific. Although there are different symptoms depending on the type of cancer, due to both disease symptoms and side effects of treatment; clinical signs and symptoms such as pain, anemia, high fever, thrombocytopenia, neutropenia, fatigue, infection, and nutritional disorders can be observed (Dommett and Morgenstern, 2018; Hackney and Welch, 2017; Rodgers et al., 2019; Erdemir and Taş Arslan, 2018; Linnard-Palmer and Coats, 2017; Kyle and Carman, 2013).

The Use of Energy Therapies in Pain Management in Pediatric Oncology

Pain; is among the frequently observed findings in children with cancer, depending on the disease, treatment, and invasive procedures (Agrawal and Feusner, 2016; Kyle and Carman, 2013). Pain is a personal experience that is affected at different levels by biological, psychological, and social variables linked to actual or prospective tissue injury. People learn the concept of pain through their past experiences, and if they express that they have pain, then there is pain. Verbal communication is only one of the methods of expressing pain. Because the individual's inability to communicate does not indicate that he/she does not have pain (International Association for the Study of Pain, 2011).

Effective management of pain in children includes a comprehensive assessment, pain management, and pain re-evaluation approach. Pain that is not properly relieved can lead to physiological, psychosocial, and behavioral problems in the long term (Agrawal and Feusner, 2016). To minimize the pain of children with cancer caused by therapy, diagnostic procedures, or disease, nurses should use a combination of pharmacological agents and many scientifically proven non-pharmacological methods (WHO, 2021; Rodgers, 2017; Agrawal and Feusner, 2016). To reduce pain in children with cancer, nurses can use many non-pharmacological complementary and integrative methods such as; vibration and cold application (Baxter et al., 2011; Canbulat et al., 2015), balloon inflation (Mutlu and Balcı, 2015), virtual reality glasses (Hundert et al., 2022), reiki therapy (Demir, 2022; Demir and Birsen, 2022; Zucchetti et al., 2019), acupuncture (Bettini et al., 2023), music therapy (Ghanbari et al., 2021). It is very important that all nurses and other health professionals working with children increase their knowledge about appropriate pain management and non-pharmacological methods and apply complementary and integrative methods with a high level of evidence to increase the comfort level and quality of life of children.

Complementary and integrative therapies; It is defined as evidence-based healthcare approaches developed outside of traditional medicine and used together with traditional care. (McClafferty et al., 2017). Today, many complementary and integrative methods have been integrated into pediatric care in clinics and hospitals. These methods are not used to replace traditional medicine, but rather to support traditional medical care (Plotnikoff et al., 2017). Complementary and integrated therapies used in patients with cancer address the integrity of the patient's mind, body, and spirit and include a multidisciplinary approach. Complementary and integrative therapies can improve pain and quality of life in pediatric oncology patients. These therapies are effective in assisting with both procedural and cancer pain. Evidence-based complementary and integrative therapies without any side effects can be routinely provided to children with cancer and their families along with pharmacological methods to reduce pain (NCI, 2023; Rodgers et al., 2019; Agrawal and Feusner, 2016). Nurses have a significant role in providing supportive care in addition to medical care that can reduce pain and improve the quality of life of children with cancer (Rodgers et al., 2019; Agrawal and Feusner, 2016).

Energy therapies are a complementary therapy accepted by WHO and NCCAM. (NCCAM, 2018; Shaybak et al., 2017). Nurses and other healthcare professionals are increasingly interested in energy therapies applied without the need for expensive technologies considering the needs of individuals/patients. International nursing research on energy therapies dates back to ancient times (Miles and True, 2003). Pioneers of modern nursing, such as Martha Rogers and Jean Watson and the American Holistic Nurses Association have recognized the use of energy therapies in the field (Natale, 2010; Vitale, 2007). The nursing diagnosis expressed as an "Imbalanced Energy Field" defines energy therapies. This diagnosis refers to the disruption that occurs in the normally continuous, unique, dynamic, creative, and holistic human energy flow (North American Nursing Diagnosis Association, 2021).

Energy therapies are based on the belief in balancing the flow of energy in the patient/individual. These are reiki, therapeutic touch, and healing touch (Shaybak et al., 2017; Natale, 2010). Energy therapies are a non-pharmacological method that is cost-effective and allows nurses to use their independent functions. No side effects from energy therapies have been reported. When the literature is evaluated, it is said that energy therapies have many benefits for adults and children, such as reducing pain and anxiety and increasing the level of comfort and well-being (Plotnikoff et al., 2017; Shaybak et al., 2017). Pediatric nurses and physicians can benefit from high-evidence non-pharmacological and non-invasive energy therapies together with pharmacological methods to reduce the pain of children with cancer.

Evidence for the Benefits of Therapeutic Touch

Therapeutic Touch (TT) was developed by nursing professor Dolores Krieger and healer Dora Kunz in the 1970s (Plotnikoff et al., 2017; Tabatabaee et al., 2016; Miles and True, 2003). Krieger invented this theory, inspired by Rogers' "Holistic (Unitary) Human Theory". Therapeutic touch is a therapy method that aims to regulate disorders in the energy field. The practitioner applies healing to the person's energy fields with his/her hands (contact/non-contact) to regulate the symptoms of the disease caused by disruptions in the energy field (Erdem et al., 2018; Plotnikoff et al., 2017; Tabatabaee et al., 2016).

Therapeutic touch is used by nurses and other healthcare professionals in pediatric hospitals in many countries. Energy treatments are increasingly being integrated into nursing care through procedures for their use. Today, the energetic properties of the method are taught in nursing schools in the United States (Plotnikoff et al., 2017). At New York University, nurses were trained by developing a master's level curriculum (Plotnikoff et al., 2017; Vitale, 2007; Whelan and Wishnia, 2003). Individuals receive certification in two ways: TT practitioner and TT trainer (Efendi et al., 2018; Hanley, 2008).

Therapeutic touch has been observed to have a positive and safe effect on symptoms such as pain, anxiety, and nausea in adults with cancer (Tabatabaee et al., 2016; Aghabati et al., 2010). Studies conducted on pediatric patients are generally conducted on newborns and have small sample sizes. In a double-blind, randomized controlled pilot study conducted by Whitley and Rich (2008) with 20 premature newborns; the effect of TT on heart rate and side effects in premature newborns were examined. TT was practiced in newborns for 5 minutes for 3 consecutive days. It was found that there was a substantial shift in heart rate as a result of the relaxation response in the newborns in the experimental group and there was no adverse effect in both groups (experimental and control) (Whitley and Rich, 2008). In a study conducted with preterm infants aged 25-37 weeks, it has been reported that newborns' coordination between sucking, swallowing, and respiration is better, and their interaction with their environment increases (Hanley, 2008). In another study conducted in 2018, the effect of TT (by the mother) and maternal voice stimulation applied to preterm newborns was examined. Although not statistically significant, the study found that preterm infants' sleep patterns were more consistent (Efendi et al., 2018).

When the literature was examined, there was no randomized controlled trial that investigated the effect of TT on pain in pediatric oncology patients. There are studies showing that TT has a positive and safe effect on symptoms such as pain, anxiety, and nausea in adults with cancer (Tabatabaee et al., 2016; Aghabati et al., 2010). There is a need for studies with high evidence level examining the effect of therapeutic touch, which has no side effects and supports the independent functions of nurses, in pediatric oncology patients.

Evidence for the Benefits of Healing Touch

Healing Touch (HT) was developed by Janet Mentgen with additional techniques similar to therapeutic touch. It was integrated into nursing education in the 1980s. This theory is based on the view that if there is a blockage in the flow of energy, then the energy can spread throughout the body. Blockages in the energy field can cause physical, psychological, and mental diseases. The practitioner aims to achieve healing in the complex energy systems of the body by balancing the energy with the practitioner's hands (Erdem et al., 2018; Plotnikoff et al., 2017).

When the literature was examined, it has been stated that HT reduces pain and anxiety, accelerates wound healing, and facilitates sleep. Most of these studies have been done in adults. Although studies conducted on children are low-evidence level and small-sample studies, it has been stated in these studies that it helps reduce pain, stress, and increase the level of well-being in pediatric patients (Plotnikoff et al., 2017; Cone et al., 2014; Wong et al., 2013). In a randomized controlled prospective study conducted by Wong et al. (2013) in 9 pediatric oncology patients between the ages of 3-18; for 1 year, HT was applied to the experimental group (6 children) for 30 minutes at least once a day, and the control group (3 children) received reading and gaming activities for 30 minutes once a day. As a result of the study, it was reported that HT was effective in reducing pain in pediatric oncology patients (Wong et al., 2013). The level of evidence for this study is low due to the insufficient number of samples, the facy that the groups were not being distributed homogeneously, and the lack of a standard implementation plan. In a pilot study by Kemper et al. (2009) where they examined the effect of HT in 9 pediatric oncology patients between the ages of 1-18; they administered HT to the children for 40 minutes. They reported that HT was effective in decreasing stress and heart rate in pediatric oncology patients (Kemper et al., 2009). Although pain was not evaluated in this study, considering that pain is a major source of stress; nurses can use HT therapy, which has no side effects, as a supportive treatment to reduce stress in children with cancer who have pain.

When the literature is reviewed; although there are limited studies in pediatric oncology patients with a low level of evidence, since there are no side effects, it is recommended that HT can be used in addition to pharmacological methods to reduce pain in pediatric oncology patients, and new studies with a high level of evidence should be planned.

Evidence for the Benefits of Reiki

Reiki, a Japanese word, is an energy therapy. "Rei" means "existing everywhere" and "ki" means "life energy" (McClafferty et al., 2017; Misra et al., 2014; Usui and Grimm, 2000). It includes the "taking/giving a hand" philosophy in Turkish culture. It was discovered by Dr Mikao Usui in Japan in the late 19th century. It is known that Muhsin Doğrular brought it to Turkey in the 1980s (Yücel, 2007). There are energy fields called chakras in our body. Reiki works on the principle of sending energy to blockages in the chakras by the practitioner and healing them (NCCAM, 2018; Sahler et al., 2016; Misra et al., 2014).

There is ample evidence that Reiki reduces pain in adults (Shaybak et al., 2017; Vitale and O'Connor, 2006). In studies conducted on children; there have been reports that Reiki reduces pain, anxiety (Zucchetti et al., 2019; Thrane et al., 2017), and depression symptoms (Charkhandeh et al., 2016). Although there are limited studies examining the effect of Reiki on the pain of pediatric oncology patients, it is stated that it is effective in reducing pain. A double-blind, randomized controlled experimental study conducted by Demir (2022) in 66 children aged 5-7 years with leukemia reported that Reiki was an effective way to reduce pain and improve quality of life (Demir, 2022). In a single-group pilot study conducted with 16 children (7-16 years old) receiving palliative care at home; Reiki was applied to the children for 24 minutes twice. It has been stated that Reiki is effective in reducing pain in pediatric patients receiving palliative care (Thrane et al., 2017). In another semi-experimental pilot study, Reiki was applied to a 4-18 year-old (n=9) child patient who had a hematopoietic stem cell transplant, 3 times a week for 1 month, and the pain relief in the short, medium, and long-term was examined. As a result, it has been reported that reiki is beneficial in relieving pain in the short term (Zucchetti et al., 2019).

When the literature is examined, there are few studies evaluating Reiki's effect on the pain of pediatric oncology patients. Most of the studies were conducted with adults. It has been observed that studies conducted with children are insufficient in number and have a low level of evidence (Demir and Mutlu, 2022; Miles and True, 2003; Vitale, 2007). Although there have been few studies evaluating the impact effect of Reiki therapy on pain in pediatric oncology patients, it can be said that Reiki, which is a cost-free, non-harmful, non-invasive, and non pharmacological method, is suitable for use in dealing with pain in children. It is advised that fresh, high-quality studies be conducted to assess the effect of Reiki on pediatric oncology patients.

Conclusion

Energy therapies are a cost-effective, non-invasive, and non-pharmacological method that supports the independent functions of nurses. It is used in nursing to alleviate pain and stress, promote relaxation, and minimize the symptoms of chronic illnesses. Since energy therapies have no stated side effects, they can be used as a supportive method in the care of children with cancer. Although the effectiveness of energy therapies in adults has been proven by compiling studies on the subject, it has been observed that there are few studies evaluating the effects of energy therapies in pediatric oncology patients. It is recommended that studies with a high degree of evidence be conducted to reveal the effect of energy therapies in reducing the pain of pediatric oncology patients.

References

Aghabati, N., Mohammadi, E., & Pour, Esmaiel Z. (2010). The effect of therapeutic touch on pain and fatigue of cancer patients undergoing chemotherapy. *Evidence Based Complementary and Alternative Medicine,* 7, 375–381. https://doi.org/10.5455/medarh.2016.70.142-147.

Agrawal, A. K., & Feusner, J. (2016). Supportive care of patients with cancer. In P. Lanzkowsky, J. M. Lipton & J. D. Fish (Eds.), *Lanzkowsky's manual of pediatric hematology and oncology (*6th ed., pp. 634-640). Elsevier. ISBN: 978-0-12-801368-7.

Alqahtani, N., Oh, K. M., Kitsantas, P., & Rodan, M. (2020). Nurses' evidence-based practice knowledge, attitudes and implementation: A cross-sectional study. *Journal of Clinical Nursing*, 29(1-2), 274-283. https://doi.org/10.1111/jocn.15097.

Baxter, A. L., Cohen, L. L., Mcelvery, H. L., Lawson, M. L., & von Baeyer, C. L. (2011). An integration of vibration and cold relieves venipuncture pain in a pediatric emergency department. *Pediatric Emergency Care,* 27(12), 1151–1156. https://doi.org/10.1097/PEC.0b013e318237ace4.

Bettini, E., Idiokitas, R., Mahmood, L., Jacobs, S., & Steinhorn, D. (2023). Safety and acceptance of acupuncture and acupressure in children, adolescents, and young adults undergoing hematopoietic stem cell transplant. *Cancer Nursing*, 46(3), E204-E207. https://doi.org/10.1097/NCC.0000000000001135.

Canbulat, N., Ayhan, F., & Inal, S. (2015). Effectiveness of external cold and vibration for procedural pain relief during peripheral intravenous cannulation in pediatric patients. *Pain Management Nursing,* 16(1), 33-39. https://doi.org/10.1016/j.pmn.2014.03.003.

Charkhandeh, M., Talib, M. A., & Hunt, C. J. (2016). The clinical effectiveness of cognitive behavior therapy and an alternative medicine approach in reducing symptoms of depression in adolescents. *Psychiatry Research*, 239, 325–330. https://doi.org/10.1016/j.psychres.2016.03.044.

Cone, L., Gottschlich, M. M., Khoury, J., Simakajornboon, N., & Kagan, R. J. (2014). The effect of healing touch on sleep patterns of pediatric burn patients: A prospective pilot study. *J Sleep Disor: Treat Care*, 3(2). https://doi.org/10.4172/2325-9639.1000136.

Demir, D. (2022). The effect of reiki therapy on pain, vital signs and quality of life in pediatric oncology patients (Publication No. 777351) [Doctoral dissertation, Istanbul University-Cerrahpaşa]. Council of Higher Education Thesis Center, Turkey. https://tez.yok.gov.tr/UlusalTezMerkezi/tezSorgu SonucYeni.jsp.

Demir, D. & Mutlu., B. (2022). Reiki therapy and effects on children. *Journal of TOGU Health Sciences*, 2(2), 177-186.

Dommett, R., & Morgenstern, D. (2018). Malignant disease. In T. Lissauer & W. Carroll (Eds.), *Illustrated textbook of paediatrics* (5th ed., pp. 385-401). Elsevier. ISBN: 978-0-7234-3871-7.

Efendi, D., Caswini, N., Rustina, Y., & Iskandar, R. A. T. P. (2018). Combination of mother therapeutic touch (MTT) and maternal voice stimulus (MVS) therapies stabilize sleep and physiological function in preterm infant sreceiving minör invasive procedures. *Journal of Neonatal Nursing*, 24(6), 318-324. https://doi.org/10.1016/j.jnn.2018.08.001.

Erdem, E., Sezer Efe, Y. & Caner, N. (2018). Complementary and alternative medicine practice in children with terminal illness. In G. Cimete (Eds.), *Çocuklarda palyatif bakım; terminal dönemdeki çocuk ve aileye yaklaşım* (1st ed., pp. 79-83). Turkiye Klinikleri Pediatric Nursing-Special Topics. ISBN: 978-605-7597-02-1.

Erdemir, F., & Taş Arslan, F. (2018). Children with oncological problems and nursing care. In Z. Conk, Z. Başbakkal, H. Bal Yılmaz, & B. Bolışık (Eds.), *Pediatric nursing*, (pp. 794-802). Akademisyen Kitabevi. ISBN: 978-605-81550-2-2.

Ghanbari, N., Khankeh, H. R., Norouzi, K., & Mohammadi, A. Z. (2021). The effect of music therapy on pain and anxiety of children diagnosed with leukemia during bone marrow aspiration and lumbar puncture procedures. *Annals of The Romanian Society for Cell Biology*, 25(6), 19271-19286.

Hackney, L., & Welch, J. G. (2017). Cancers in childhood. In T. K. McInerny, H. M. Adam, D. E. Campbell, T. G. DeWitt, J. M. Foy, & D. M. Kamat (Eds.), *American academy of pediatrics textbook of pediatric care* (2nd ed., pp. 1803-1828). American Academy of Pediatrics. ISBN-13: 978-1-58110-966-5.

Hanley, M. A. (2008). Therapeutic touch with preterm infants: Composing a treatment. *Explore,* 4, 249–258. https://doi.org/10.1016/j.explore.2008.04.003.

Hundert, A. S., Birnie, K. A., Abla, O., Positano, K., Cassiani, C., Lloyd, S., Tiessen, P. H., Lalloo, C. Jibb, L. A., & Stinson, J. (2022). A pilot randomized controlled trial of virtual reality distraction to reduce procedural pain during subcutaneous port access in children and adolescents with cancer. *The Clinical Journal of Pain*, 38(3), 189-196. https://doi.org/10.1097/AJP.0000000000001017.

International Association for the Study of Pain. (2011). *Terminology-pain terms and definitions.* Retrieved March 28, 2024, from https://www.iasp-pain.org/resources/terminology/#pain.

Kapucu, S., Özer Küçük, E., & Gönderen Çakmak, H. S. (2021). Evidence-based nursing practices. In S. Kapucu & R. Kahveci (Eds.), *Evidence-Based Nursing Practices* (pp. 19-30). Hipokrat. ISBN: 978-625-7399-07-4.

Kemper, K. J., Fletcher, N. B., Hamilton, C. A., & McLean, T. W. (2009). Impact of healing touch on pediatric oncology outpatients: Pilot study. *Journal of the Society for Integrative Oncology*, 7(1), 12–18.

Kyle, T. & Carman, S. (2013). *Essentials of pediatric nursing* (2nd ed.). Lippincot Williams & Wilkins. ISBN: 978-1-60547-028-3.

Linnard-Palmer, L., & Coats, G. (2017). *Safe maternity & Pediatric nursing care.* F. A Davis Company. ISBN: 9780803624948.

McClafferty, H., Vohra, S., Bailey, M., Brown, M., Esparham, A., Gerstbacher, D., Golianu, B., Niemi, A. K., Sibinga, E., Weydert, J., Yeh, A. M., Section on İntegrative Medicine, Culbert, T., & Gold, M. (2017). Pediatric integrative medicine. *Pediatrics*, 140(3), e20171961. https://doi.org/10.1542/peds.2017-1961.

Miles, P., & True, G. (2003). Reiki-review of a biofield therapy history, theory, practice, and research. *Alternative Therapies in Health and Medicine*, 9(2), 62-72.

Misra, S. M., Kaplan, R. J., & Verissimo, A. M. (2014). Modalities of complementary and alternative medicine. In S. M. Misra & A. M. Verissimo (Eds.), *A guide to integrative pediatrics for the healthcare professional* (pp. 53-69). Springer. https://doi.org/10.1007/978-3-319-06835-0.

Mutlu, B., & Balcı, S. (2015). Effects of balloon inflation and cough trick methods on easing pain in children during the drawing of venous blood samples: A randomized controlled trial. *Journal for Specialists in Pediatric Nursing*, 20(3), 178-186. https://doi.org/10.1111/jspn.12112.

Natale, G. W. (2010). Reconnecting to nursing through Reiki. *Creative Nursing,* 16(4), 171–176. https://doi.org/10.1891/1078-4535.16.4.171.

National Cancer Institute (NCI). (2022). *Annual report to the nation 2022: Overall cancer statistics.* Retrieved March 28, 2024, from https://seer.cancer.gov/report_to_nation/statistics.html.

North American Nursing Diagnosis Association. (2021). *NANDA international nursing diagnoses: Definitions and classification 2021–2023.* Thieme Medical Publishers. ISBN: 9781684204540.

Plotnikoff, G. A., Kemper K. J., & Culbert, T. P. (2017). Complementary and intefrative medical therapies. In T. K. McInerny, H. M. Adam, D. E. Campbell, T. G. DeWitt, J. M. Foy, & D. M. Kamat (Eds), *American academy of pediatrics textbook of pediatric care* (2nd ed., pp. 411-419). American Academy of Pediatrics. ISBN-13: 978-1-58110-966-5, 411-419.

Republic of Türkiye Ministry of Health General Directorate of Public Health. (2022). *Türkiye cancer statistics* 2018. Retrieved March 28, 2024, from https://hsgm.saglik.gov.tr/tr/kanser-istatistikleri.html.

Robbins, B. W. (2017). Evidence-based medicine. American academy of pediatrics textbook of pediatric care. In T. K. McInerny, H. M. Adam, D. E. Campbell, T. G. DeWitt, J. M. Foy, & D. M. Kamat (Eds), *American academy of pediatrics textbook of pediatric care* (2nd ed., pp.29-32). American Academy of Pediatrics. ISBN-13: 978-1-58110-966-5, 29-32.

Rodgers, C. C. (2017). The child with cancer. In M. J. Hockenberry, & D. Wilson, C. C. Rodgers (Eds.), *Wong's essentials of pediatric nursing* (pp. 1616-1620). Elsevier. ISBN: 978-0-323-35316-8.

Rodgers, C. C., Hooke, M. C., Taylor, O. A., Koerner, K. M., Mitby, P. A., Moore, I. M., Scheurer, M. E., Hockenberry, M. J., & Pan, W. (2019). Childhood cancer symptom cluster: Leukemia and health-related quality of life. *Oncology Nursing Forum*, 46(2), 228–237. https://doi.org/10.1188/19.ONF.228-237.

Sahler, O. J. Z., McClafferty, H., & Rosen, M. A. (2016). Integrative care in pediatric oncology. In A. N. Abrams, A. C. Muriel, L. Wiener (Eds.), *Pediatric psychosocial oncology: Textbook for multidisciplinary care* (pp. 299). Springer International Publishing. ISBN: 978-3-319-21373-6.

Siegel, R. L., Miller, K. D., Fuchs, H. E., & Jemal, A. (2022). Cancer statistics, 2022. *CA: A cancer journal for clinicians*, 72, 7–33. https://doi.org/10.3322/caac.21708.

Shaybak, E., Abdollahimohammad, A., Rahnama, M., Masinaeinezhad, N., Azadi-Ahmadabadi, C., & Firouzkohi, M. (2017). The effect of reiki energy healing on CABG postoperative chest pain caused by coughing and deep breathing. *Indian Journal of Public Health Research and Development*, 8(2), 305-310. https://doi.org/10.5958/0976-5506.2017.00131.0.

Tabatabaee, A., Tafreshi, M. Z., Rassouli, M., Aledavood, S. A., AlaviMajd, H., & Farahmand, S. K. (2016). Effect of therapeutic touch in patients with cancer: A literature review. *Medical Archives,* 70(2), 142–147. https://doi.org/10.5455/medarh.2016.70.142-147.

The National Center of Complementary and Alternative Medicine (NCCAM). (2018). *Reiki.* Retrieved March 28, 2024, from https://www.nccih.nih.gov/health/reiki.

Thrane, S. E., Maurer, S. H., Ren, D., Danford, C. A., & Cohen, S. M. (2017). Reiki therapy for symptom management in children receiving palliative care: A pilot study. *The American Journal of Hospice & Palliative Care*, 34(4), 373–379. https://doi.org/10.1177/1049909116630973.

Usui, M., & Grimm, C. M. (2000). *The original Reiki handbook of Dr. Mikao Usui: The traditional Usui Reiki ryoho treatment positions and numerous Reiki techniques for health and well-being (*2nd ed.). Lotus Press.

Vitale, A. (2007). An integrative review of Reiki touch therapy research. *Holistic Nursing Practice*, 21(4), 167–179. https://doi.org/10.1097/01.HNP.0000280927.83506.f6.

Vitale, A. T., & O'Connor, P. C. (2006). The effect of Reiki on pain and anxiety in women with abdominal hysterectomies. *Holistic Nursing Practice*, 20(6), 263-272.

Whelan, K. M., & Wishnia, G. S. (2003). Reiki therapy: The benefits to a nurse/Reiki practitioner. *Holistic Nursing Practice*, 17(4), 209–217.

Whitley, J. A., & Rich, B. L. (2008). A double-blind randomized controlled pilot trial examining the safety and efficacy of therapeutic touch in premature infants. *Advances in Neonatal Care,* 8(6), 315–333. https://doi.org/10.1097/01.ANC.0000342764.71864.28.

Wong, J., Ghiasuddin, A., Kimata, C., Patelesio, B., & Siu, A. (2013). The impact of healing touch on pediatric oncology patients. *Integrative Cancer Therapies*, 12(1), 25–30. https://doi.org/10.1177/1534735412446864.

World Health Organization (WHO). (2021). *Global Initiative for Childhood Cancer. Increasing access, advancing quality, saving lives. Geneva: World Health Organization.* https://creativecommons.org/licenses/by-nc-sa/3.0/igo/.

Yücel, D. (2007). Arise and development of reiki and reflections of it in Turkey (Publication No. 220297) [Master dissertation, Dokuz Eylül University]. Council of Higher Education Thesis Center, Turkey. https://tez.yok.gov.tr/UlusalTezMerkezi/tezSorguSonucYeni.jsp.

Zucchetti, G., Candela, F., Bottigelli, C., Campione, G., Parrinello, A., Piu, P., Vassallo, E., & Fagioli, F. (2019). The power of reiki: Feasibility and efficacy of reducing pain in children with cancer undergoing hematopoietic stem cell transplantation. *Journal Pediatric Oncology Nursing,* 36(5), 361-368. https://doi.org/10.1177/1043454219845879.

Chapter 17

Evidence-Based Nursing Practices for Nausea and Vomiting in Pediatric Oncology

Fatma Dinç*, PhD

Department of Nursing, Faculty of Health Sciences, Bartın University, Türkiye

Abstract

In pediatric oncology patients, nausea and vomiting secondary to chemotherapy and radiotherapy can lead to fluid electrolyte imbalance, increased risk of infection, delayed recovery, and reduced childhood activities. For pediatric oncology patients, severe nausea and vomiting can also lead to an increased need for parenteral nutrition support and place an additional burden on care. Despite the existence of guidelines published by The Multinational Association for Supportive Care in Cancer, the European Society of Medical Oncology, and the Pediatric Oncology Group of Ontario, the assessment of nausea and the lack of a standardized scoring system remain a challenge. Therefore, it is important to implement innovative and age-appropriate interventions to prevent and manage chemotherapy-induced nausea and vomiting. In addition to pharmacological interventions such as serotonin receptor antagonists, anticholinergics, antiemetics, aromatherapy, relaxation techniques, acupressure, acupuncture, massage, storytelling, hypnosis, yoga, and video games, child distraction methods, music, painting, non-pharmacological interventions are used in the treatment of nausea and vomiting that may develop secondary to chemotherapy. Accurate and timely assessment of symptoms in pediatric oncology patients can lead to more effective treatment and management of nausea and vomiting and have a positive impact on overall treatment processes. Pediatric nurses can provide symptom recognition of children through standardized assessment tools and provide education and counseling to children and their parents regarding the identification of signs and symptoms of nausea and vomiting. In this section, we will discuss evidence-based nursing interventions for nausea and vomiting in pediatric oncology patients.

Keywords: nausea, vomiting, pediatric nursing, pediatric oncology

---

* Corresponding Author's Email: fatmadinccocuk@hotmail.com.

In: Evidence-Based Care Practices in Pediatric Nursing
Editors: Feyza Küçük and Serap Özdemir
ISBN: 979-8-89530-304-7

Introduction

Childhood Cancers

Cancer remains a formidable and life-altering condition globally, particularly affecting children, with over 400,000 new cases diagnosed annually (World Health Organization, 2018). Cancers occurring from birth up to the age of 19 are collectively referred to as Childhood Cancers (Esbenshade et al., 2023). The most prevalent cancers among children include acute leukemia, brain tumors, bone and soft tissue sarcomas, germ cell tumors, and lymphomas. Advances in access to treatment and innovative, evidence-based therapeutic methods have improved children's survival rates (Radossi et al., 2018). With the increase in survival rates among pediatric oncology patients, there is a critical need to address symptoms that can occur during their treatment (Mora et al., 2023). The World Health Organization's Global Initiative for Childhood Cancer, established in 2018, aims to increase the global survival rate of pediatric oncology patients to at least 60% by 2030 while also striving to reduce their pain, alleviate suffering, and enhance their quality of life (World Health Organization, 2018).

Symptoms of Childhood Cancers

The treatment for childhood cancers encompasses vital and effective methods such as chemotherapy, radiotherapy, surgery, immunotherapy, and stem cell transplantation (Flank et al., 2017; Kovacevic et al., 2019). Despite the innovation in therapeutic advancements, pediatric oncology patients still face numerous symptoms, including oral mucositis, pain, fatigue, nausea and vomiting, insomnia, hair loss, and peripheral neuropathy (Cheng et al., 2022; Lavasidis et al., 2022). Even with the advent of more effective antiemetic regimens in recent years, chemotherapy-induced nausea and vomiting (CINV) remains prevalent, especially among pediatric oncology patients undergoing highly emetogenic chemotherapy regimens (Kestler & Lobiondo-Wood, 2012).

Nausea and Vomiting Symptoms

Nausea is an intermittent and unpleasant sensation in the epigastrium or abdomen that may lead to an impending feeling of vomiting (Hooke & Linder, 2019). Conversely, vomiting occurs when the stomach's contents are expelled through the mouth, accompanied by the contraction of the abdominal and chest wall muscles and an increase in salivation (Clark-Snow et al., 2018; Zhao et al., 2023). These symptoms can be triggered by the use of chemotherapy, opioids, increased intracranial pressure, gastritis, anxiety, infections, and constipation (Ameringer et al., 2015). In pediatric oncology patients receiving cytotoxic chemotherapy, factors such as damage to the blood-brain barrier, the emergence of adrenal hormones, and disrupted gastrointestinal motility can lead to symptoms of nausea and vomiting (Esbenshade et al., 2023). CINV typically occurs within the first 24 hours of chemotherapy treatment in pediatric oncology patients, while delayed nausea and vomiting appear more than 24 hours post-chemotherapy, and anticipatory nausea and vomiting precede the chemotherapy based on previous experiences, anxiety, and stress responses (Yurdakul et al., 2021). Studies have indicated that the sight and smell of treatment rooms can act as stimuli that exacerbate anticipatory nausea and vomiting (Kamen et al., 2014).

Nausea and Vomiting Incidences

A previous study with pediatric oncology patients revealed that those experiencing nausea and vomiting within the first 24 hours of chemotherapy treatment were more likely to encounter anticipatory nausea and vomiting during the infusion process (Dupuis et al., 2017). Research observing pediatric oncology patients aged 4-18 years who received prophylaxis with intrathecal methotrexate and either ondansetron or granisetron reported that while the majority had control over acute and delayed vomiting, nausea control was found to be inadequate (Vol et al., 2016). Another study highlighted that nausea was the most frequently reported symptom within the first 96 hours following chemotherapy treatment among pediatric oncology patients (Esbenshade et al., 2023). It was identified that children diagnosed with acute lymphoblastic leukemia or osteosarcoma and treated with medium doses of methotrexate experienced uncontrollable nausea and vomiting in 60% of cases, whereas those treated with high doses reported these symptoms in 30% of cases (Vol et al., 2016). Further research found that acute nausea and vomiting occurred in 25% to 42% of pediatric oncology patients (Rodgers et al., 2012). Those receiving radiotherapy, especially with abdominal and whole-body irradiation, also presented higher rates of nausea and vomiting symptoms (Green et al., 2010). Despite antiemetic treatment, high and medium-emetogenic chemotherapy can negatively impact the quality of life of pediatric oncology patients (Antill Keener, 2019; Awwad et al., 2023).

Effects of Nausea and Vomiting

The Pediatric Oncology Group of Ontario (POGO) defines the control of antineoplastic induced nausea and vomiting in pediatric patients as the absence of the sensation of nausea, vomiting, and retching, without change in appetite or dietary patterns due to nausea (Dupuis et al., 2019). Symptoms of nausea and vomiting in childhood cancers can lead to dehydration, fluid-electrolyte imbalance, weight loss, nutritional deficiency, acute renal failure, aspiration pneumonia, gastrointestinal bleeding, developmental delays, metabolic imbalance, and weakened immune systems. Additionally, these symptoms can disrupt social life and childhood activities such as school attendance (Ewig et al., 2022). This situation may lead to further complications, such as postponement of treatment protocols and reduced medication doses (Evans et al., 2018). The treatment processes of pediatric oncology patients can negatively affect their desire to eat and quality of life, potentially extending hospital stays (Dupuis et al., 2019). Severe nausea and vomiting in pediatric oncology patients can also increase the need for parenteral nutritional support, adding a burden on care. If not adequately controlled, nausea and vomiting can lead to treatment refusal and compliance issues among pediatric patients (Walsh et al., 2021).

An Assessment of Nausea and Vomiting Symptoms

The frequency of vomiting symptoms can be quantified, and its severity can be more easily measured. However, due to the subjective nature of nausea, the use of self-assessment tools is beneficial to convey the experience (Awwad et al., 2023). Nonetheless, the interpretation and expression symptoms can be more challenging for pediatric oncology patients due to their age, cognitive level, and language development. A study examining the experiences of pediatric oncology patients aged five to seven years during their treatment found that children could not directly express "nausea" but instead described it using metaphors (Cheng et al., 2022). Therefore, the use of a standardized nausea assessment tool is a crucial component of effective nursing intervention to reccognize, alleviate, and manage symptoms (Evans et al., 2018; Navari, 2017). Despite the availability of guidelines published by The Multinational Association for Supportive Care in Cancer, the European Society of Medical Oncology, and the Pediatric Oncology Group of Ontario, challenges persist due to the lack of a standard scoring system to assess nausea. Few validated tools are specifically designed for pediatric oncology patients' clinical care, and those validated may not be fully understood by healthcare professionals or may be limited by age range (Donaghey et al., 2022). Therefore, implementing innovative and age-appropriate interventions to prevent and manage chemotherapy-induced nausea and vomiting is of significant importance. Commonly used measurement tools in pediatrics include the Pediatric Nausea Assessment Tool, the Visual Analog Scale, and the Baxter Animated Retching Faces (BARF) scale.

The Visual Analog Scale has been validated as an evidence-based method to assess pain and nausea symptoms in medicine. However, its reliability in pediatric evaluations is less consistent (Hendey et al., 2005). The Pediatric Nausea Assessment Tool employs a modified facial scale with four measurement points to assess nausea, but its specificity is limited due to only four options to indicate severity (Dupuis et al., 2006). The Baxter Animated Retching Faces (BARF) scale, validated for children aged 4-18, uses a 10-point modified facial scale depicting progressively worsening nausea symptoms, with the final face indicating active vomiting (Baxter et al., 2011). An evidence-based study among nurses examined the impact of the BARF scale on nursing assessments in pediatric oncology patients, finding it user-friendly and effective for symptom feedback (Donaghey et al., 2022). Additionally, the Nausea and Vomiting Thermometer Scale (NVTS) has been developed as a valid and reliable tool for pediatric oncology patients and the Adapted Rhodes Index of Nausea and Vomiting for Pediatrics provides another perspective-based assessment tool for nausea and vomiting in this demographic (Akdeniz Kudubeş & Bektaş, 2022).

Researches

Pharmacological and Non-pharmacological Interventions for Nausea and Vomiting Symptoms

The Children's Oncology Group has been working to standardize the evaluation of symptoms in pediatric oncology patients within a conceptual framework. In 2009, the Multinational Association of Supportive Care in Cancer (MASCC) and the European Society for Medical

Oncology (ESMO) developed clinical practice guidelines to prevent acute nausea and vomiting in this patient group, which were updated in 2016 by the Pediatric Oncology Group of Ontario (POGO) and MASCC, including evidence-based recommendations for treatment, non-pharmacological adjunct therapies, and antiemetic agent dosages (Sherani et al., 2019). Implementing these guidelines could improve adherence to antiemetic protocols, prevent delays in chemotherapy, and reduce hospital admissions (Awwad et al., 2023).

Pharmacological Interventions for Nausea and Vomiting Symptoms

From the start of treatment protocols, it is crucial to use anti-nausea medication in appropriate doses and intervals in pediatric oncology patients (Jacobs et al., 2022). Treatment for CINV includes neurokinin-1 receptor antagonists, serotonin receptor antagonists, corticosteroids, and anticholinergics aimed at blocking receptors before the onset of emetic stimuli (Diorio et al., 2022; Ruggiero et al., 2018). The American Society of Clinical Oncology (ASCO) and the National Comprehensive Cancer Network (NCCN) classify chemotherapy agents by their emetogenic potential. Currently, the combination of 5-HT3 serotonin antagonists and dexamethasone is a widely used and effective pharmacological treatment for nausea in pediatric oncology patients (Hesketh et al., 2020). However, the addition of steroids continues to be debated in terms of risk versus benefit, with long-term use of dexamethasone potentially leading to side effects such as epigastric discomfort, hyperglycemia, insomnia, weight gain, and agitation (Phillips et al., 2016; Ruggiero et al., 2018). A meta-analysis of randomized controlled trials examining the efficacy of palonosetron in preventing delayed chemotherapy-induced nausea and vomiting found it effective in prophylaxis against delayed CINV (Yamaguchi et al., 2024). The Pediatric Oncology Group of Ontario (POGO) recommends the use of 5-HT3 serotonin antagonists such as ondansetron or granisetron to prevent acute chemotherapy-induced nausea and vomiting in patients receiving low, moderate, or high emetogenic chemotherapy (Esbenshade et al., 2023).

Non Pharmacological Interventions for Nausea and Vomiting Symptoms

Understanding and effectively managing early nausea in pediatric oncology patients receiving chemotherapy is vital, as both expected and delayed nausea and vomiting can be reduced through effective and evidence-based nursing approaches (Reis et al., 2019). Pharmacological interventions alone may not be sufficient to prevent nausea and vomiting in these patients. Nutrition issues during treatment for patients experiencing nausea and vomiting highlight the importance of integrating non-pharmacological interventions. The Oncology Nursing Society (ONS) recommends various non-pharmacological methods such as massage, aromatherapy, guided imagery, cognitive-behavioral therapies, progressive muscle relaxation, yoga, acupuncture-acupressure, animal-assisted therapy, mind-body practices, creative arts therapy, music, and fantasy to prevent nausea and vomiting (Abdulah & Abdulla, 2018; Miladinia et al., 2015). Previous studies have also used non-pharmacological interventions such as storytelling, imagination, hypnosis, music listening, video games, acupuncture, acupressure, and distraction techniques to manage chemotherapy-related nausea and vomiting in pediatric oncology patients (Bradt et al., 2021; Chong et al., 2022; Momani & Berry, 2017; Robb et al., 2017; Velez-Florez et al., 2018).

Aromatherapy

Aromatherapy, endorsed by the National Institutes of Health, involves inhaling or applying essential oils extracted from aromatic plants. It operates by stimulating olfactory receptors and transmitting signals along the olfactory nerve, interacting in a neuropsychological manner to diminish nausea and vomiting (Radossi et al., 2018). As a non-invasive holistic nursing intervention, aromatherapy has been used to provide comfort, manage stress, and reduce pain and anxiety in pediatric oncology patients. In one study examining the management of chemotherapy-induced nausea and vomiting, the experimental group received inhalation aromatherapy with peppermint-lemon in addition to antiemetic treatment, resulting in a lower frequency of nausea and vomiting compared to placebo and control groups (Şancı et al., 2023). Another study found that ginger aromatherapy reduced CINV in pediatric oncology patients (Evans et al., 2018).

Acupuncture

Acupuncture and acupressure, traditional Chinese medicine techniques, aim to improve health by regulating the body's vital energy. Acupressure, similar to acupuncture but using pressure instead of needles, is an accessible, safe, economical, and nurse-independent intervention to alleviate chemotherapy-induced nausea and vomiting in pediatric oncology patients (Lown et al., 2019). The Children's Oncology Group emphasizes the potential benefits of acupuncture and acupressure in minimizing nausea and vomiting related to chemotherapy. However, the recommendations are made with weak strength and very low-quality evidence. A placebo-controlled randomized study compared the efficacy of manual acupuncture and wristband acupressure, finding that manual acupuncture is more effective in reducing the severity and frequency of nausea and vomiting (Altuntaş & Dalgiç, 2022). A systematic review concluded that acupuncture significantly reduced the frequency of acute vomiting in pediatric oncology patients compared to antiemetics alone (McKeon et al., 2013). In another study, laser acupuncture was also found to be effective in alleviating nausea and reducing the number of nausea episodes within five days post-chemotherapy (Varejão & Santo, 2019). However, a placebo-controlled randomized study applying acupressure wristbands to pediatric oncology patients undergoing high-dose chemotherapy found them safe but ineffective in improving chemotherapy-induced nausea and vomiting (Dupuis et al., 2019).

Hypnosis

Hypnosis is among the mind-body therapies used to induce relaxation in children. It is mentioned as a non-pharmacological intervention with a conditional recommendation and low-quality evidence to prevent expected CINV (Patel et al., 2023). A systematic review of a meta-analysis of randomized controlled trials, including hypnosis and acupuncture, found these complementary and alternative medicine interventions to reduce chemotherapy-induced nausea and vomiting in pediatric oncology patients (Mora et al., 2022).

Massage Therapy

Massage therapy, a body-based practice within complementary and alternative medicine, was found to reduce chemotherapy-related nausea and vomiting in pediatric oncology patients aged 4-18 in a randomized controlled trial. The treatment group received Swedish massage 0.5 hours before and 24 hours after chemotherapy sessions, demonstrating a significant reduction in nausea and vomiting (Mazlum et al., 2013). Another study applying Slow-stroke Back Massage to children with acute lymphoblastic leukemia undergoing chemotherapy showed effectiveness in controlling CINV (Miladinia et al., 2015).

Yoga

Yoga, a meditation practice that enhances physical strength, balance, and mental well-being through stretching and breathing exercises, can significantly impact symptoms such as nausea and vomiting in pediatric oncology patients (Diorio et al., 2016). The Pediatric Oncology Group of Ontario's (POGO's) Guideline Program, updated in 2016, suggests that dietary counseling and yoga for pediatric oncology patients experiencing resistant chemotherapy-related nausea and vomiting have a conditional recommendation strength and low evidence quality (Patel et al., 2023). A study of hospitalized children receiving intensive chemotherapy found that a yoga program focusing on relaxation, breathing, strength, flexibility, and balance reduced nausea (Diorio et al., 2016). However, there is insufficient research to evaluate yoga's effectiveness in pediatric oncology patients fully (Velez-Florez et al., 2018).

Creative Arts Therapy

Creative arts therapy, encompassing dance, music, art, and drama, facilitates self-expression and enhances coping skills through externalizing emotions (Raybin et al., 2020; Robb et al., 2014). In pediatric oncology patients, creative arts therapies contribute to mitigating the severity of nausea and vomiting throughout their treatment process (Madden et al., 2010). Listening to familiar music, singing, and improvising can regulate emotions and impact vital functions such as heart rate and breathing by affecting the amygdala (Bradt et al., 2021). A randomized controlled trial on the distressing symptoms in pediatric oncology patients administered music therapy twice a week for 45 minutes over 4-6 weeks finding it effective in reducing symptoms of pain and vomiting (Uggla et al., 2018).

Mobile Technology-Based Applications

Modern mobile technology applications, such as phones and tablets, have become increasingly popular for the management and evaluation of chemotherapy-related nausea and vomiting in pediatric oncology patients (Bruggers et al., 2018). Video games, text messaging, and other mobile applications can improve patients' resilience, coping skills, and self-management regarding their treatment (Semerci et al., 2022). The integration of nausea assessment into electronic health records and the potential for increased use of mobile applications show positive outcomes (McKinnon & Jupp, 2020; Ward et al., 2020). A randomized study demonstrated that distraction and relaxation-based virtual reality are effective, feasible, and acceptable for the management of anxiety and acute nausea (Lee Wong et al., 2022).

The widespread use of digital health tools and the durability of electronic diaries drive the use of mobile health applications (Evans et al., 2020). Mobile applications and electronic health records contribute to monitoring and evaluating nausea in pediatric oncology patients (McKinnon et al., 2019). A systematic review of twenty-four studies on pediatric nausea and vomiting found that structured questionnaires and patient diaries were the most commonly used assessment tools (Ewig et al., 2022). Smartphones enable pediatric oncology patients to manage their symptoms effectively (Jibb et al., 2017). The development of smartphone applications to monitor nausea severity has increased due to the frequent need for patients to travel between hospital and home and the potential for losing or forgetting paper diaries. For instance, a user-friendly application, PeNAT's electronic version, has been developed for pediatric oncology patients undergoing chemotherapy. Researchers and clinicians can overview patients' chemotherapy dates and responses through a secure, web-based portal (Eliasen et al., 2020). Mobile applications are needed to track symptoms arising from chemotherapy in pediatric oncology patients. A study introduced an interactive mobile app called inD, featuring mandalas, puzzles, Tetris, music, and blowing activities, which was found to be effective in reducing chemotherapy-related nausea and vomiting in children (Semerci et al., 2022). Digital mobile games that enhance exercise have been effective as a distraction method in reducing CINV in children (Bruggers et al., 2018). Another randomized controlled trial involved sending daily text message reminders to parents in the experimental group to reduce nausea and vomiting for three weeks. Text message reminders effectively reduced nausea and vomiting levels and improved health-related quality of life in children (Akdeniz Kudubes et al., 2022).

Nursing Approaches in Nausea-Vomiting Symptoms

Pediatric nurses have the huge task of assessing nausea in pediatric oncology patients and deciding which intervention to provide. It is important for them to recognize the symptoms of nausea and vomiting, listen to the child, observe, and use standardized assessment tools to identify symptoms (Cheng et al., 2022). Pediatric nurses should try to build a partnership with the child, allowing the child to guide their own preferences in interventions to reduce nausea (Akçay Didişen et al., 2018). Pediatric nurses should consider the subjective words and age period characteristics of pediatric oncology patients in their evaluations of nausea. Pediatric nurses should be aware that the nausea and vomiting in pediatric oncology patients may be in the expected, acute, and delayed phase during their treatment (Yurdakul et al., 2021). It is important to decide on a care plan with measurable goals for the treatment of nausea in pediatric oncology patients in collaboration with the child (Evans et al., 2018). Pediatric nurses should benefit from and implement guidelines and models on how to assess and treat nausea and vomiting (Karaman & Yilmaz, 2023). In addition, it may be a valuable practice to develop care plans with a holistic care approach for patients established within the framework of evidence-based guidelines (Nogéus et al., 2023). Pediatric nurses can use nonpharmacological interventions in the Nursing Intervention Classification (NIC) to alleviate chemotherapy-related nausea and vomiting in children (Kestler & Lobiondo-Wood, 2012). Additionally, pediatric oncology patients should plan interventions and evaluations for nursing diagnoses such as "fluid volume deficiency", "risk of fluid-electrolyte imbalance", "imbalance in nutrition: less nutrition than needed", "disturbance in sleep pattern" (Hooke & Linder, 2019).

Conclusion

The primary goal in managing nausea and vomiting in pediatric oncology patients is to achieve complete symptom control during treatment, increase comfort, and improve quality of life. Combining pharmacological methods with various non-pharmacological interventions is vital for more effective management of CINV. Preventing CINV in pediatric oncology patients involves maintaining fluid-electrolyte balance, oral mucosal integrity, and nutritional patterns, enhancing treatment compliance and motivation.

Pediatric nurses must be informed about current guidelines and protocols to optimally manage nausea and vomiting (Momani & Berry, 2017). They should administer prescribed antiemetics according to the treatment protocol and assist pediatric oncology patients in developing active coping strategies for nausea and vomiting symptoms (Rodgers et al., 2012). Furthermore, nurses should evaluate the effectiveness of the administered treatment at regular intervals. Pediatric nurses can advocate for the availability of music and art supplies in the hospital and infusion rooms and use non-pharmacological interventions such as dance and yoga that patients can perform at their bedside (Nogéus et al., 2023). They can provide individualized care to pediatric oncology patients at risk for nausea and vomiting who need additional care services and create an environment that reduces nausea and vomiting. Pediatric nurses can facilitate the recognition of symptoms in children through standardized assessment tools. A holistic care approach enables nurses to educate and counsel children and their parents about the management of nausea and vomiting symptoms (Karaman & Yilmaz, 2023). Future research should focus on developing and implementing up-to-date guidelines and models to assess and treat nausea in pediatric oncology patients.

References

Abdulah, D. M., & Abdulla, B. M. O. (2018). Effectiveness of group art therapy on quality of life in paediatric patients with cancer: A randomized controlled trial. *Complementary Therapies in Medicine*, *41*, 180–185. https://doi.org/10.1016/j.ctim.2018.09.020.

Akçay Didişen, N., Yavuz, B., Yardimci, F., & Basbakkal, D. Z. (2018). Validity and reliability of the Turkish version of the adapted rhodes index of nausea and vomiting for pediatrics by child (ARINVc) and by parent (ARINVp). *Journal of Pediatric Oncology Nursing*, *35*(5), 353–360. https://doi.org/10.1177/1043454218765173.

Akdeniz Kudubeş, A., & Bektaş, M. (2022). Developing the nausea and vomiting thermometer scale in children with cancer. *Turkish Journal of Medical Sciences*, *52*(1), 166–174. https://doi.org/10.3906/sag-2005-88.

Akdeniz Kudubes, A., Bektas, M., İnce, D., & Olgun, N. (2022). The effect of text message reminders on nausea, vomiting and quality of life in children with cancer receiving cisplatin. *Journal of Pediatric Nursing*, *64*, e109–e118. https://doi.org/10.1016/j.pedn.2021.12.011.

Altuntaş, D., & Dalgiç, A. İ. (2022). The effects of acupressure in the prevention of nausea and vomiting related to chemotherapy in children: A randomized double-blinded placebo-controlled study. *Journal of Pediatric Hematology/Oncology Nursing*, *39*(6), 386–395. https://doi.org/10.1177/27527530221092324.

Ameringer, S., Erickson, J. M., Macpherson, C. F., Stegenga, K., & Linder, L. A. (2015). Symptoms and symptom clusters identified by adolescents and young adults with cancer using a symptom heuristics app. *Research in Nursing and Health*, *38*(6), 436–448. https://doi.org/10.1002/nur.21697.

Antill Keener, T. (2019). Childhood cancer-related fatigue and day-to-day quality of life. *Journal of Pediatric Oncology Nursing*, *36*(2), 74–85. https://doi.org/10.1177/1043454218818062.

Awwad, S., Ali, A., Alshaikh, F., & Alomtari, M. (2023). Assessment of chemotherapy-induced nausea and vomiting in pediatrics: Adequacy of control and adherence to guidelines. *Pediatric Hematology Oncology Journal*, *8*(3), 171–178. https://doi.org/10.1016/j.phoj.2023.07.003.

Baxter, A. L., Watcha, M. F., Baxter, W. V., Leong, T., & Wyatt, M. M. (2011). Development and validation of a pictorial nausea rating scale for children. *Pediatrics*, *127*(6), e1542–e1549. https://doi.org/10.1542/peds.2010-1410.

Bradt, J., Dileo, C., Myers-Coffman, K., & Biondo, J. (2021). Music interventions for improving psychological and physical outcomes in people with cancer. *Cochrane Database of Systematic Reviews*, *10*, CD006911. https://doi.org/10.1002/14651858.CD006911.pub4.

Bruggers, C. S., Baranowski, S., Beseris, M., Leonard, R., Long, D., Schulte, E., Shorter, A., Stigner, R., Mason, C. C., Bedrov, A., Pascual, I., & Bulaj, G. (2018). A prototype exercise-empowerment mobile video game for children with cancer, and its usability assessment: Developing digital empowerment interventions for pediatric diseases. *Frontiers in Pediatrics*, *6*, 69. https://doi.org/10.3389/fped.2018.00069.

Cheng, L., Zhao, X., Ge, Y., Wang, Y., & Kang, Q. (2022). The experiences of chinese children 5-to 7-year-old during cancer treatment reflected through interviews and drawings. *Journal of Pediatric Hematology/Oncology Nursing*, *39*(2), 88–98. https://doi.org/10.1177/10434542211041919.

Chong, W. W., Abd Rahman, F. N., & Harun, N. A. (2022). Screen time of children with speech delay: a cross-sectional study in a tertiary center in Kuantan, Malaysia. *Pediatrics International*, *64*(1). https://doi.org/
10.1111/ped.15105.

Clark-Snow, R., Affronti, M. Lou, & Rittenberg, C. N. (2018). Chemotherapy-induced nausea and vomiting (CINV) and adherence to antiemetic guidelines: results of a survey of oncology nurses. *Supportive Care in Cancer*, *26*(2), 557–564. https://doi.org/10.1007/s00520-017-3866-6.

Diorio, C., Celis Ekstrand, A., Hesser, T., O'Sullivan, C., Lee, M., Schechter, T., & Sung, L. (2016). Development of an individualized yoga intervention to address fatigue in hospitalized children undergoing intensive chemotherapy. *Integrative Cancer Therapies*, *15*(3), 279–284. https://doi.org/10.1177/
1534735416630806.

Diorio, C., Vardaro, J., Wei, Y., Mauro, J., Croy, C., Oranges, K. E., Flanagan, L., Reilly, A. F., Bailey, L. C., Jubelirer, T., Elgarten, C. W., & Freedman, J. L. (2022). Improving guideline-congruent care for chemotherapy-induced nausea and vomiting prophylaxis in pediatric oncology patients. *JCO Oncology Practice*, *18*(3), e412–e419. https://doi.org/10.1200/op.21.00476.

Donaghey, C. T., Bowerrs, C., & Kiefer, J. (2022). Evaluation of a nausea assessment tool in the pediatric oncology population. *Journal for Specialists in Pediatric Nurisng*, *27*, e12394.

Dupuis, L. L., Sung, L., Molassiotis, A., Orsey, A. D., Tissing, W., & van de Wetering, M. (2017). 2016 updated MASCC/ESMO consensus recommendations: Prevention of acute chemotherapy-induced nausea and vomiting in children. *Supportive Care in Cancer*, *25*(1), 323–331. https://doi.org/10.1007/s00520-016-3384-y.

Dupuis, L. L., Taddio, A., Kerr, E. N., Kelly, A., & MacKeigan, L. (2006). Development and validation of the pediatric nausea assessment tool for use in children receiving antineoplastic agents. *Pharmacotherapy*, *26*(9 I), 1221–1231. https://doi.org/10.1592/phco.26.9.1221.

Dupuis, L. L., Tamura, R. N., Kelly, K. M., Krischer, J. P., Langevin, A. M., Chen, L., Kolb, E. A., Ullrich, N. J., Sahler, O. J. Z., Hendershot, E., Stratton, A., Sung, L., & McLean, T. W. (2019). Risk factors for chemotherapy-induced nausea in pediatric patients receiving highly emetogenic chemotherapy. *Pediatric Blood and Cancer*, *66*(4), e27584. https://doi.org/10.1002/pbc.27584.

Eliasen, A., Abildtoft, M. K., Krogh, N. S., Rechnitzer, C., Brok, J. S., Mathiasen, R., Schmiegelow, K., & Dalhoff, K. P. (2020). Smartphone app to self-monitor nausea during pediatric chemotherapy treatment: User-centered design process. *JMIR MHealth and UHealth*, *8*(7), e18564. https://doi.org/10.2196/18564.

Esbenshade, A. J., Sung, L., Brackett, J., Dupuis, L. L., Fisher, B. T., Grimes, A., Miller, T. P., Ullrich, N. J., & Dvorak, C. C. (2023). Children's Oncology Group's 2023 blueprint for research: Cancer control and supportive care. *Pediatric Blood and Cancer*, *70*(Suppl 6), 1e30568. https://doi.org/10.1002/pbc.30568.

Evans, A., Malvar, J., Garretson, C., Pedroja Kolovos, E., & Baron Nelson, M. (2018). The use of aromatherapy to reduce chemotherapy-induced nausea in children with cancer: A randomized, double-blind, placebo-controlled trial. *Journal of Pediatric Oncology Nursing*, *35*(6), 392–398. https://doi.org/10.1177/
1043454218782133.

Evans, A., Vingelen, M. B., Yu, C., Baird, J., Murray, P., & Bryant, P. (2020). Nausea in numbers: Electronic medical record nausea and vomiting assessment for children with cancer. *Journal of Pediatric Oncology Nursing*, *37*(3), 195–203. https://doi.org/10.1177/1043454219900467.

Ewig, C. L., Yung, W. Y., Ng, H. H. M., Wong, C. L., Leung, A. W. K., Li, C., & Cheung, Y. T. (2022). A scoping review of nausea, vomiting and retching measurement methods in children with cancer. *Pediatrics and Neonatology*, *63*(4), 331–340. https://doi.org/10.1016/j.pedneo.2021.12.010.

Flank, J., Nadeem, K., Moledina, S., Khanna, M., Schindera, C., Punnett, A., & Dupuis, L. L. (2017). Nausea and vomiting in children and adolescents receiving intrathecal methotrexate: A prospective, observational study. *Pediatric Blood and Cancer*, *64*(10), e26603. https://doi.org/10.1002/pbc.26603.

Green, R., Horn, H., & Erickson, J. M. (2010). Eating experiences of children and adolescents with chemotherapy-related nausea and mucositis. *Journal of Pediatric Oncology Nursing*, *27*(4), 209–216. https://doi.org/10.1177/1043454209360779.

Hendey, G. W., Donner, N. F., & Fuller, K. (2005). Clinically significant changes in nausea as measured on a visual analog scale. *Annals of Emergency Medicine*, *45*(1), 77–81. https://doi.org/10.1016/j.annemergmed.2004.07.446.

Hesketh, P. J., Kris, M. G., Basch, E., Bohlke, K., Barbour, S. Y., Clark-Snow, R. A., Danso, M. A., Dennis, K., Dupuis, L. L., Dusetzina, S. B., Eng, C., Feyer, P. C., Jordan, K., Noonan, K., Sparacio, D., & Lyman, G. H. (2020). Antiemetics: ASCO guideline update. *Journal of Clinical Oncology*, *38*(24), 2782–2797. https://doi.org/10.1200/JCO.20.01296.

Hooke, M. C., & Linder, L. A. (2019). Symptoms in children receiving treatment for cancer—part I: Fatigue, sleep disturbance, and nausea/vomiting. *Journal of Pediatric Oncology Nursing*, *36*(4), 244–261. https://doi.org/10.1177/1043454219849576.

Jacobs, S. S., Dome, J. S., Gai, J., Gross, A. M., Postell, E., Hinds, P. S., Davenport, L., van den Anker, J. N., & Mowbray, C. (2022). Pharmacogenetic and clinical predictors of ondansetron failure in a diverse pediatric oncology population. *Supportive Care in Cancer*, *30*(4), 3513–3520. https://doi.org/10.1007/s00520-022-06818-9.

Jibb, L. A., Cafazzo, J. A., Nathan, P. C., Seto, E., Stevens, B. J., Nguyen, C., & Stinson, J. N. (2017). Development of a mHealth real-time pain self-management app for adolescents with cancer: an iterative usability testing study. *Journal of Pediatric Oncology Nursing*, *34*(4), 283–294. https://doi.org/10.1177/1043454217697022.

Kamen, C., Tejani, M. A., Chandwani, K., Janelsins, M., Peoples, A. R., Roscoe, J. A., & Morrow, G. R. (2014). Anticipatory nausea and vomiting due to chemotherapy. *European Journal of Pharmacology*, *722*(1), 172–179. https://doi.org/10.1016/j.ejphar.2013.09.071.

Karaman, N., & Yilmaz, P. (2023). Current status of pediatric oncology clinics and nursing practices in Turkey. *Journal of Pediatric Hematology/Oncology Nursing*, *40*(5), 351–355. https://doi.org/10.1177/27527530231197221.

Kestler, S. A., & Lobiondo-Wood, G. (2012). Review of symptom experiences in children and adolescents with cancer. *Cancer Nursing*, *35*(2), 31–49. https://doi.org/10.1097/NCC.0b013e3182207a2a.

Kovacevic, A., Sivananthan, A., Patel, R., Patel, P., Vennettilli, A., Sing, E. P. C., Zupanec, S., Alexander, S., Sung, L., & Dupuis, L. L. (2019). Chemotherapy-induced nausea and vomiting from oral chemotherapy for childhood acute lymphoblastic leukaemia: feasibility study. *BMJ Supportive and Palliative Care*, *12*(e5), e646–e649. https://doi.org/10.1136/bmjspcare-2019-002022.

Lavasidis, G., Markozannes, G., Voorhies, K., Trikalinos, N. A., Petridou, E. T., Panagiotou, O. A., & Ntzani, E. E. (2022). Supportive interventions for childhood cancer: An umbrella review of randomized evidence. *Critical Reviews in Oncology/Hematology*, *180*, 103845. https://doi.org/10.1016/j.critrevonc.2022.103845.

Lee Wong, C., Li, C. K., Choi, K. C., Wei So, W. K., Yan Kwok, J. Y., Cheung, Y. T., & Chan, C. W. H. (2022). Effects of immersive virtual reality for managing anxiety, nausea and vomiting among paediatric cancer patients receiving their first chemotherapy: An exploratory randomised controlled trial. *European Journal of Oncology Nursing*, *61*, 102233. https://doi.org/10.1016/j.ejon.2022.102233.

Lown, E. A., Banerjee, A., Vittinghoff, E., Dvorak, C. C., Hartogensis, W., Melton, A., Mangurian, C., Hu, H., Shear, D., Adcock, R., Morgan, M., Golden, C., & Hecht, F. M. (2019). Acupressure to reduce treatment-related symptoms for children with cancer and recipients of hematopoietic stem cell transplant: protocol for a randomized controlled trial. *Global Advances In Health and Medicine*, *8*, 2164956119870444. https://doi.org/10.1177/2164956119870444.

Madden, J. R., Mowry, P., Gao, D., McGuire Cullen, P., & Foreman, N. K. (2010). Creative arts therapy improves quality of life for pediatric brain tumor patients receiving outpatient chemotherapy. *Journal of Pediatric Oncology Nursing*, *27*(3), 133–145. https://doi.org/10.1177/1043454209355452.

Mazlum, S., Chaharsoughi, N. T., Banihashem, A., & Vashani, H. B. (2013). The effect of massage therapy on chemotherapy-induced nausea and vomiting in pediatric cancer. *Iranian Journal of Nursing and Midwifery Research*, *18*(4), 280–284. http://www.ncbi.nlm.nih.gov/pubmed/24403922%0A http://www.pubmedcentral.nih.gov/articlerender.fcgi?artid=PMC3872861.

McKeon, C., Smith, C. A., Hardy, J., & Chang, E. (2013). Acupuncture and acupressure for chemotherapy-induced nausea and vomiting: A systematic review. *Australian Journal of Acupuncture and Chinese Medicine*, *8*(1), 2–27.

McKinnon, K., & Jupp, J. (2020). Integration of a nausea and vomiting assessment tool into antineoplastic management of pediatric oncology patients. *Journal of Oncology Pharmacy Practice*, *26*(6), 1353–1360. https://doi.org/10.1177/1078155219892666.

McKinnon, K., Jupp, J., Ghosh, S., Digout, C., Eason, S., & Romanick, M. (2019). Adherence to pediatric acute chemotherapy-induced nausea and vomiting guidelines in Canadian hospitals. *Pediatric Blood and Cancer*, *66*(1), e27488. https://doi.org/10.1002/pbc.27488.

Miladinia, M., Baraz, S., Nouri, E. M., & Baeis, M. G. (2015). Effects of slow-stroke back massage on chemotherapy-induced nausea and vomiting in the pediatrics with acute leukemia: a challenge of controlling symptoms. *International Journal of Pediatrics*, *3*(24), 1145–1152.

Momani, T. G., & Berry, D. L. (2017). Integrative therapeutic approaches for the management and control of nausea in children undergoing cancer treatment: a systematic review of literature. *Journal of Pediatric Oncology Nursing*, *34*(3), 173–184.

Mora, D. C., Jong, M. C., Quandt, S. A., Arcury, T. A., Kristoffersen, A. E., & Stub, T. (2023). Supportive care for cancer-related symptoms in pediatric oncology: a qualitative study among healthcare providers. *BMC Complementary Medicine and Therapies*, *23*, 104. https://doi.org/10.1186/s12906-023-03924-x.

Mora, D. C., Overvåg, G., Jong, M. C., Kristoffersen, A. E., Stavleu, D. C., Liu, J., & Stub, T. (2022). Complementary and alternative medicine modalities used to treat adverse effects of anti-cancer treatment among children and young adults: a systematic review and meta-analysis of randomized controlled trials. *BMC Complementary Medicine and Therapies*, *22*(1), 97. https://doi.org/10.1186/s12906-022-03537-w.

Navari, R. M. (2017). Management of chemotherapy-induced nausea and vomiting in pediatric patients. *Pediatric Drugs*, *19*, 213–222. https://doi.org/10.1007/s40272-017-0228-2.

Nogéus, M., Nilsson, S., & Björk, M. (2023). Pediatric nurses' person-centered approach to nausea management in children with cancer. *Journal of Pediatric Hematology/Oncology Nursing*, *40*(2), 91–99. https://doi.org/10.1177/27527530221140056.

Patel, P., Robinson, P. D., Phillips, R., Baggott, C., Devine, K., Gibson, P., Guilcher, G. M. T., Holdsworth, M. T., Neumann, E., Orsey, A. D., Spinelli, D., Thackray, J., van de Wetering, M., Cabral, S., Sung, L., & Dupuis, L. L. (2023). Treatment of breakthrough and prevention of refractory chemotherapy-induced nausea and vomiting in pediatric cancer patients: Clinical practice guideline update. *Pediatric Blood and Cancer*, *70*(8), e30395. https://doi.org/10.1002/pbc.30395.

Phillips, R. S., Friend, A. J., Gibson, F., Houghton, E., Gopaul, S., Craig, J. V., & Pizer, B. (2016). Antiemetic medication for prevention and treatment of chemotherapy-induced nausea and vomiting in childhood. *Cochrane Database of Systematic Reviews*, *2016*(2), CD007786. https://doi.org/10.1002/14651858.CD007786.pub3.

Radossi, A. L., Taromina, K., Marjerrison, S., Diorio, C. J., Similio, R., Njuguna, F., Afungchwi, G. M., & Ladas, E. J. (2018). A systematic review of integrative clinical trials for supportive care in pediatric oncology: a report from the International Society of Pediatric Oncology, T&CM collaborative. *Supportive Care in Cancer*, *26*(2), 375–391. https://doi.org/10.1007/s00520-017-3908-0.

Raybin, J. L., Barr, E., Krajicek, M., & Jones, J. (2020). How does creative arts therapy reduce distress for children with cancer? A metasynthesis of extant qualitative literature. *Journal of Pediatric Oncology Nursing*, *37*(2), 91–104.

Reis, D., Güthlin, C., Schildmann, J., Zuzak, T. J., Hilje, C. C., & Längler, A. (2019). Information and training needs of pediatric oncologists in complementary and integrative medicine: A cross-sectional study. *Journal of Pediatric Hematology/Oncology*, *41*(7), 551–556. https://doi.org/10.1097/MPH.0000000000001578.

Robb, S. L., Burns, D. S., Stegenga, K. A., Haut, P. R., Monahan, P. O., Meza, J., Stump, T. E., Cherven, B. O., Docherty, S. L., Hendricks-Ferguson, V. L., Kintner, E. K., Haight, A. E., Wall, D. A., & Haase, J. E. (2014). Randomized clinical trial of therapeutic music video intervention for resilience outcomes in adolescents/young adults undergoing hematopoietic stem cell transplant: A report from the Children's Oncology Group. *Cancer*, *120*(6), 909–917. https://doi.org/10.1002/cncr.28355.

Robb, S. L., Haase, J. E., Perkins, S. M., Haut, P. R., Henley, A. K., Knafl, K. A., & Tong, Y. (2017). Pilot randomized trial of active music engagement intervention parent delivery for young children with cancer. *Journal of Pediatric Psychology*, *42*(2), 208–219. https://doi.org/10.1093/jpepsy/jsw050.

Rodgers, C., Kollar, D., Taylor, O., Bryant, R., Crockett, K., Gregurich, M. A., & Hockenberry, M. (2012). Nausea and vomiting perspectives among children receiving moderate to highly emetogenic chemotherapy treatment. *Cancer Nursing*, *35*(3), 203–210. https://doi.org/10.1097/NCC.0b013e3182281493.

Ruggiero, A., Rizzo, D., Catalano, M., Coccia, P., Triarico, S., & Attiná, G. (2018). Acute chemotherapy-induced nausea and vomiting in children with cancer: Still waiting for a common consensus on treatment. *Journal of International Medical Research*, *46*(6), 2149–2156. https://doi.org/10.1177/0300060518765324.

Şancı, Y., Yıldız, S., Ayçiçek, A., & Möhür, N. (2023). Effect of peppermint-lemon aromatherapy on nausea-vomiting and quality of life in pediatric patients with leukemia: A randomized controlled trial. *Journal of Pediatric Nursing*, *72*, e217–e227. https://doi.org/10.1016/j.pedn.2023.07.001.

Semerci, R., Akgün Kostak, M., & Taşkın, C. (2022). The effect of using an interactive mobile application for the management of chemotherapy-induced nausea and vomiting in children: Randomized controlled study. *European Journal of Oncology Nursing*, *58*, 102121. https://doi.org/10.1016/j.ejon.2022.102121.

Sherani, F., Boston, C., & Mba, N. (2019). Latest update on prevention of acute chemotherapy-induced nausea and vomiting in pediatric cancer patients. *Current Oncology Reports*, *21*(10), 89. https://doi.org/10.1007
/s11912-019-0840-0.

Uggla, L., Bonde, L. O., Hammar, U., Wrangsjö, B., & Gustafsson, B. (2018). Music therapy supported the health-related quality of life for children undergoing haematopoietic stem cell transplants. *Acta Paediatrica, International Journal of Paediatrics*, *107*(11), 1986–1994. https://doi.org/10.1111/apa.14515.

Varejão, C. da S., & Santo, F. H. d. E. (2019). Laser acupuncture for relieving nausea and vomiting in pediatric patients undergoing chemotherapy: A single-blind randomized clinical trial. *Journal of Pediatric Oncology Nursing*, *36*(1), 44–54. https://doi.org/10.1177/1043454218810140.

Velez-Florez, G., Velez-Florez, M. C., Mantilla-Rivas, J. O., Patarroyo-Rodríguez, L., Borrero-León, R., & Rodríguez-León, S. (2018). Mind-body therapies in childhood cancer. *Current Psychiatry Reports*, *20*(8), 58. https://doi.org/10.1007/s11920-018-0927-6.

Vol, H., Flank, J., Lavoratore, S. R., Nathan, P. C., Taylor, T., Zelunka, E., Maloney, A. M., & Lee Dupuis, L. (2016). Poor chemotherapy-induced nausea and vomiting control in children receiving intermediate or high dose methotrexate. *Supportive Care in Cancer*, *24*(3), 1365–1371. https://doi.org/10.1007/s00520-015-2924-1.

Walsh, A. M., Hess, J., Rees, M., Wetmore, C., & Vadiya, V. (2021). Creation of a chemotherapy-induced nausea/vomiting dashboard to improve outcomes for pediatric cancer patients. *Supportive Care in Cancer*, *29*(3), 1549–1555. https://doi.org/10.1007/s00520-020-05652-1.

Ward, J. A., Balian, C., Gilger, E., Raybin, J. L., Li, Z., & Montgomery, K. E. (2020). Electronic symptom assessment in children and adolescents with advanced cancer undergoing hematopoietic stem cell transplantation. *Journal of Pediatric Oncology Nursing : Official Journal of the Association of Pediatric Oncology Nurses*, *37*(4), 255–264. https://doi.org/10.1177/1043454220917686.

World Health Organization. (2018). *The Global Initiative for Childhood Cancer*. https://www.who.int/initiatives/the-global-initiative-for-childhood-cancer.

Yamaguchi, A., Saito, Y., Takekuma, Y., & Sugawara, M. (2024). Palonosetron for prevention of delayed chemotherapy-induced nausea and vomiting in pediatric patients: a meta-analysis. *Supportive Care in Cancer*, *32*, 58. https://doi.org/10.1007/s00520-023-08283-4.

Yurdakul, Z., Sezer, T. A., & Esenay, F. I. (2021). The effect of concealing the hydration fluid on anticipatory nausea-vomiting in pediatric hematology-oncology patients undergoing chemotherapy treatment: A randomized controlled study. *Journal of Pediatric Nursing*, *59*, 181–187. https://doi.org/10.1016/
j.pedn.2021.04.021.

Zhao, H., Weng, J., Shi, W., Pan, L., Lin, C., Wang, N., Zhu, J., & Shen, Z. (2023). Age of pediatric patients affects delayed chemotherapy–induced vomiting. *Clinical Pediatrics*, *26*, 99228231206708. https://doi.org/10.1177/00099228231206708.

Chapter 18

Evidence-Based Nursing Practices in Mucositis in Pediatric Oncology

Aysel Topan[1], PhD
and Betül Akkoç[2,*], MSc
[1]Department of Pediatric Nursing, Faculty of Health Sciences, Bülent Ecevit University, Zonguldak, Türkiye
[2]Department of Pediatric Service, Bartın Maternity and Children's Hospital, Bartın, Türkiye

Abstract

Evidence-based practices solidify the management of care provided by pediatric nurses, who are responsible for the care of child patients, making it both valid and reliable. It is within the roles and responsibilities of pediatric nurses to ensure universal care management through the application of current, scientifically supported, evidence-based care practices. Evidence-based approaches are particularly crucial in managing oral mucositis, one of the most common treatment complications encountered by pediatric cancer patients. Alongside their fundamental roles and responsibilities as researchers, educators, counselors, and providers of care based on scientific data, pediatric nurses must be knowledgeable about the pathophysiology of oral mucositis, its risk factors, grading systems, and care practices to prevent its occurrence. This book chapter discusses evidence-based practices for the management of oral mucositis in pediatric cancer patients, illuminated by scientific data and literature.

Keywords: children, evidence-based practices, nurse, oral mucositis, pediatric oncology

Introduction

Globally, approximately 160,000 children under the age of 14 receive a cancer diagnosis for the first time each year. Treatment of pediatric cancer and its associated side effects significantly impact the lives of the child and their family negatively (Gardner et al., 2017). Among the side effects encountered in clinical settings due to cancer treatment methods such as chemotherapy, radiotherapy, and stem cell transplantation is oral mucositis, a painful and

* Corresponding Author's Email: betulakkoc89@hotmail.com.

In: Evidence-Based Care Practices in Pediatric Nursing
Editors: Feyza Küçük and Serap Özdemir
ISBN: 979-8-89530-304-7

distressing condition. Managing care for pediatric cancer patients with oral mucositis, planning care based on evidence-based practices, and reducing their pain and discomfort are among the roles and responsibilities of pediatric nurses (Chan & Ismail, 2014; Çakır, Altay & Kılıçarslan Törüner, 2022).

Definition of Oral Mucositis

Oral mucositis is an inflammation observed in the oral mucosa of patients undergoing cancer treatment with chemotherapy or radiotherapy. It is characterized by erythema in the oral cavity, edema on the tongue, dry mouth, burning and bleeding on the lips, and a white superficial inflammation (Bell & Kasi, 2023).

Epidemiology of Oral Mucositis

The incidence of oral mucositis varies based on the individual's age, diagnosis, oral hygiene, and the chemotherapeutic drug. The prevalence of oral mucositis among patients receiving standard chemotherapy treatment is approximately 15-40% (Çakmak & Nural, 2019).

According to a study using the World Health Organization (WHO) oral toxicity grading scale, 63.1% of patients developed Stage 1, 38.5% developed Stage 2, and 15.6% developed Stage 3-4 oral mucositis (Marcadante, 2015). Particularly in childhood cancers such as lymphoma and leukemia, 35-76% of treated children develop oral mucositis (Miranda-Silva et al., 2021). The frequency of oral mucositis in children is three times higher than in adult patients (Devi & Allenidekania, 2019).

Etiology and Symptoms of Oral Mucositis

Oral mucositis can develop due to the chemotherapeutic drugs used by the patient, as well as factors such as the patient's age, gender, body mass index, nutrition, adequacy of oral hygiene, genetic factors, and whether they have acute or chronic illnesses (Karadakovan, 2014). The initial signs and symptoms of oral mucositis include ulceration accompanied by dryness, redness, bleeding, and pain in the mouth and lips (Hong, Gueiros, Fulton et al., 2019). Additionally, patients may experience loss of appetite, loss of taste and smell, difficulty swallowing, and edema on the tongue (Erdem & Güngörmüş, 2014).

Pathophysiology of Oral Mucositis

The primary objective of cancer treatment is to destroy or damage cancerous cells. However, this treatment also adversely affects healthy cells, a notable example being the destruction of epithelial cells in the oral cavity. Following the deformation of cells in the oral mucosa, their regeneration time is typically rapid. Nevertheless, exposure to chemotherapeutic agents results in a delay in the renewal and repair of these cells (Bell & Kasi, 2023).

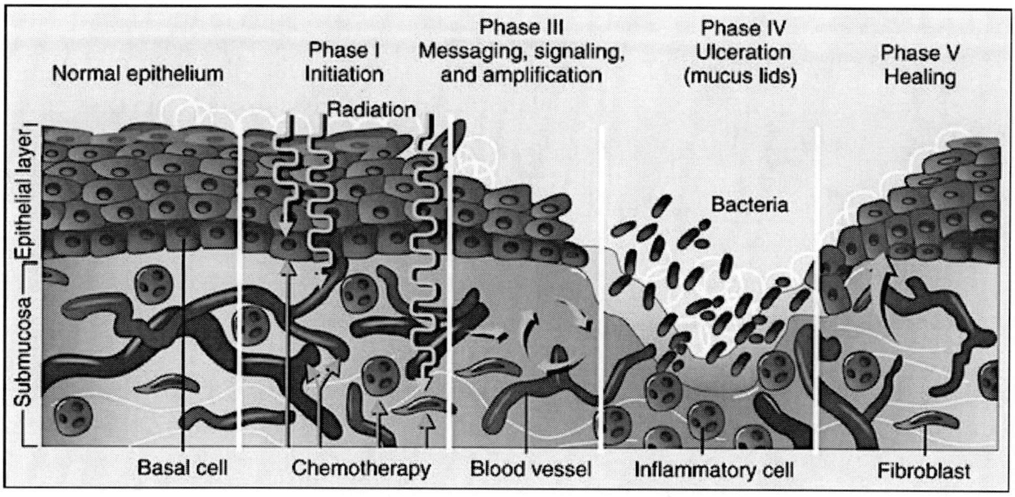

Figure 1. Pathophysiology of Oral Mucositis.

The pathophysiology of oral mucositis unfolds in five stages.

- *Stage 1: Initiation*
  Following chemotherapy treatment, rapid tissue damage occurs. In the basal epithelium and submucosa, the destruction of deoxyribonucleic acid (DNA) and non-DNA damage leads to the formation of reactive oxygen species (ROS). These cells cause damage to healthy tissues and increase the release of nuclear factor-kB (NF-kB), leading to secondary damage. At this stage, the mucosa appears normal (Karadakovan, 2014; Bell & Kasi, 2023).
- *Stage 2: Damage Response and Signal Generation*
  The destruction of DNA and the resulting reactive oxygen species activate transcription factors, initiating the damage response mechanism. Such activation leads to an increase in inflammatory cytokines and further tissue damage. The integrity of the oral mucosa is compromised, and erythema may be observed, although patients may not report discomfort (Karadakovan, 2014; Bell & Kasi, 2023).
- *Stage 3: Signal Amplification*
  The compromised integrity of the oral mucosa creates an entry point for bacteria, viruses, and fungi, accumulating microorganisms that cause damage. Colonies formed in this area initiate the wound formation process by causing further tissue damage with the substances they secrete (Karadakovan, 2014; Bell & Kasi, 2023).
- *Stage 4: Ulceration*
  The disruption of the oral mucosa's integrity and the settlement of microorganisms into the submucosa lead to the development of lesions. This process typically occurs between days 5 and 8, while patients may experience difficulties meeting needs such as oral care and nutrition between days 6 and 12 (Karadakovan, 2014; Bell & Kasi, 2023).

- *Stage 5: Healing*
  The healing process of the oral mucosa begins with the stimulation of the extracellular matrix and mesenchymal cells in the submucosa. Damaged epithelial cells migrate to the area, covering and proliferating on the surface to repair the mucosa. Healing occurs between days 12 and 16 following the treatment (Karadakovan, 2014; Bell & Kasi, 2023).

Assessment of Oral Mucositis

The primary objective of pediatric nurses in assessing oral mucositis is to identify the care needs of children with cancer for oral mucositis, to prevent the development of oral mucositis, and to provide appropriate care under the guidance of care guidelines for any mucositis that occurs (Yurdakul & Esenay, 2018; Çakir & Altay, 2022).

Different scales are used to administer care in the assessment and classification of oral mucositis. The most commonly used scales include the World Health Organization's (WHO) scale, based on objective signs of mucositis, such as erythema and ulceration, alongside the ability to eat and drink. Another significant tool is the adverse event reporting system used by the National Cancer Institute (NCI-CTC) (Yavuz, Yılmaz & Karaman, 2011; Jacobs et al., 2013).

However, the number of validated scales to assess oral mucositis in children is insufficient. The International Children's Mucositis Evaluation Scale (ChIMES), which has international validity and reliability, is used specifically for children (Jacobs et al., 2013).

Table 1. World Health Organization Mucositis Classification

Grade	Erythema	Inflammation	Edema	Ulceration	Bleeding and Necrosis
Stage 0	-	-	-	-	-
Stage 1	+	+	-	-	-
Stage 2	+	+/-	+/-	+/-	-
Stage 3	+	+	+/-	+/-	-
Stage 4	+	+	+	+	+

Table 2. Adverse Event Reporting System Used by the National Cancer Institute (NCI-CTC)

Grade	Erythema	Inflammation	Edema	Ulceration	Nutrition
Stage 0	-	-	-	-	+
Stage 1	+	+	-	-	+
Stage 2	+	+	+	+	+ (liquid and solid food)
Stage 3	+	+	+	+	- (liquid nutrition)
Stage 4	+	+	+	+	- Enteral nutrition if oral intake is not possible

The International Children's Mucositis Assessment Scale (ChIMES) was developed by Tomlinson et al. (2010) to evaluate oral mucositis in children receiving chemotherapy. The scale is designed to determine the presence or absence of oral mucositis, the intensity of pain, and the difficulty due to pain caused by swallowing. It comprises questions rated on a scale from 0 to 5, with 0 being the lowest score and 5 the highest possible score, and the maximum total score from all items being 23. A higher total score on the scale indicates an increased severity of oral mucositis (Tomlinson et al., 2010).

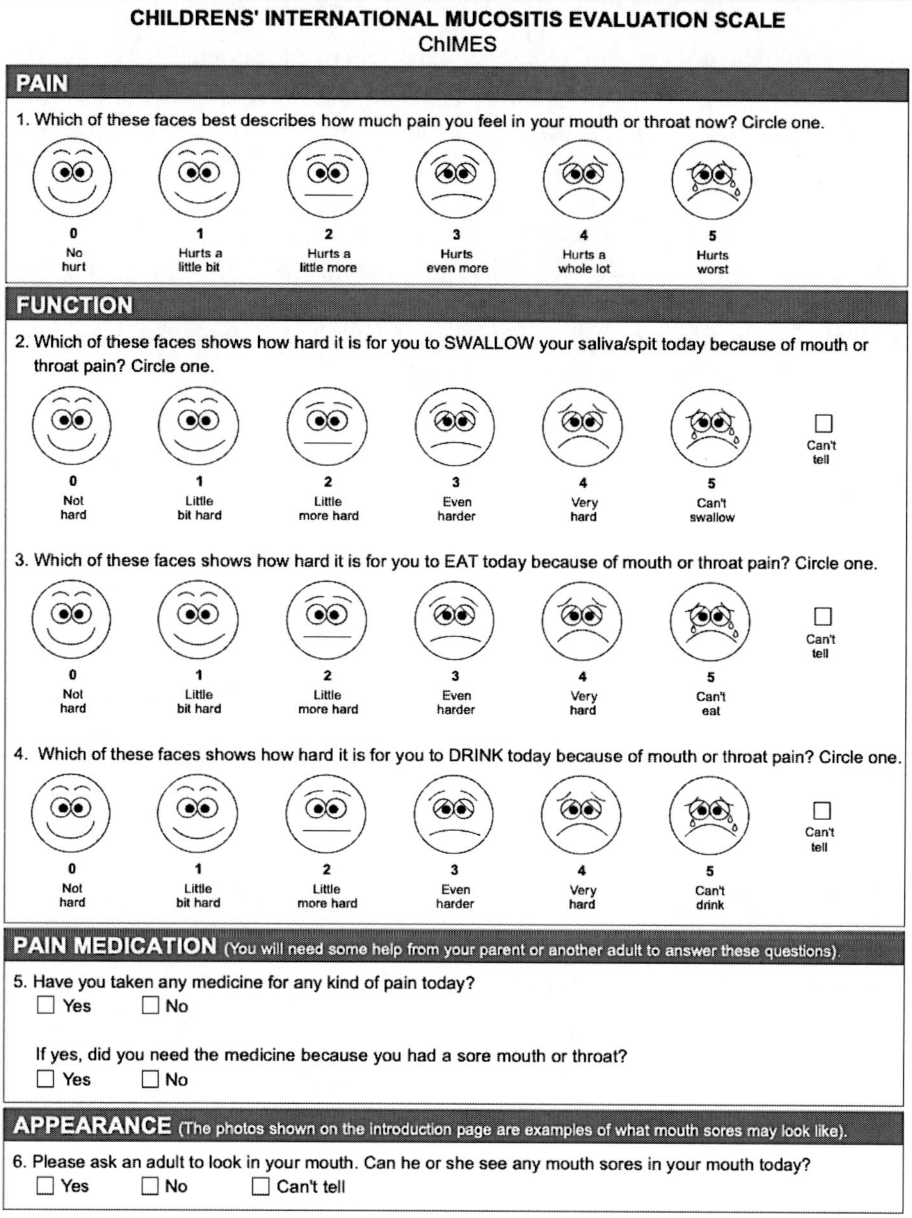

CHILDRENS' INTERNATIONAL MUCOSITIS EVALUATION SCALE
ChIMES

PAIN

1. Which of these faces best describes how much pain you feel in your mouth or throat now? Circle one.

0 No hurt | 1 Hurts a little bit | 2 Hurts a little more | 3 Hurts even more | 4 Hurts a whole lot | 5 Hurts worst

FUNCTION

2. Which of these faces shows how hard it is for you to SWALLOW your saliva/spit today because of mouth or throat pain? Circle one.

0 Not hard | 1 Little bit hard | 2 Little more hard | 3 Even harder | 4 Very hard | 5 Can't swallow | ☐ Can't tell

3. Which of these faces shows how hard it is for you to EAT today because of mouth or throat pain? Circle one.

0 Not hard | 1 Little bit hard | 2 Little more hard | 3 Even harder | 4 Very hard | 5 Can't eat | ☐ Can't tell

4. Which of these faces shows how hard it is for you to DRINK today because of mouth or throat pain? Circle one.

0 Not hard | 1 Little bit hard | 2 Little more hard | 3 Even harder | 4 Very hard | 5 Can't drink | ☐ Can't tell

PAIN MEDICATION (You will need some help from your parent or another adult to answer these questions).

5. Have you taken any medicine for any kind of pain today?
☐ Yes ☐ No

If yes, did you need the medicine because you had a sore mouth or throat?
☐ Yes ☐ No

APPEARANCE (The photos shown on the introduction page are examples of what mouth sores may look like).

6. Please ask an adult to look in your mouth. Can he or she see any mouth sores in your mouth today?
☐ Yes ☐ No ☐ Can't tell

Figure 2. International Children's Mucositis Assessment Scale (ChIMES).

The Role and Responsibilities of Pediatric Nurses in the Management of Oral Mucositis

Oral mucositis is among the highest morbidity outcomes following treatment with chemotherapy, radiotherapy, or stem cell transplantation in pediatric patients. The significance of pediatric nurses' roles as caregivers, educators, and counselors becomes apparent in the management of oral mucositis. The experience of pain and intense treatment due to oral mucositis causes psychological and physiological stress in pediatric patients (Yavuz & Bal Yılmaz, 2015). The prevention of mucositis and the provision of evidence-based care practices to manage oral mucositis, if it occurs, place significant roles and responsibilities on nurses to use appropriate evidence-based care guidelines and scales (Çakır, Altay & Kılıçarslan Törüner, 2022). While the literature is full of numerous care practices, nutritional approaches, and guidelines, they are often insufficient. The crucial role of nurses as researchers and developers in improving and updating these guidelines and in their monitoring is undeniable (Özdemir & Zülfikar, 2022).

Evidence-Based Approaches in Managing Oral Mucositis

Globally accepted care practices significantly contribute to ensuring patient safety in medical treatments. Implementing evidence-based practices aims to provide effective patient care, assess the quality of care, and elevate the patient's psychological, physical, and mental well-being to the highest level. Research indicates that there are effective, evidence-based care practices for managing oral mucositis. Despite the scarcity of studies based on the level of evidence and effectiveness, experimental research on oral mucositis management has been conducted (Friend, Rubagumya, & Cartledge, 2017).

Principal methods to prevent oral mucositis include:

Basic Oral Hygiene

Oral care protocols in pediatric cancer patients represent a critical approach to preventing oral mucositis. Health institutions implement standardized care practices. The objective of basic oral care is to maintain healthy oral mucosa and prevent inflammation. It is recommended that pediatric cancer patients engage in basic oral hygiene practices, including brushing their teeth at least twice daily and using oral care solutions. The most commonly recommended solutions are normal saline, sodium bicarbonate, chlorhexidine, and benzydamine (Çakır, Altay & Kılıçarslan Törüner, 2022).

1. *Normal Saline*: Although it has minimal side effects, its effectiveness is considered insufficient when used alone or in combination, rendering it an option with inadequate evidence (Hong et al., 2019).
2. *Sodium Bicarbonate*: It is often preferred in clinical settings for children and adults due to its lack of side effects. However, its efficacy in treating oral mucositis lacks sufficient evidence; therefore, its evidence level is considered low (Al Jaouni et al., 2017).

3. *Chlorhexidine Gluconate*: An antiseptic agent that is effective against microorganisms. Studies support its use in reducing the severity and pain associated with oral mucositis (Mallick, Benson & Rath, 2016; Papadopoulou et al., 2014). However, it is not recommended for patients undergoing cancer treatments such as radiotherapy, chemotherapy, and bone marrow transplantation due to insufficient evidence. More research is needed to prevent and treat oral mucositis with chlorhexidine gluconate (Konuk Sener et al., 2019; Gholizadeh et al., 2016).
4. *Benzydamine:* A non-steroidal anti-inflammatory agent (Chaveli-López & Bagán-Sebastián, 2016). The Multinational Association of Supportive Care in Cancer (MASCC) and the International Society of Oral Oncology (ISOO) have indicated in their current guidelines for pediatric patients that there is no high-level evidence for the efficacy of benzydamine solutions (Sydor, 2019; Elad et al., 2020; Miranda-Silva et al., 2021). Nicolatou-Galitis et al. (2013) revealed that it effectively reduces pain and prevents oral mucositis in children over 6 years of age (Nicolatou-Galitis et al., 2013). However, a study by Hashemi et al. (2015) found the efficacy of benzydamine limited in pediatric patients (Hashemi et al., 2015). Nevertheless, for cancer patients receiving radiotherapy, benzydamine solutions have shown significant evidence to prevent oral mucositis (Sydor, 2019). Further studies with larger sample sizes and higher levels of evidence are needed to address contradictions and confirm its efficacy.

Cryoprotective Agents

Cryoprotective agents assist in the production of mucus secretion and the stimulation of blood flow within the gastrointestinal system. Evidence-based practices primarily involve using vitamin E and glutamine as cryoprotective agents (Yarom et al., 2019).

1. *Vitamin E* protects the cell membrane, thereby reducing the severity of oral mucositis. With their anti-inflammatory properties, vitamin E supplements can be used in the treatment of pediatric patients undergoing radiotherapy and chemotherapy (He et al., 2018). A study by Khurana et al. (2013) compared the efficacy of vitamin E and pine bark extract with chlorhexidine, finding that both vitamin E and pine bark extract are effective in healing, with no significant differences between them (Khurana et al., 2013). Topical treatment with vitamin E in pediatric cancer patients is considered more effective than systemic vitamin E treatments, recognizing it as an effective therapy in reducing the severity of oral mucositis (Chaitanya et al., 2017; Slade, 2019).
2. *Glutamine* is an amino acid that plays an active role in cell proliferation and is the most abundant in plasma (Chaitanya et al., 2017). A study by Ward et al. (2009) noted that high-dose oral glutamine did not reduce oral mucositis's severity or pain intensity, whereas intravenous application significantly decreased it. Chang et al. (2017) indicated that intravenous glutamine administration could prevent oral mucositis without side effects (Chang et al., 2017). The MASCC/ISOO guidelines mention that intravenous glutamine application in pediatric patients undergoing stem cell transplantation is not effective, but oral glutamine administration can effectively reduce pain (Elad et al., 2020; Miranda-Silva et al., 2021). Due to insufficient evidence, more research is needed to prevent and treat oral mucositis.

Palifermin (Biological Response Modifier)

Palifermin is a protein produced by mesenchymal cells that stimulates cellular responses, preventing mucositis through the proliferation and differentiation of cells along the gastrointestinal tract. Its effectiveness in preventing oral mucositis in pediatric cancer patients, especially those undergoing stem cell transplantation, is supported by studies (Vadhan-Raj et al., 2013; Vitale et al., 2014; Lauritano et al., 2014; Gholizadeh et al., 2016; Morris et al., 2016). However, due to the lack of sufficient evidence, further research is warranted.

Natural Products

Honey, propolis, and beeswax are natural products that prevent oral mucositis. Honey creates an acidic environment in the oral cavity, inhibiting bacterial growth, and is known for its antioxidant and anti-inflammatory properties due to its polyphenol content (Bulut & Tüfekçi 2016). Its low cost, natural composition, accessibility, and lack of side effects support its use in pediatric cancer patients (Bulut & Tüfekçi, 2016; Kobya-Bulut & Guducu-Tufekci, 2016; Al Jaouni et al., 2017; Singh et al., 2019). However, the level of evidence to reduce the severity of oral mucositis is considered insufficient.

Physical Therapies

Physical interventions to treat oral mucositis include laser therapy and the application of ice cubes (cryotherapy).

1. *Laser Therapy*: Laser therapy, using wavelengths of 630-650 nm and 780-900 nm, stimulates collagen structure, promotes cell proliferation, and prevents mucositis formation. It has been found to have anti-inflammatory and analgesic effects, particularly beneficial for wounds that do not heal over a long period (He et al., 2018; Elad et al., 2020). A study by Kuhn et al. (2009) with pediatric cancer patients aged 3-18 years showed an acceleration in the healing of oral mucositis (Kuhn et al., 2009). It has been observed that the use of laser as a preventative method in pediatric cancer patients reduces the risk of oral mucositis (Castro et al., 2013), weekly sessions of low-intensity laser therapy heal lesions in the oral cavity (Cauwels & Martens, 2011), and it prevents the development of stages 3 and 4 oral mucositis in patients undergoing bone marrow transplantation (Eduardo et al., 2015), proving to be an effective method of pain reduction (Amadori et al., 2016; Silva et al., 2018). While MASCC/ISOO recommends its use for adults, limited studies and small pediatric populations render the evidence level insufficient (Elad et al., 2020).
2. *Cryotherapy*: Involves the application of ice cubes or chips. Ice cubes reduce blood flow through vasoconstriction, thereby decreasing the severity of oral mucositis (Marin, 2019; Chaveli-López & Bagán-Sebastián, 2016). The MASCC/ISOO Clinical Practice Guidelines recommend 30 minutes of oral cryotherapy during chemotherapy (Elad et al., 2020). Studies support cryotherapy as an effective method in adult cancer patients (Peterson et al., 2013; Riley et al., 2015; Marchesi et al., 2017; Park & Lee, 2019; Lu et al., 2020). For pediatric cancer patients, the literature indicates its efficacy. Sato et al. (2006) found that the combined use of propantheline and cryotherapy reduced the risk of oral mucositis in pediatric cancer patients,

decreasing the oral cavity temperature to 20°C and effectively preventing oral mucositis (Walladbegi et al., 2018), and flavored ice cubes proved to be more effective than plain ones (Mishra & Nayak, 2017). Cryotherapy is a cost-effective, minimally invasive, and accessible treatment for pediatric cancer patients who are conscious during chemotherapy. However, the scarcity of studies in the pediatric population does not provide a strong level of evidence (Sung et al., 2017).

Conclusion

The treatment and approaches to oral mucositis in pediatric cancer patients vary depending on the type of disease and the treatment method. Although the methods used in oral mucositis care approaches vary, there are studies with high and insufficient evidence levels. Pediatric nurses should adopt care protocols prepared according to universally accepted, evidence-based practice guidelines. They are advised to stay abreast of current developments and integrate them into their care practices. Studies that will contribute to advancing care practices should be conducted based on high-level evidence studies.

Disclaimer

None.

References

Al Jaouni SK, Al Muhayawi MS, Husssein A, Elfiki I, Al Raddadi R, Al Muhayawi S. et al. (2017). Effects of honey on oral mucositis among pediatric cancer patients undergoing chemo/radiotherapy treatment at King Abdulaziz University Hospital in Jeddah, Kingdom of Saudi Arabia. *Evid Based Complement Aternat Med.*, 2017:5861024.

Amadori F, Bardellini E, Conti G, Pedrini N, Schumacher RF, Majorana A. (2016). Low-level laser therapy for treatment of chemotherapy-induced oral mucositis in childhood: a randomized double-blind controlled study. *Lasers Med Sci.*, Aug;31(6):1231-6. doi: 10.1007/s10103-016-1975-y. Epub 2016 Jun 6. PMID: 27272517.

Bell A, Kasi A. (2023) Oral Mucositis. May 29. In: StatPearls [Internet]. Treasure Island (FL): StatPearls Publishing; 2024 Jan–. PMID: 33351407.

Bulut HK, Tüfekçi FG. (2016). Honey prevents oral mocositis in children undergoing chemotherapy: A quasi-experimental study with a control group. *Complement Ther Med.*, 29:132-40.

Castro JFL, Abreu EGF, Correia AVL, Mota Vasconcelos Brasil C, Cruz Perez DE,Paula Ramos Pedrosa F. (2013). Low-level laser in prevention and treatment of oral mucositis in pediatric patients with acute lymphoblastic leukemia. *Photomed Laser Surg.*, 31(12):613-8.

Cauwels RG, Martens LC. (2011). Low level laser therapy in oral mucositis: a pilot study. *Eur Arch Paediatr Dent.,* 12(2):118-23.

Chaitanya NC, Muthukrishnan A, Babu DBG, Kumari CS, Lakshmi MA, Palat G, et al. (2017). Role of vitamin E and vitamin A in oral mucositis induced by cancer chemo/radiotherapy- a meta-analysis. *J Clin Diagn Res.*, 11(5):6-9.

Chan, HK., & Ismail, S. (2014). Side Effects of Chemotherapy among Cancer Patients in a Malaysian General Hospital: Experiences, Perceptions and Informational Needs from Clinical Pharmacists. *Asian*

Pacific Journal of Cancer Prevention, 15(13), 5305–5309. https://doi.org/10.7314/apjcp.2014.15.13.5305.

Chang YH, Yu MS, Wu KH, Hsu MC, Chiou YH, Wu HP, et al. (2017). Effectiveness of parenteral glutamine on methotrexate-induced oral mucositis in children with acute lymphoblastic leukemia. *Nutr Cancer*, 69(5):751-65.

Chaveli-López, B, & Bagán-Sebastián, J V. (2016). "Treatment of oral mucositis due to chemotherapy." *Journal of Clinical and Experimental Dentistry*, 8 (2), e201.

Çakir G, Altay N, Kiliçarslan Törüner E. (2022). Kemoterapi Alan Pediatrik Onkoloji Hastalarında Oral Mukozit Yönetimi: Kanıt Temelli Uygulamaların Değerlendirilmesi. *Johufon,* 9(2):225-32.

Çakmak S, Nural N. (2019). Incidence of and risk factors for development of oral mucositis in outpatients undergoing cancer chemotherapy. *Int J Nurs Pract*., 25(1):e12710.

Devi KS, Allenidekania A. (2019). The Relationship of Oral Care Practice at Home with Incidence in Children with Acute Lymphoblastic Leukemia. *Comprehensive Child and Adolescent Nursing*, 42(1): 56-64.

Eduardo FP, Bezinelli LM, Carvalho DL, Lopes RM, Fernandes JF, Brumatti M, et al. (2015). Oral mucositis in pediatric patients undergoing hematopoietic stem cell transplantation: clinical outcomes in a context of specialized oral care using low-level laser therapy. *Pediatr Transplant*., 19(3):316-25.

Elad S, Cheng KKF, Lalla RV, Yarom N, Hong C, Logan RM, Bowen J, Gibson R, Saunders DP, Zadik Y, Ariyawardana A, Correa ME, Ranna V, Bossi P. (2020). Mucositis Guidelines Leadership Group of the Multinational Association of Supportive Care in Cancer and International Society of Oral Oncology (MASCC/ISOO). MASCC/ISOO clinical practice guidelines for the management of mucositis secondary to cancer therapy. *Cancer*, Oct 1;126(19):4423-4431. doi: 10.1002/cncr.33100. Epub 2020 Jul 28. Erratum in: Cancer. 2021 Oct 1;127(19):3700. PMID: 32786044; PMCID: PMC7540329.

Erdem B, Güngörmüş Z. (2014) Kanser Hastalarında Oral Mukozit ve Yaşam Kalitesi. *Acıbadem Üniversitesi Sağlık Bilimleri Dergisi*, 25-29.

Friend, A, Rubagumya, F, & Cartledge, P. (2017). "Global Health Journal Club: Is Honey Effective as a Treatment for Chemotherapy-induced Mucositis in Paediatric Oncology Patients?." *Journal of Tropical Pediatrics,* 64 (2), 162-168.

Gardner, M. H., Mrug, S., Schwebel, D. C., Phipps, S., Whelan, K., & Madan-Swain, A. (2017). Demographic, medical, and psychosocial predictors of benefit finding among caregivers of childhood cancer survivors. *Psycho-Oncology*, 26(1), pon.4014 125–132. https://doi.org/10.1002/

Gholizadeh N, Mehdipoor M, Sajadi H, Moosavi MS. (2016). Palifermin and hlorhexidine mouthwashes in prevention of chemotherapy-ınduced mucositis in children with acute lymphocytic leukemia: a randomized controlled trial. *J Dent.,* 17(4):343-7.

Hashemi A, Bahrololoumi Z, Khaksar Y, Saffarzadeh N, Neamatzade H, Foroughi E. (2015). Mouth-rinses for the prevention of chemotherapy induced oral mucositis in children: A systematic review. *Iran J Ped Hematol Oncol*., 5(2):106-12.

He M, Zhang B, Shen N, Wu N, Sun J. (2018). A systematic review and meta-analysis of the effect of low-level laser therapy (LLLT) on chemotherapy-induced oral mucositis in pediatric and young patients. *Eur J Pediatr*., 177(1):7-17.

Hong CHL, Gueiros LA, Fulton JS, Cheng KKF, Kandwal A, Galiti D, et al. (2019). Systematic review of basic oral care for the management mucositis in cancer patients and clinical of oral practice guidelines. *Support Care Cancer*., 27(10):3949 67.

Jacobs S, Baggott C, Agarwal R et al. (2013). Validation of the Children's International Mucositis Evaluation Scale (ChIMES) in Paediatric Cancer and SCT. *British Journal of Cancer*, 109(10): 2515.

Karadakovan A. (2014). Semptom Yönetimi: Mukozit. In: Can G. editor. Onkoloji Hemşireliği. İstanbul, Nobel Tıp Kitabevi s: 371-383.

Khurana H, Pandey RK, Saksena AK, Kumar A. (2013). An evaluation of Vitamin E and Pycnogenol in children suffering from oral mucositis during cancer chemotherapy. *Oral Dis.,* 19(5):456-64.

Kobya-Bulut H, Guducu-Tufekci F. (2016). Honey prevents oral mucositis in children undergoing chemotherapy: A quasi-experimental study with a control group. Complement Ther Med. 2016; 29:132-40.

Konuk Sener D, Aydin M, Cangur S, Guven E. (2019). The effect of oral care with chlorhexidine, vitamin e and honey on mucositis in pediatric intensive care patients: A randomized controlled trial. *J Pediatr Nurs.*, 45: 95-101.

Lauritano D, Petruzzı M, Dı Stasıo D, Lucchese A. (2014). Clinical effectiveness of palifermin in prevention and treatment of oral mucositis in children with acute lymphoblastic leukaemia: a case–control study. *Int J Dent Oral Sci.,* 6(1):27-30.

Lu Y, Zhu X, Ma Q, et al. (2020). Oral cryotherapy for oral mucositis management in patients receiving allogeneic hematopoietic stem cell transplantation: a prospective randomized study. *Support Care Cancer*. 28:1747-1754.

Mallick, S, Benson, R, & Rath, G K. (2016). "Radiation induced oral mucositis: a review of current literature on prevention and management." *European Archives of Oto Rhino-Laryngology*, 273 (9), 2285-2293.

Marcadante T. (2015). Prevalence of oral mucositis, dry mouth, and dysphagia in advanced cancer patients. *Support Care Cancer*, 34-41. 66 78. 79. 80. 81. 82. 83.

Marchesi F, Tendas A, Giannarelli D, et al. (2017). Cryotherapy reduces oral mucositis and febrile episodes in myeloma patients treated with high-dose melphalan and autologous stem cell transplant: a prospective, randomized study. *Bone Marrow Transplant.*, 52:154-156.

Marin T. (2019b). Oral mucositis: Cryotherapy. *JBI Evidence Summary*. 1-2.

Miranda-Silva W, Gomes-Silva W, Zadik Y, Yarom N, Al-Azri AR, Hong CHL, Ariyawardana A, Saunders DP, et al. (2021). MASCC/ISOO clinical practice guidelines for the management of mucositis: sub-analysis of current interventions for the management of oral mucositis in pedaitric cancer patients. *Support Care Cancer*. 29(7):3539-62.

Mishra L. Nayak G. (2017). Effect of flavoured ice chips in reduction of oral mucositis among children receiving chemotherapy. International Journal of Pharmaceutical Sciences *Review and Research*. 43(107):25-8.

Morris J, Rudebeck M, Neudorf S, Moore T, Graham M, Aquino V, et al. (2016). Safety, pharmacokinetics, and efficacy of palifermin in children and adolescents with acute leukemias undergoing myeloablative therapy and allogeneic hematopoietic stem cell transplantation: a pediatric blood and marrow transplant consortium trial. *Biol Blood Marrow Transplant.*, 22(7):1247-56.

Nicolatou-Galitis, O, Sarri, T, Bowen, J, Di Palma, M, Kouloulias, V E, Niscola, P, et al. (2013). "Systematic review of anti-inflammatory agents for the management of oral mucositis in cancer patients." *Supportive Care in Cancer*, 21 (11), 3179-3189.

Ozdemir, S., & Zülfikar, O. B. (2022). Kemoterapi alan lösemili çocuklarda hasta ailesi ve bakım veren hemşireye yapılan eğitimin oral mukozitlerin kontrolüne etkisi. *Göbeklitepe Sağlık Bilimleri Dergisi*, 5(8), 88-97.

Papadopoulou, K, Perdikaris, P, Patiraki, E, Giannakopoulou, M, Stamoulara, A, & Matziou, V. (2014). "Stomatitis in children with cancer." *Nursing Care & Research/Nosileia Kai Ereuna*, (40)

Park SH, Lee HS. (2019). Meta-analysis of oral cryotherapy in pre venting oral mucositis associated with cancer therapy. *Int J Nurs Pract.*, 25: e12759.

Peterson DE, Ohrn K, Bowen J, et al. (2013). Systematic review of oral cryotherapy for management of oral mucositis caused by cancer therapy. *Support Care Cancer*, 21:327-332.

Riley P, Glenny AM, Worthington HV, Littlewood A, Clarkson JE, McCabe MG. (2015). Interventions for preventing oral muco sitis in patients with cancer receiving treatment: Oral cryo therapy. *Cochrane Database Syst Rev.*,12):CD011552. doi:10.1002/14651858.CD011552.pub2.

Sato A, Saisho-Hattori T, Koizumi Y, Minegishi M, Iinuma K, Imaizumi M. (2006). Prophylaxis of mucosal toxicity by oral propantheline and cryotherapy in children with malignancies undergoing myeloablative chemo-radiotherapy. *Tohoku J Exp Med.*, 210: 315–20.

Silva VCR, Motta Silveira FM, Lima GS, Cruz MMD, Júnior ADFC, Godoy GP. (2018). Photodynamic therapy for treatment of oral mucositis: pilot study with pediatric patients undergoing chemotherapy. *Photodiagnosis Photodyn Ther.*,21:115-20.

Singh R, Sharma S, Kaur S, Medhi B, Trehan A, Bijarania SK. (2019). Effectiveness of topical application of honey on oral mucosa of children for the management of oral mucositis associated with chemotherapy. *Indian J Pediatr.*, 86(3):224 8.

Slade S. (2019). Oral mucositis: Treatment. *JBI Evidence Summary*.2.

Sung L, Robinson P, Treister N, Baggott T, Gibson P, Tissing W, et al. (2017). Guideline for the prevention of oral and oropharyngeal mucositis in children receiving treatment for cancer or undergoing haematopoietic stem cell transplantation. *BMJ Support Palliat Care*., 7(1):7-16.

Sydor A. (2019). Oral mucositis prevention: Benzydamine. *JBI Recommendation Practice*.3.

Tomlinson D, Gibson F, Treister N, Baggott C, Judd P, Hendershot E, et al. (2010). Refinement of the Children's International Mucositis Evaluation Scale (ChIMES): child and parent perspectives on understandability, content validity and acceptability. *Eur J Oncol Nurs.*, 14(1):29-41.

Vadhan-Raj S, Goldberg JD, Perales MA, Berger DP, Brink MR. (2013). Clinical applications of palifermin: amelioration of oral mucositis and other potential indications. *J Cell Mol Med.,* 17(11):1371-84.

Vitale KM, Violago L, Cofnas P, Bishop J, Jin Z, Bhatia M, et al. (2014). Impact of palifermin on incidence of oral mucositis and healthcare utilization in children undergoing autologous hematopoietic stem cell transplantation for malignant diseases. *Pediatr Transplant.,* 18(2):211-6.

Walladbegi J, Smith SA, Grayson AK, Murdoch C, Jontell M, Colley HE. (2018). Cooling of the oral mucosa to prevent adverse effects of chemotherapeutic agents: an in vitro study. *J Oral Pathol Med*., 47(5):477 83.

Ward E, Smıth M, Henderson M, Reıd U, Lewıs I, Kınsey S, et al. (2009). The effect of high-dose enteral glutamine on the incidence and severity of mucositis in paediatric oncology patients. *Eur J Clin Nutr*., 63(1):134-40.

Yarom N, Hovan A, Bossi P, Ariyawardana A, Jensen SB, Gobbo M, et al. (2019). Systematic review of natural and miscellaneous agents for the management of ora mucositis in cancer patients and clinical practice guidelines-part 1: vitamins, minerals, and nutritional supplements. *Supportive Care in Cancer*, 27:3997–4010.

Yavuz B, Yılmaz HB, Karaman N. (2011). Kanserli Çocuklarda Uluslararası Çocuk Mukozit Değerlendirme Ölçeği Türkçe Formunun Geçerlilik Güvenilirlik Çalışması. *Türk Onkoloji Dergisi*, 26(4): 157-162. doi: 10.5505/tjoncol.2011.688.

Yavuz, B, & Bal Yılmaz, H. (2015). "Investigation of the effects of planned mouth care education on the degree of oral mucositis in pediatric oncology patients." *Journal of Pediatric Oncology Nursing*, 32 (1), 47-56.

Yurdakul OZ, Esenay F. (2018). Kanserli Çocuklarda Oral Mukozit İçin Kullanılan Kanıta Dayalı Yöntemler: Sistematik Derleme. *Güncel Pediatri,* 16(3): 51-78.

Chapter 19

Evidence-Based Nursing Practices in Non-Pharmacological Procedural Pain Management in Children

Selver Mete İzci*, PhD

Department of Paediatric Clinic, Servergazi State Hospital, Ministry of Health, Türkiye

Abstract

As defined by the International Association for the Study of Pain, pain is an unpleasant sensory and emotional experience associated with, or similar to, actual or potential tissue damage. Hospital-based health monitoring, medical examinations, and treatments are often painful procedures. Pain associated with examinations, treatments, and procedures to which children are often exposed is called procedural pain. Procedural pain is common in children. Procedures such as the insertion of a peripheral venous catheter, blood sampling, heel-stick blood sampling in infants, finger-stick blood sampling in children, vaccinations, injections, lumbar puncture in children with cancer, and bone marrow aspiration may cause procedural pain. In the recognition, assessment, and management of pain, children are a special and vulnerable group. Pain is a factor that affects the satisfaction of children's and parents with healthcare services. Inadequate pain management in children can have both short- and long-term negative consequences. It can cause pain, anxiety, and stress, making it difficult to cope and delaying recovery. Exposure to pain in infancy may increase the risk of psychological problems (anxiety, depression) in later life. Non-pharmacological methods are used to manage and control procedural pain in children. Non-pharmacological methods can be used by children parents or nurses. Nurses have an important role to play in the management of procedural pain in children. Nurses should be aware of and use evidence-based non-pharmacological methods in clinical practice.

In this section, non-pharmacological methods such as non-nutritive sucking, positioning (swaddling, skin-to-skin contact), maternal voices, touch and massage intervention, age-appropriate distraction, and parental participation used to reduce procedural pain will be examined.

Keywords: procedural pain, non-pharmacological methods, children

* Corresponding Author's Email: selvermete50@gmail.com.

In: Evidence-Based Care Practices in Pediatric Nursing
Editors: Feyza Küçük and Serap Özdemir
ISBN: 979-8-89530-304-7

Introduction

Pain is a universal experience. Pain is with humans from birth to death (Arnstein, 2010). Pain is a subjective feeling of discomfort and a comprehensive response process consisting of sensation, emotion, cognition, and behavior (Jin et al., 2023). In 2020, the International Association for the Study of Pain updated the definition of pain. According to the new definition, pain is defined as "an unpleasant sensory and emotional experience associated with or defined by actual or potential tissue damage" (Raja et al., 2020). People need health services throughout their lives. Procedures required within the scope of health services can commonly cause pain (Wrona et al., 2022).

Newborns, babies, and children admitted to the hospital may be exposed to painful procedures during their examination and treatment, and such pains associated with medical care are defined as procedure pain (Wilson-Smith, 2011). The procedure pain is applied at a point in time and is expected to be in short duration. The techniques used to reduce pain should be teachable and practicable at the moment, not requiring time to learn and practice (Wrona et al., 2022).

Acute pain during medical procedures is common in children and adolescents and is often underestimated by healthcare professionals. In fact, pain that occurs during medical practice is very common, and it both burdens people economically and impairs their quality of life. Pain, the importance of which has only recently begun to be recognized, has not reached the value it deserves by healthcare professionals as other vital signs. All branches, including nursing, should be included in serious education on the assessment and management of pain (Hurley-Wallace et al., 2018). The American Pain Society coined the phrase "pain as a vital sign" to emphasize to healthcare professionals that pain is as important as other vital signs. Thus, the importance of pain for a complete and thorough evaluation of patients was emphasized. (American Pain Society,2000).

Although innovative and effective pain treatments are available for pain management, they are generally not well translated into practice. In current practice, pain is not treated, or inadequate analgesia is provided (Arnstein, 2010; Hurley-Wallace et al., 2018). The following may be reasons for inadequate pain management:

- Professional barriers- personal prejudices or a lack of knowledge
- Patient barriers- fears, misconceptions, poor communication, passivity
- Systemic obstacles- restricting policies and legislation, limited access to treatment

A common concern in all these barriers is inadequate pain assessment and misconceptions about pain and current treatments (Arnstein, 2010). In a descriptive and cross-sectional study in which nurses' perceptions of procedural pain assessment were examined, nurses participating in the study stated that pain assessment of infants was necessary for nursing care and was effective in reducing pain. However, it was reported that nurses did not routinely use pain assessment tools in their working practices and did not perform pain assessment regularly (Treiman-Kiveste et al., 2022).

Children want to feel safe and not lose control during medical procedures involving needles. Developing coping skills for medical procedures that cause pain is a personal experience. It is important to develop the child's personal coping strategies for managing medical procedures. It is important to both the child and the parents that health professionals are aware of the child's personal coping strategies. This awareness can improve the identification of the appropriate coping strategy and the compliance with the coping strategy (Segers et al., 2023). Using non-pharmacological distraction techniques based on children's personal preferences is more effective in managing procedure-related pain and providing better medical care (T. Shen et al., 2023).

Procedural pain management is a practice that is not used enough today in children. There are effective methods that can be used in the management of painful applications. However, despite all this, many nurses cannot provide adequate analgesia during painful procedures. In cases where conventional treatments are insufficient for pain management, additional non-pharmacological applications are also required (Bice et al., 2014). Non-pharmacological methods to reduce procedural pain should be known and applied by nurses (Yilmaz & Canbulat Sahiner, 2023).

Pain interferes with healing, immunity, and function. It can increase the risk of complications (Arnstein, 2010). Acute pain and distress are common in infants. Pain and distress that are not relieved in infancy can have lifelong consequences (Riddell et al., 2023). Effective pain management in healthcare affects both child and family satisfaction (Lambert et al., 2020).

Pain Mechanism and Classification

Pain can be broadly classified into 3 groups: nociceptive, neuropathic, or nociciplastic. As a result of the stimulation of pain receptors in the peripheral nervous system with various stimuli, afferent sensory neurons are activated and transmit the message to the cerebral cortex where pain is felt through the medulla spinalis, brain stem, and thalamus by making various synapses (Eccleston et al., 2021).

- *Nociceptive pain*: "Pain caused by actual or potential damage to non-neural tissue and resulting from the activation of nociceptors (nerves that sense pain). This is the mechanism at work in most everyday painful experiences and, when it is the result of an injury or damage, should be resolved when healing takes place". The mechanisms of nociceptive pain change as we progress with age.
- *Nociceptive pain*: "It occurs within an intact and normally functioning somatosensory nervous system and can therefore, to some extent, be considered normal pain because this is the mechanism of common everyday pain experienced after injury. This type of pain is usually predictable in duration and intensity and is the most common experience".
- *Neuropathic pain:* "Pain caused by a lesion or disease in the somatosensory nervous system.
- *Nociplastic pain*: Pain resulting from altered nociception despite no evidence of actual or threatened tissue damage causing activation of peripheral nociceptors or disease or lesion in the somatosensory system causing the pain".
- *Acute pain:* Pain lasting 3 months or less. Needle-related medical procedures are examples of acute pain (Eccleston et al., 2021).

Recognition and Assessment of Pain

Nurses communicate with patients more than other healthcare professionals due to nursing care. Therefore, nurses are in a good position to identify and evaluate patients' pain. The nurse should screen every patient for pain with a simple question. If pain is present, a more detailed assessment should be conducted. Nurses should be aware of pain assessment tools and be able to perform an appropriate pain assessment for the patient they care for (Arnstein, 2010).

- *Effective pain assessment tool characteristics*
  - It is easy to use.
  - It is sensitive enough to detect changes over time and responses to interventions.
  - Provides clinically meaningful data (Arnstein, 2010).
- *Characteristics of a multidimensional pain assessment tool*
  - Determine the underlying cause and mechanism of the pain.
  - Monitoring of the general condition and progress of the patients.
  - Explore the psychosocial factors associated with pain.
  - Identify risks and strategies by identifying prior responses to pain or treatment.
  - Identify patient barriers to pain relief (Arnstein, 2010).

Nurse's Role and Responsibilities

Pain management is an important part of nursing practice. Nurses have a responsibility to reduce or relieve pain. For the nurse to fulfill her/his responsibilities in relation to pain, she/he must be knowledgeable and skilled in pain management.

- Protection of patients against injury and the development and progression of disease.
- Relieve the pain.
- To be an advocate for the care that individuals, families, communities, and societies need.
- Working in collaboration with patients, families, and other healthcare providers.
- Apply the nursing process independently and use nursing guidelines when planning the nursing process (Arnstein, 2010).

Research

For the purposes of this chapter, the focus is on non-pharmacological approaches used to reduce procedural pain and pain-related distress associated with medical examination and treatment in healthcare practices.

Pain is a subjective symptom that is difficult to recognize and assess (Obeidat et al., 2021). Blood sampling, intravenous cannula insertion, tracheal aspiration, and tape removal are the most common painful procedures routinely performed in neonatal intensive care units (Sawleshwarkar et al., 2022). Premature babies, who are known to have a lower pain threshold, are exposed to many painful procedures in intensive care units (Obeidat et al., 2021). Early exposure of the newborn to uncontrolled pain can lead to several adverse long-term consequences, including the development of hypersensitivity to pain, harmful psychological symptoms, and altered neurological development. These findings emphasize the critical role of pain management in neonatal care. Pain assessment should be performed systematically and regularly (Bucsea & Riddell, 2019; Obeidat et al., 2021).

The first principle in pain management should be not to perform a painful procedure if it is unnecessary (Bucsea & Riddell, 2019; Obeidat et al., 2021). If it is medically necessary to perform the painful procedure, the first goal should be to reduce pain by appropriately managing the painful procedure. Examples include choosing the correct injection site for an injection procedure, administering the vaccine with the least pain potential first if more than one vaccine is to be administered, and leaving the vaccine with the highest pain potential last (Bucsea & Riddell, 2019). If painful procedures are necessary, the non-pharmacological methods to be used should be planned in advance (Obeidat et al., 2021).

In a prospective observational study, 143 infants admitted to the neonatal intensive care unit were exposed to an average of 93.1 invasive medical procedures per newborn in the first 14 days of admission to the unit. This indicates that an infant is exposed to 8.2 painful medical procedures per day. Babies with the shortest gestational age, the lowest birth weight, and those on respiratory support experienced the most procedural pain. It is known that exposure to pain during the neonatal period can cause some negative consequences in the future. Non-pharmacological pain reduction (proximal, distal, and procedural) methods in neonatal care have been shown to be effective in reducing pain and its negative consequences in the neonatal period. Additionally, the combined use of methods used for pain management can provide more effective analgesia compared to using them alone (Bucsea & Riddell, 2019).

Parental Participation/Parental Touch

Newborns are exposed to painful procedures from the first week of life. Repeated painful procedures such as routine health screenings after birth, heel prick, blood tests for jaundice, etc. are necessary (Bucsea & Riddell, 2019; Avan Antepli et al., 2022; Cobo et al., 2022; Sawleshwarkar et al., 2022; Shoghi et al., 2023). The pain experienced by newborns can negatively affect acute physiological life indicators, and can also lead to neurodevelopmental deficits in the long term (Sawleshwarkar et al., 2022). Repeated painful procedures negatively affect the neurological, behavioral, and cognitive development of preterm infants (Obeidat et al., 2021).

In a study conducted to compare procedural and non-pharmacological methods used by parents to reduce pain in neonatal intensive care units, most participants reported that they frequently used methods such as positioning the baby comfortably and holding the baby. Parents indicated that they would like to be involved in more care to relieve their baby's pain. However, it was reported that this was somehow prevented by health professionals during painful procedures. As health professionals, within the scope of family-centered care principles, it should be ensured that families participate in care (Treiman-Kiveste et al., 2023).

Pain experienced by newborns can have long-term negative consequences. It may have neurodevelopmental consequences on the newborn, as well as cause parents to increase anxiety and avoid future health care services. Cobo et al. (2022), in their study conducted with 112 newborns and investigating whether harmful stimulated brain activity decreases with parental caressing, stated that caressing can reduce pain by activating tactile fibers in the brain (Cobo et al., 2022).

Maternal Voice

The meta-analysis conducted by Jin et al. in 2023 included 584 newborns and 8 randomized controlled trials. The meta-analysis showed that the maternal voice decreased the pain score and heart rate and increased comfort level and blood oxygen saturation during the procedure. The mother's voice has been stated as a simple and effective practice that provides a reduction in procedural pain in newborns, resulting in better physiological indicators of the newborn (Jin et al., 2023).

Positioning

Positioning can be used as a non-pharmacological technique to reduce procedural pain in neonates. Positioning can be classified as prone, supine, and lateral decubitus. According to a systematic review, facilitated parental tucking should be used for 30 minutes during painful procedures in preterm neonates. Positioning should be used for 15 minutes before the painful procedure and a further 15 minutes during and after the procedure. Effective positioning allows the neonate to stabilize vital signs and stress (Francisco et al., 2021). In a cross-sectional study describing nurses' perceptions of the use of non-pharmacological analgesic methods, it was reported that they used touch (83%) and positioning the baby (78%) as the most useful non-pharmacological pain relief method. (Treiman-Kiveste et al., 2022).

Breastfeeding, Non-Nutritive Sucking, Skin-to-Skin Contact and Facilitated Compression

Breastfeeding is effective in reducing procedural pain in newborns. Breastfeeding after painful procedures increases comfort by calming the baby (Bektas et al., 2023). Breastfeeding is a practical, easily applicable and economical non-pharmacological method (Yang et al., 2022; Bektas et al., 2023). Breastfeeding strengthens the bond between mother and baby. It provides both physical and psychological relaxation to babies. The lactose secreted by the mother during breastfeeding has a sweetening effect. Although the sweetening effect of lactose is not as great as that of glucose and sucrose, breastfeeding is effective in pain management because of the benefits of taste and skin contact (Yang et al., 2022). A descriptive cross-sectional study reported that infants rarely used breastfeeding (34%) and skin-to-skin contact (12%) as non-pharmacological practices in procedural pain management. (Treiman-Kiveste et al., 2022).

In their 2023 study, Bektaş et al. investigated the effect of breastfeeding on procedural pain during heel stick blood collection. Breastfeeding during the procedure reduced the newborn's pain and allowed them to settle down more quickly after the procedure (Bektas et al., 2023).

Non-nutritive sucking, skin-to-skin contact, and facilitated compression interventions have been shown to reduce pain in newborns (Obeidat et al., 2021; Yang et al., 2022). Using these non-pharmacological interventions in combination rather than as single interventions can increase the analgesic effect (Obeidat et al., 2021). Non-nutritive sucking is a practice to increase the sucking movement of the newborn using a pacifier (Yang et al., 2022). The moderate to severe pain in preterm infants during heel prick blood collection was reduced by combined dual interventions. These interventions were: non-nutritive sucking, breast milk, and facilitated tucking; non-nutritive sucking, and breast milk. Facilitated tucking facilitated the stabilization of preterms (Peng et al., 2018).

A systematic review of the efficacy and safety of non-pharmacological methods used to prevent pain in neonates included 29 published systematic reviews. Non-pharmacological techniques such as small volumes of sweet solutions, facilitated compression, kangaroo care, familiar scent or sucrose, and non-nutritive suctioning have been proven to be effective in reducing procedural pain in neonates (Q. Shen et al., 2022).

Sensory Stimulation

Sensory stimulation is one of the leading non-pharmacological methods of pain relief in neonates. The combined use of sensory stimulation has been shown to be more effective than oral sucrose alone (Yang et al., 2022). 108 babies were enrolled in a randomized controlled trial to assess the effect of sensory stimulation from breast milk on procedural pain in newborns. Neonates undergoing intravenous access were randomized into three groups: Sensory saturation and sucrose, sensory saturation, and breast milk, and finally the group that received oral sucrose only. The analgesic effect was compared between the groups. Sensory saturation is a non-pharmacological pain relief technique that uses touch and sound as distractors. Breast milk can be a safe and natural sweetener. Pain was reduced more effectively in neonates who received multiple sensory stimulations (sensory saturation and breast milk, sensory saturation, and oral sucrose groups) than in those who received a single application (oral sucrose). Breast milk can be used in sensory stimulation to reduce procedural pain. Breast milk is a natural sweetener. In the trial, breast milk became an effective, cheap, and reliable method of replacing sucrose in sensory stimulation (Fitri et al., 2020).

Distraction/Virtual Reality (VR)

Hospital procedures such as health checks and examinations, blood draws, vaccinations, and injections can cause pain in children. It is important to reduce the pain and distress experienced during these procedures. Distraction techniques can be used to help children cope with these difficult procedures (Lambert et al., 2020). Distraction techniques can block pain signals from reaching the brain (Phuttamas Chanthong & Jirapaet, 2017). Practices that allow children to actively engage in distraction (e.g., video games) are defined as active distraction, and practices that allow children to passively engage in distraction (e.g., watching videos, listening to music) are defined as passive distraction (T. Shen et al., 2023). Even simple distraction techniques, such as talking to the child and asking questions, can be used by nurses to reduce the pain and anxiety of the procedure (Yıldırım & Gerçeker, 2023). Innovative applications continue to be included in distraction techniques as technology develops. Nurses can effectively manage procedural pain using distraction techniques in the medical procedures they perform during the nursing care process. (Birnie et al., 2014).

A meta-analysis and systematic review of 13 randomized controlled trials in 2023 investigated the effect of active and passive distraction interventions on procedural pain in children. There was evidence that active distraction was more effective than passive distraction in reducing procedural pain and anxiety. However, it was reported that there was no significant difference between the two distraction techniques in terms of procedural pain reported by the children themselves (T.Shen et al., 2023).

One of the innovative distraction techniques that can be used as technology advances is the application of virtual reality (Lambert et al., 2020). Virtual reality is the technology that allows users to separate themselves from the current environment and enter an alternative computer-generated environment, providing a three-dimensional artificial experience that closely resembles reality (Lambert et al., 2020; Addab et al., 2022; Li et al., 2022). The use of virtual reality can target emotional and cognitive pain pathways, reducing the severity and distress of pain by altering the way it is perceived in the central nervous system (Lambert et al., 2020). Virtual reality is both a visual and an auditory technology. It may be more beneficial for children because it can activate both senses. The use of virtual reality can enhance pain management by allowing children in the hospital to spend time in a virtual world, effectively reducing pain and anxiety (Addab et al., 2022).

Nurses can use VR distraction, a medical innovation, to provide effective pain management during medical procedures routinely performed in the pediatric setting (Addab et al., 2022). By reducing the anxiety associated with medical procedures, the use of virtual reality can prevent increased pain sensitivity, anxiety, and subsequent avoidance of healthcare. Nurses can play an important role in supporting the technology and the use of virtual reality as a distraction technique (Addab et al., 2022).

The Cochrane Database of Systematic Reviews included 17 randomized controlled trials that looked at the effect of virtual reality on procedural pain. They included 1008 children between the ages of 4 and 18 who were undergoing medical procedures. The medical procedures in the trials included bloodletting, injections, dressing changes, and physiotherapy sessions. The review found that the immersive virtual reality application was effective compared to other distraction techniques that did not use a virtual reality application. Virtual reality applications can effectively reduce pain in children (Lambert et al., 2020).

In the study conducted by Yıldırım and Gerçeker in 2023 in children between the ages of 4 and 10, it was found that in the intervention group where the virtual reality application was used as a distraction technique, children reported less pain and anxiety during intravenous catheter placement (Yıldırım & Gerçeker, 2023).

Another study looked at the effect of participants' chosen distraction technique (listening to music or playing computer games) on reducing procedural pain during vascular access procedures in adolescents with cancer. The participants' self-selected distraction technique allowed them to feel less procedural pain. The adolescents' choice of distraction technique may have increased their focus on the chosen technique, increased their sense of control, and affected their perception of pain. (Phuttamas Chanthong & Jirapaet, 2017).

Children undergoing pediatric wound manipulation experience pain. The meta-analysis of the effect of virtual reality on procedural pain in pediatric wounds looked at 39 trials involving 273 patients. The use of virtual reality as a non-pharmacological distraction technique was shown to significantly reduce pain and discomfort during wound manipulation in children. Virtual reality is an innovative approach to reducing procedural pain (Li et al., 2022).

Vibration/Buzzy

Buzzy is a motorized, battery-powered device in the shape of a bee that provides a combination of cold and vibration effects. The inventor of the device is Dr. Amy Baxter, a pediatric emergency physician. The purpose of the device is to reduce the procedural pain caused by the effects of needles in children. It is a method that is quick, easy, and can be used repeatedly (Baxter et al., 2011).

The principle of the Buzzy intervention is that it reduces the pain signal transmitted to the brain by vibration and cold stimuli, according to the gate control theory, and it is believed that it can reduce pain by suppressing the harmful stimulus caused by the needle (Ballard et al., 2019).

The wings of the bee-shaped Buzzy device contain 18 grams of ice. The ice bags that form the wings can be removed and kept in the freezer between operations. Buzzy's wings can stay frozen at room temperature for 10 minutes (Ballard et al., 2019). The ice packs must be removed from the freezer immediately before use. The ice wings are attached to the device and made ready for use. Buzzy should be placed 5 cm above the area where the needle will be inserted. The device is then activated, and the vibration is started. After 30-60 seconds, the invasive procedure can begin. The device must remain active until the procedure is complete (Baxter et al., 2011; Ballard et al., 2019).

A systematic review and meta-analyzed study that synthesized evidence from 9 RCTs involving 1,145 children and adolescents aged 3 to 18 years found that Buzzy application reduced needle-related procedural pain in children (Ballard et al., 2019). In their 2023 study, Bilgen Sivri et al. found that Buzzy was the best method for reducing procedural pain during blood sampling in children aged 6-12 years. It was found that children who used the Buzzy method experienced less procedural pain than children who used distraction cards (Bilgen Sivri et al., 2023).

In another study, the analgesic effect of the virtual reality application and the Buzzy application on the pain experienced by children aged 7-12 during blood collection was compared and it was found that both the Buzzy and the virtual reality applications were more effective in reducing procedure pain in children and that the procedure pain was least in the virtual reality group. It has been reported that (Yilmaz & Canbulat Sahiner, 2023). In a study comparing the effects of ShotBlocker and distraction cards on procedure pain during blood collection in children aged 9-12, it was found that Buzzy and distraction cards were more effective in reducing procedure pain (Sivri et al., 2023).

In the study, a mechanical vibrator device was used to investigate the effect of vibration on pain during heel stick blood sampling in term newborns. In the group that used the mechanical vibrator device, the device was placed before the procedure to affect the afferent nerve fibers on the back of the babies' legs and vibration was applied for 30 seconds. The blood was then taken by a heel prick. When pain was assessed during and 2 minutes after the procedure, the non-vibrated group reported more pain than the vibrated group. It has been found that mechanical vibration application reduces pain in babies (Shoghi et al., 2023). In another similar study, it was found that procedural pain scores were lower in the group that received vibration 15-20 seconds and 5 minutes after the procedure than in the control group (Avan Antepli et al., 2022). The results of the studies showed that the use of vibration as a non-pharmacological method during heel blood sampling is effective in procedural pain management (Avan Antepli et al., 2022; Shoghi et al., 2023).

Hypnosis

Distraction and hypnosis can reduce procedural pain in children. Systematic reviews and meta-analyses have reported that distraction significantly reduces self-reported and observer-reported pain and distress in children. The use of hypnosis has been found to reduce self-reported pain and distress in children during injection-related procedures. (Birnie et al., 2014, 2018).

In a study investigating the effect of virtual reality hypnosis compared to medical hypnosis to reduce pain during medical procedures, it was reported that virtual reality hypnosis reduced procedural pain in children to a similar level as medical hypnosis. The use of virtual reality is an effective tool for reducing procedural pain-related distress and increasing comfort in children with lower levels of anxiety (van den Berg et al., 2023).

Massage

Massage therapy is the practical application of soft tissue manipulation and massage. A systematic review of the effects of massage therapy on procedural pain in newborns found that massage reduced procedural pain in newborns. It was also effective in improving vital signs, improving crying status, and stabilizing the newborn (Sharma et al., 2023).

Conclusion

Children remember the pain they had experienced. It has been found that children with higher levels of trait anxiety may remember more pain in their painful experiences than they initially reported. What is considered a minor and simple procedure by healthcare professionals can be remembered as distressing to a child.

What children remember should be considered as part of the pain management intervention. Healthcare professionals can provide effective personalized interventions by assessing children's previous health experiences, fears, and anxieties (Rocha et al., 2009). Children's views on pediatric pain management should be considered, and they should be encouraged to share their own pain experiences. Nurses should collaborate with children for effective pain management. More research should be conducted to include children's views to provide child-centered care in pain management and better understand children's expectations (Kortesluoma et al., 2008). In this way, negativity such as anxiety, fear, and avoidance of health care can be reduced by ensuring that the child is better able to cope with the next health experience (Rocha et al., 2009).

There is a growing interest and curiosity in non-pharmacological applications to reduce procedural pain in infants and children. With the advancement of science and technology, innovative approaches are being added to applications used to reduce procedural pain. Virtual reality applications, the scope of which is gradually expanding, are one of them. Virtual reality technology is open to development in areas such as personalization, humanistic approach, meeting patients' needs, and hardware development of virtual devices (Li et al., 2022).

Effective use of procedural pain reduction approaches requires good pain management, including pain recognition and good pain assessment. It is important to select appropriate pain assessment tools according to the age and clinical characteristics of children and to use them systematically in pain monitoring. Effective pain assessment tools can measure the analgesic effect of non-pharmacological methods. Objective pain assessment should be used to understand whether or not the intervention being used is effective. Evidence-based pain assessment tools should be known to nurses and used in practice. Nurses should be aware that pain assessment is the important first step in recognizing and preventing pain. Nurses should increase their interest in procedural pain pursue evidence-based, innovative non-pharmacological interventions, and be able to use this evidence appropriately by developing their own clinical practice.

References

Addab, S., Hamdy, R., Thorstad, K., Le May, S., & Tsimicalis, A. (2022). Use of virtual reality in managing paediatric procedural pain and anxiety: An integrative literature review. *Journal of clinical nursing*, 31(21-22), 3032-3059. https://doi.org/10.1111/jocn.16217.

Arnstein, P. (2010). Clinical Coach for Effective Pain Management. F.A. Davis.

American Pain Society, (2000). *Pain as the 5th Vital Sign Toolkit.* Retrived from http://www.va.gov/painmanagement/docs/toolkit.pdf . Retrieved February 23, 2024.

Avan Antepli, N., Bilsin Kocamaz, E., & Güngörmüş, Z. (2022). The Effect of Vibration on Pain During Heel Lance Procedures in Newborns: A Randomized Controlled Trial. *Advances in Neonatal Care,* 22(2), E43. https://doi.org/10.1097/ANC.0000000000000918.

Ballard, A., Khadra, C., Adler, S., Trottier, E. D., & Le May, S. (2019). Efficacy of the Buzzy Device for Pain Management During Needle-related Procedures: A Systematic Review and Meta-Analysis. *The Clinical Journal of Pain*, 35(6), 532-543. https://doi.org/10.1097/AJP.0000000000000690.

Baxter, A. L., Cohen, L. L., McElvery, H. L., Lawson, M. L., & von Baeyer, C. L. (2011). An Integration of Vibration and Cold Relieves Venipuncture Pain in a Pediatric Emergency Department. *Pediatric Emergency Care*, 27(12), 1151. https://doi.org/10.1097/PEC.0b013e318237ace4.

Bektas, İ., Oktay, S. Ş., Köylü, P., Ulu, H., & Akdeniz Kudubeş, A. (2023). The Effect of Breastfeeding on the Newborn's Comfort and Pain Levels During Heel Blood Collection. *Comprehensive Child and Adolescent Nursing,* 0(0), 1-11. https://doi.org/10.1080/24694193.2023.2259991.

Bice, A. A., Gunther, M., & Wyatt, T. (2014). Increasing Nursing Treatment for Pediatric Procedural Pain. *Pain Management Nursing*, 15(1), 365-379. https://doi.org/10.1016/j.pmn.2012.06.004.

Bilgen Sivri, B., Feng, Y. S., Michler, C., Kuemmerle-Deschner, J., & Mahler, C. (2023). The effect of buzzy®, DistrACTION® cards on reducing pediatric pain and fear during blood collection in the rheumatology polyclinic: A randomized controlled trial. *Journal of Pediatric Nursing*, 73, e446-e454. https://doi.org/10.1016/j.pedn.2023.10.013.

Birnie, K. A., Noel, M., Chambers, C. T., Uman, L. S., & Parker, J. A. (2018). Psychological interventions for needle-related procedural pain and distress in children and adolescents. *Cochrane Database of Systematic Reviews,* 10. https://doi.org/10.1002/14651858.CD005179.pub4.

Birnie, K. A., Noel, M., Parker, J. A., Chambers, C. T., Uman, L. S., Kisely, S. R., & McGrath, P. J. (2014). Systematic Review and Meta-Analysis of Distraction and Hypnosis for Needle-Related Pain and Distress in Children and Adolescents. *Journal of Pediatric Psychology*, 39(8), 783-808. https://doi.org/10.1093/jpepsy/jsu029.

Bucsea, O., & Riddell, R. (2019). Non-pharmacological pain management in the neonatal intensive care unit: Managing neonatal pain without drugs. *Semınars in Fetal & Neonatal Medıcıne*, 24(4). https://doi.org/10.1016/j.siny.2019.05.009.

Cobo, M., Moultrie, F., Hauck, A., Crankshaw, D., Monk, V., Hartley, C., Fry, R., Robinson, S., van der Vaart, M., Baxter, L., Adams, E., Poorun, R., Bhatt, A., & Slater, R. (2022). Multicentre, randomised controlled trial to investigate the effects of parental touch on relieving acute procedural pain in neonates (Petal). *Bmj Open*, 12(7). https://doi.org/10.1136/bmjopen-2022-061841.

Eccleston, C., Fisher, E., Howard, R. F., Slater, R., Forgeron, P., Palermo, T. M., Birnie, K. A., Anderson, B. J., Chambers, C. T., Crombez, G., Ljungman, G., Jordan, I., Jordan, Z., Roberts, C., Schechter, N., Sieberg, C. B., Tibboel, D., Walker, S. M., Wilkinson, D., & Wood, C. (2021). Delivering transformative action in paediatric pain: A Lancet Child & Adolescent Health Commission. *The Lancet Child & Adolescent Health*, 5(1), 47-87. https://doi.org/10.1016/S2352-4642(20)30277-7.

Fitri, S., Lusmilasari, L., Juffrie, M., & Bellieni, C. (2020). Modi fied Sensory Stimulation Using Breastmilk for Reducing Pain Intensity in Neonates in Indonesia: A Randomized Controlled Trial. *Journal Of Pediatric Nursing-Nursing Care Of Children & Families*, 53, 199-203. https://doi.org/10.1016/j.pedn.2020.04.004.

Francisco, A. S. P. G., Montemezzo, D., Ribeiro, S. N. dos S., Frata, B., Menegol, N. A., Okubo, R., Sonza, A., & Sanada, L. S. (2021). Positioning Effects for Procedural Pain Relief in NICU: Systematic Review. *Pain Management Nursing*, 22(2), 121-132. https://doi.org/10.1016/j.pmn.2020.07.006.

Hurley-Wallace, A., Wood, C., Franck, L. S., Howard, R. F., & Liossi, C. (2018). Paediatric pain education for health care professionals. *Pain Reports*, 4(1), e701. https://doi.org/10.1097/PR9.0000000000000701.

Ivancsó, J., Fejes, M., Fürjész, D., Kelen, M., Megyeri, T., Váradi, K., & Szucs, I. (2021). Number of painful procedures and pain management in a neonatal intensive care unit. *Orvosı Hetılap*, 162(48), 1931-1939. https://doi.org/10.1556/650.2021.32284.

Jin, L., Zhang, J., Yang, X., & Rong, H. (2023). Maternal voice reduces procedural pain in neonates: A meta-analysis of randomized controlled trials. *Medicine,* 102(12), e33060. https://doi.org/10.1097/MD.0000000000033060.

Kortesluoma, R.-L., Nikkonen, M., & Serlo, W. (2008). "You just have to make the pain go away"—Children's experiences of pain management. Pain Management Nursing: *Official Journal of the American Society of Pain Management Nurses*, 9(4), 143-149, 149.e1-5. https://doi.org/10.1016/j.pmn.2008.07.002.

Lambert, V., Boylan, P., Boran, L., Hicks, P., Kirubakaran, R., Devane, D., & Matthews, A. (2020). Virtual reality distraction for acute pain in children. *Cochrane Database of Systematic Reviews*, 10. https://doi.org/10.1002/14651858.CD010686.pub2.

Li, T., Fu, Y., Yang, Y., & Zhou, Y.-E. (2022). Control effect of virtual reality technology on procedural pain in children's wound: A meta-analysis. *Medicine,* 101(40), e30961. https://doi.org/10.1097/MD.0000000000030961.

Obeidat, H., Dwairej, D., & Aloweidi, A. (2021). Pain in Preterm Infants: Different Perspectives. *Journal Of Perinatal Education,* 30(4), 185-195. https://doi.org/10.1891/J-PE-D-20-00032.

Peng, H.-F., Yin, T., Yang, L., Wang, C., Chang, Y.-C., Jeng, M.-J., & Liaw, J.-J. (2018). Non-nutritive sucking, oral breast milk, and facilitated tucking relieve preterm infant pain during heel-stick procedures: A prospective, randomized controlled trial. *International Journal of Nursing Studies*, 77, 162-170. https://doi.org/10.1016/j.ijnurstu.2017.10.001.

Phuttamas Chanthong, & Jirapaet, V. (2017). The Effect of Self-Selected Distraction Technique on the Pain Caused by Venipuncture in Early Adolescents with Cancer. Journal of Health Research, 31, 3. https://doi.org/10.14456/JHR.2017.21.

Raja, S. N., Carr, D. B., Cohen, M., Finnerup, N. B., Flor, H., Gibson, S., Keefe, F. J., Mogil, J. S., Ringkamp, M., Sluka, K. A., Song, X.-J., Stevens, B., Sullivan, M. D., Tutelman, P. R., Ushida, T., & Vader, K. (2020). The revised International Association for the Study of Pain definition of pain: Concepts, challenges, and compromises. *Pain,* 161(9), 1976-1982. https://doi.org/10.1097/j.pain.0000000000001939.

Riddell, R. R. P., Bucsea, O., Shiff, I., Chow, C., Gennis, H. G., Badovinac, S., DiLorenzo-Klas, M., Racine, N. M., Kohut, S. A., Lisi, D., Turcotte, K., Stevens, B., & Uman, L. S. (2023). Non-pharmacological management of infant and young child procedural pain. *Cochrane Database of Systematic Reviews,* 2023(6). https://doi.org/10.1002/14651858.cd006275.pub4.

Rocha, E. M., Marche, T. A., & Von Baeyer, C. L. (2009). Anxiety Influences Children's Memory for Procedural Pain. *Pain Research and Management*, 14(3), 233-237. https://doi.org/10.1155/2009/535941.

Sawleshwarkar, K., Singh, M., Bajaj, R., Loya, S., Chikhlondhe, R., & Bhave, S. (2022). Implementing use of sucrose analgesia (non-pharmacological management of neonatal pain) in a standalone private facility level 3 neonatal care unit using point of care quality improvement methodology. *Bmj Open Quality*, 11(SUPPL_1). https://doi.org/10.1136/bmjoq-2022-001830.

Segers, E., Ketelaar, M., de Man, M., Schoonhoven, L., van de Putte, E., & van den Hoogen, A. (2023). How to support children to develop and express their coping preferences around minor invasive medical procedures: Children's and parents' perspectives. *European Journal Of Pediatrics*. https://doi.org/10.1007/s00431-023-05222-7.

Sharma, A., Sharma, N., & Sharma, A. (2023). Soft tissue therapy in managing neonatal procedural pain: A Systematic Review. Journal of Neonatal Nursing, 29(6), 815-824. https://doi.org/10.1016/j.jnn.2023.02.011.

Shen, Q., Huang, Z., Leng, H., Luo, X., & Zheng, X. (2022). Efficacy and safety of non-pharmacological interventions for neonatal pain: An overview of systematic reviews. *Bmj Open,* 12(9). https://doi.org/10.1136/bmjopen-2022-062296.

Shen, T., Wang, X., Xue, Q., & Chen, D. (2023). Active versus passive distraction for reducing procedural pain and anxiety in children: A meta-analysis and systematic review. *Italian Journal of Pediatrics*, 49(1), 109. https://doi.org/10.1186/s13052-023-01518-4.

Shoghi, M., Dehghan, A., & Bozorgzad, P. (2023). The effect of vibration on pain intensity during neonatal heel-blood sampling. *Anaesthesia Pain & Intensive Care*, 27(2), 191-197. https://doi.org/10.35975/apic.v27i2.2183.

Sivri, B. B., Balci, S., & Dolgun, G. (2023). The Effect of 3 Methods (Buzzy, ShotBlocker, and DistrACTION Cards) Used While Taking Blood Samples From Children with Pain and Anxiety: A Randomized Controlled Trial. *Pediatric Emergency Care*, 39(8), 600. https://doi.org/10.1097/PEC.0000000000002866.

Treiman-Kiveste, A., Kangasniemi, M., Kalda, R., & Pölkki, T. (2023). Parental Participation in Their Infants' Procedural Pain Alleviation with Nonpharmacologic Methods in Estonia. *Pain Management Nursing*, 0(0). https://doi.org/10.1016/j.pmn.2023.02.008.

Treiman-Kiveste, A., Pölkki, T., Kalda, R., & Kangasniemi, M. (2022). Nurses' perceptions of infants' procedural pain assessment and alleviation with non-pharmacological methods in Estonia. *Journal of Pediatric Nursing-Nursing Care Of Children & Families,* 62, E156-E163. https://doi.org/10.1016/j.pedn.2021.09.006.

van den Berg, S., Hoogeveen, M. O., van Winden, T. M. S., Chegary, M., Genco, M. S., & Jonkman, N. H. (2023). Virtual reality hypnosis for needle-related procedural pain and fear management in children: A non-inferiority randomized trial. *European journal of pediatrics*, 182(10), 4421-4430. https://doi.org/10.1007/s00431-023-05116-8.

Wilson-Smith, E. M. (2011). Procedural Pain Management in Neonates, Infants and Children. *Reviews in Pain*, 5(3), 4-12. https://doi.org/10.1177/204946371100500303.

Wrona, S. K., Quinlan-Colwell, A., Brown, L., & Jannuzzi, R. G. E. (2022). Procedural Pain Management: Clinical Practice Recommendations American Society for Pain Management Nursing. *Pain Management Nursing,* 23(3), 254-258. https://doi.org/10.1016/j.pmn.2021.11.008.

Yang, Z., Fu, Y., & Wang, Y. (2022). Summary and Analysis of Relevant Evidence for Nondrug Nursing Programs in Neonatal Operational Pain Management. *Emergency Medicine International*, 2022, 7074500. https://doi.org/10.1155/2022/7074500.

Yıldırım, B. G., & Gerçeker, G. Ö. (2023). The Effect of Virtual Reality and Buzzy on First Insertion Success, Procedure-Related Fear, Anxiety, and Pain in Children during Intravenous Insertion in the Pediatric Emergency Unit: A Randomized Controlled Trial. *Journal of Emergency Nursing*, 49(1), 62-74. https://doi.org/10.1016/j.jen.2022.09.018.

Yilmaz, D., & Canbulat Sahiner, N. (2023). The effects of virtual reality glasses and external cold and vibration on procedural pain and anxiety in children during venous phlebotomy: Randomized controlled trial. *Virtual Reality*, 27(4), 3393-3401. https://doi.org/10.1007/s10055-022-00714-7.

Chapter 20

Evidence-Based Nursing Practices to Prevent Home Accidents in Children

Feyza Küçük*, PhD
Department of Nursing, Faculty of Health Sciences, Usak University, Usak, Türkiye

Abstract

Home accidents are unintentional injuries that occur at and around the home and are a major cause of serious health problems and disability. The three most important risk groups in home accidents are children, the elderly, and the disabled. Home accidents occur because children in the 0-6 age group are open and sensitive to the dangers in the environment, they are curious to search and learn, they are not physically strong and competent enough to protect themselves from accidents that may occur, their concepts of depth, height, and width are not fully developed, and the home environment is not organized according to the developmental levels of children. The most common home accidents in children occur due to falls, drowning, burns, cuts, and poisoning. Today, home accidents still maintain their importance due to their high incidence. It is the responsibility of parents who provide primary care for children to live in safe environments in terms of accidents, to take protective measures, to ensure the safety of their living spaces, and to supervise them. Parental education plays an important role in preventing childhood accidents and protecting children. Nurses have the responsibility of educating children, families, teachers, and society in preventing home accidents that may occur by using their roles such as caregiving, active observer, researcher, consultant, educator, policy-making, manager, and advocate. Protective measures for possible home accidents that may occur, considering the physical and cognitive development characteristics of children according to their age groups; when an accident occurs, it is important to provide guidance and counseling to parents and other caregivers about first aid.

This paper, includes evidence-based nursing approaches to preventing home accidents.

Keywords: child, home accident, nursing, parents

* Corresponding Author's Email: feyza.kucuk@usak.edu.tr.

In: Evidence-Based Care Practices in Pediatric Nursing
Editors: Feyza Küçük and Serap Özdemir
ISBN: 979-8-89530-304-7

Introduction

Home accidents are accidents that occur inside the house or in the immediate surroundings of the house, such as balconies, gardens, pools, and garages (Silva et al., 2016). Home accidents experienced in childhood are a worldwide health problem and an important cause of accidents and injuries (Piffer et al., 2021; Sabea et al., 2019; Villar et al., 2021). Children are open and sensitive to the dangers in the environment, not having the physical strength and competence to protect themselves from possible accidents, the concepts of depth, height, and width not being fully developed, and the home environment not being arranged according to the developmental levels of children may cause home accidents (Nageh et al., 2020; Pathak et al., 2020). Children in the 0-6 age group are very vulnerable to home accidents due to reasons such as their psychomotor skills are not yet sufficiently developed, their visual field is narrow, they cannot interpret sounds well, they are active, they want to imitate adults, and they are curious (Çiçek et al., 2022; Kurt et al., 2022; Yorulmaz & Hisar 2020). In a study on home accidents, the incidence of home accidents in the 1-4 year old group was reported to be 21.8% (Patchala et al., 2020). The most common home accidents in children are occur due to falls, drowning, burns, cuts, and poisoning (Ahmedov & Ortabağ, 2023; Rumhi et al., 2020).

Accidents affect the child's health as a whole, physically, socially, and psychologically, and can cause illness, disability, and death. For this reason, childhood injuries are a health problem that requires attention (Abbassinia et al., 2019). Today, there are many safety products that help parents take precautions against home accidents. Increasing the use of these products (locks that prevent the opening of cabinets, drawer holders that prevent fingers from being pinched and drawers from opening too much, child locks that prevent windows from being opened, safety barriers to prevent walking downstairs and falling, bed borders, door stoppers, corner protectors that can be used on sharp-edged furniture, electrical outlet covers (locks, stove button safeties, playground fences, pool safety net), and increasing families' awareness of safety measures are effective measures to reduce injury rates resulting from home accidents (Çiçek et al., 2022). Preventing, monitoring, recording, and maintaining home accidents requires a multi-disciplinary team service. Initiatives to protect and improve health are among the duties of the nurse, who is an important member of the healthcare team (Çapık & Gürol, 2014). To prevent home accidents, nurses need to provide conscious and positive attitudes preventing home accidents for all family members, especially those who care for the child.

Common Home Accidents in Children and Precautions

The types of accidents that children may frequently encounter at home are known as falls, injuries, drowning, burns, and poisoning (Ahmedov & Ortabağ, 2023; Rumhi et al., 2020; Şentepe & Kahriman, 2022).

Falls

Children's experiences of exploring the environment through activities such as learning to walk, climbing, running, and jumping are important for children to develop their motor skills, gain balance, and discover their bodies, and the falls that occur in this process are considered a natural part of child development. Falls occur in many different ways within the home. At home, it is usually caused by high furniture, stairs and balconies, and uneven and wet floors (Chaudhary et al., 2018). Children under one year of age have the highest rate of fall-related injuries and deaths among all childhood age groups. These can be listed as falls from a height, such as babies falling from the lap, falling while walking, or falling from the bed. Due to the fact that the grasping abilities and coordination of children in the play period are not sufficiently developed, falling while running, falling on slippery and unsuitable ground, falling as a result of trying to climb on furniture, and falling from the walker are among the common situations (Fidancı et al., 2021).

Falls are considered the second cause of unintentional injury-related deaths in the world, according to the WHO. An estimated 684,000 people die from falls every year, and more than 80% of them are stated to be in low- and middle-income countries (WHO, 2018). In the study by Rumhi et al. (2020) in which 1333 children who had home accidents were examined; it was reported that 53.7% of home accidents occurred due to falling. The severity of falls varies depending on the distance/height the child falls, the ground on which he falls (concrete, gravel, soil, etc.), and the way he falls (falling on his head, falling on his limbs). However, regarding child falls, factors such as inadequate adult supervision, leaving children alone, and a crowded home environment also increase the likelihood of children encountering falls. According to a study, factors such as low socioeconomic level, being in the 0-6 age group, male gender, education level of the mother and caregiver, cognitive disorders of the caregiver, and housing conditions are shown as risk factors for falls. Falls are an important public health problem in that they are preventable, cause death and disability, and are costly (WHO, 2018).

As precautions to be taken against falls:

- Preferring furniture suitable for the age of the child
- Having security locks on windows
- Mounting furniture with a risk of falling to the floor or wall
- There are handrails on the sides of the stairs and a door to prevent small children from falling
- Do not place heavy objects on objects that can be pulled, such as tablecloths
- Children's clothes should not be too big or loose, which could cause them to fall
- Children under the age of six should not sleep in bunk beds
- Using car seats and seat belts for young children
- Wearing non-slip socks, slippers or slippers
- The child should not be left unsupervised (Gür & Kılınç, 2023; Rumhi et al., 2020; Watson & Errington, 2016).

Burns

The second most common type of home accident after falls is burns. Burns are injuries to the skin or other body tissues that occur as a result of exposure to factors such as heat, hot liquids, hot solid objects, or flames. It can also occur as a result of contact with radiation, electricity, or chemicals. Scald burns, flame burns, electrical burns, and chemical burns are more common in children. Burns can cause permanent sequelae and cause large expenses in the healthcare system due to the types of care and treatment (Kawalec & Pawlas, 2020). The American Burn Association (ABA) National Burn Unit (2019) reports that overall, flame burns account for the majority of injuries in the United States (41%), with scalds second with 31%. Chemical (3.5%) and electrical burn injuries (3.6%) occur much less frequently (ABA, 2019). In the study by Javaid et al. (2021), where they examined accidental scald burn cases of 1041 children under the age of 5 years, it was found that these injuries occurred as a result of pulling down a cup or mug of hot drink and scalding the head or torso. In a study conducted with caregivers of 200 children under the age of 18 in Poland, it was found that 85.5% of burns occurred most frequently at home and 84.5% of thermal burns were scalds. In the study, in the analysis of the room where the burn occurred, it was determined that 59% of the burns were in the kitchen (Soori & Khodakarim, 2016).

Burns can be classified in two different ways, depending on the surface area of the body and the depth of the burn. If it is less than 15% of the body surface area, it is considered a minor burn. Burns between 15% and 49% are called moderate burns, while burns between 50% and 69% are considered extensive burns. Burns with more than 70% of body surface area are classified as extensive burns (Özkaya et al., 2014). In the classification based on burn depth; First-degree burns are burns that are marked only by swelling and redness on the skin. While second-degree burns are characterized by the complete loss of the epidermis layer, third-degree burns are deep burns that occur with the complete loss of the skin layer. Fourth-degree burns are deep burns that affect the musculoskeletal system. This classification gives an idea of the prevalence and impact of burns and plays an important role in treatment planning (Jeschke et al., 2020).

It is stated that the rate of burn-related injuries is higher in women than in men. Death cases due to burns are more common, especially among infants and the elderly. However, it is reported that burn-related deaths in children under 5 years of age are 1.5 times higher than in the general population. The risk of fire and burns increases in regions with low sociocultural levels, poverty, and unemployment (Esen et al., 2021). In a study by Kawalec and Pawlas (2020) in which they examined the relationship between the home environment and parameters such as burn location, severity, depth, and area, it was found that the average burn area of children in rural areas was larger than the burn area of children in urban areas.

Precautions that can be taken against burns:

- Removing accessible electrical appliances (television, iron, charger, etc.) and lamps
- Electrical cables are not exposed
- Covering cables with plastic protectors against biting
- Covering sockets with plastic protectors
- Cooking food on the stove in the back and the handles of pans facing inward
- Keeping flammable materials such as matches/lighters out of reach of children
- Do not leave hot drinks such as tea or coffee around

- Protection of children against sunburns
- Presence of smoke detectors in all bedrooms and the kitchen
- Having a fire extinguisher at home
- No smoking at home
- These include conducting fire drills at home and having a fire escape plan (Jeschke et al., 2020; Kawalec & Pawlas, 2020; Price et al., 2021).

Penetrating, Cutting, and Contusion Injuries

Injury is defined as the disruption of the integrity of the skin or mucosa due to trauma. In addition to the skin, other tissues such as vessels, muscles, and nerves may also be affected by injury formation. The injured skin loses its protective properties, and this increases the risk of infection. Common features of injuries include pain, bleeding, and separation of injury edges (Gündüz & Aytekin, 2015). In a study examining childhood penetrating injuries, the objects that caused the injuries were found at home: scissors, knife, door handle, seat edge, and on the street; It was seen that there were stones, iron, and wire. It has been reported that injuries are more common in preschool boys than in girls (Büyük & Şerefoğlu, 2020).

Etiologically, injuries are considered in 5 categories.

- *Cut Injuries:* They are defined as injuries caused by cutting tools such as knives, pocketknives, and glass. These types of injuries usually occur as a result of sharp and pointed objects penetrating the skin. The most distinctive feature of cut injuries is that they are usually simple injuries, and their depth can be easily determined.
- *Bruised Injuries*: These types of injuries are injuries that occur as a result of violent impact on the body by factors such as stones, fists, or sticks. These types of injuries often cause tissue damage and tenderness in the affected area. Injury edges may appear bruised. The amount of bleeding in bruised injuries is generally not too great.
- *Penetrating Injuries*: Penetrating injuries are injuries caused by sharp-pointed objects, such as knives, needles, and nails penetrating the skin. Depth is generally effective in such injuries. There is also a risk of tetanus infection in such injuries.
- *Split Injuries:* These types of injuries occur due to the pulling effect of tissues. In such injuries, ruptures and injuries may occur between the tissues. Split injuries can affect all tissue-related organs and even the scalp.
- *Infected Injuries*: Infected injuries are injuries that are at high risk of contracting germs. Infected injuries include injuries that have been crossed, injuries with separated stitches, injuries with irregular edges, very dirty and deep injuries, gunshot injuries, and injuries resulting from bites and stings (Gosain et al., 2004).

Two-fifths of stab injuries occur while children play at home or outside. The presence of glass doors, glass ornaments, and windows increases injuries (Gündüz & Aytekin, 2015). Injuries to children's hands and fingers are common, and children's abilities such as playing with their fingers, examining the environment, and satisfying their curiosity cause them to experience these accidents (Liu et al., 2015). In another study, it was determined that the rate of injuries caused by sharp objects among home accidents that children frequently experience was 13.6% (Kayıran et al., 2022).

To prevent stabbing and crushing injuries:

- Corner protectors should be placed on sharp edges of furniture
- Television or other heavy objects should be placed so that they do not fall
- Unbreakable glass should be used on doors and windows
- The garbage bin containing kitchen garbage should be kept locked
- Glassware such as glasses and bottles should not be given to the child
- Cutting tools such as scissors and razors should be kept out of reach of the child
- Sewing materials should be kept out of reach of children
- Tables, chairs, and similar items with missing nails should be repaired immediately
- Broken items should be repaired by experts in these works (Büyük & Şerefoğlu, 2020; Mytton et al., 2014).

Drowning

While the situation of not being able to breathe as a result of immersing one's face in water while breathing is called drowning, the emergency that occurs when some or all parts of the airways are blocked and can result in early death if intervention is delayed is defined as drowning with a foreign object (Kim et al., 2015). Drowning is the third cause of unintentional injury-related deaths worldwide, accounting for 7% of all injury-related deaths (WHO, 2021), and the sixth cause of death in children aged 5-14 years (WHO, 2014). Drowning cases in children generally occur in the form of obstruction of the respiratory tract or drowning in water as a result of a foreign object entering the respiratory tract (Doğan, 2019).

Drownings in water usually occur in bathrooms and garden pools during the summer months in children under the age of 5 (Banks, 2014). Although it usually occurs as a result of an accident, the possibility of suicide, and alcohol and drug intake should be considered, especially in adolescent cases. Underlying diseases such as epilepsy and cardiac arrhythmia should be considered. In a study evaluating 736 autopsied child deaths, it was reported that drowning in water constituted approximately half of the asphyxia cases determined as the most common cause of death (Canturk et al., 2007). In another study, the deaths of children aged 0-14 years who were autopsied over a 5-year period were examined, and drowning was reported as the main cause of death in deaths due to asphyxia (Väli et al., 2007). Drownings due to foreign body aspiration occur more frequently between 6 months and under 5 years of age (Dereci et al., 2015).

Children tend to put objects they hold in their mouths, causing foreign body aspiration. The most commonly swallowed objects are batteries, coins, small hard parts and needles, nuts, and hard foods with small grains (Sutherland & Bowen, 2023). In the case of foreign body aspiration, one of the most common symptoms is cough. However, in addition to this symptom, symptoms such as wheezing, changes in respiratory sounds, chronic cough, and recurrent lung infections can also be observed (Kipiki et al., 2023). If the person frequently has lung infections with unknown causes or if there are differences in voice and breathing, a foreign body in the lung should be considered. If foreign bodies remain in the lungs for a long time, conditions such as atelectasis (partial or complete collapse of the lung), chronic lung infections, abscess (accumulation of pus), and bronchiectasis (permanent expansion of the bronchi) may occur. In another study, it was determined that the average age of children with foreign body aspiration was 24 months and that their gender was mostly male (66.2%). The most common symptom was found to be a cough (Pacheco et al., 2021). In case of suspected drowning, it is important to intervene quickly and effectively (Sutherland & Bowen, 2023).

Regarding precautions that can be taken against drowning:

- Be careful with hanging objects with strings such as baby bibs
- If there is a swimming pool at home, it should be completely surrounded and protected
- Keeping toilet seats closed
- Children from the age of 4 years receive swimming training
- Using flotation devices in children
- Training adults or caregivers on cardiopulmonary resuscitation
- Children under one year of age should not be placed on their backs
- Removing objects that pose a risk of suffocation in their beds
- Keeping small or detachable objects away from children
- Babies should sleep in the same room with caregivers for up to 12 months
- Avoid giving foods with small, hard pieces
- Do not leave objects that prevent air, such as plastic bags and stretch film, lying around
- It is important not to use powder (DeGeorge et al., 2020; Tobin et al., 2017).

Poisoning

Poisoning is a situation that occurs as a result of substances entering the organism through breathing, digestion, absorption through the skin, or injection, disrupting the physiological systems in the body. With poisoning, events that cause damage and death at the cellular level can occur (Kırcı et al., 2023). While the majority of poisoning cases that occur in childhood occur as a result of accidents, a small number are caused by intentional actions. Factors that increase the risk of poisoning include the young age of the parents, the male gender, and the child's past poisoning experience. Additionally, it is stated that poisoning cases are more common when parents are busy with different jobs other than their children or when the child is cared for by a grandmother, grandmother, or sibling (Schwebel et al., 2017).

Substances that cause poisoning in childhood: cleaning agents, cosmetics and personal care products, analgesics such as acetaminophen, cardiovascular drugs, alcohol, and carbon monoxide gas (Gummin et al., 2017). While poisoning is more common in boys at a young age, it increases in girls during adolescence (Orton et al., 2016). In addition to the substance that causes poisoning, the amount of exposure, the route of entry, the duration of exposure, and the time that has passed are also important (Emeksiz & Perk, 2020).

Precautions That Can Be Taken Against Poisoning:

- Be sure to read the labels of cleaning products
- Removing toxic substances from the environment
- Substances or drugs that may cause poisoning should be kept in their own packaging and never placed in beverage bottles

- Packages of substances, such as medicines and detergents, must be durable and childproof
- Keeping cleaning products and disinfectants in locked cabinets out of reach of children
- Preparing and placing single doses of medicines to be given to children
- Batteries large enough to be swallowed by children should not be left lying around
- Adults should not use medicines by showing them to children
- Medicines should never be introduced to children by comparing them to foods and drinks such as candy, milk, or fruit juice
- Not growing poisonous plants at home
- Installing carbon monoxide detectors in homes
- Parents and caregivers are willing to take a first-aid course
- Ventilation of the environment when substances that cause inhalation poisoning are used, such as bleach and salt spirits (Gür & Kılınç, 2023; Kırcı et al., 2023; Küçük & Balcı, 2011; Schwebel et al., 2017).

Nursing Approaches to Prevent At-Home Accidents in Children

Reducing deaths and disabilities due to home accidents in childhood is important to protect and improve the health of society. Preventing, monitoring, recording, and maintaining home accidents requires a multi-disciplinary team service. Initiatives to protect and improve health are among the duties of the nurse, who is an important member of the healthcare team (Çapık & Gürol, 2014). The roles of the nurse in childhood injuries include; identifying, reducing, and eliminating dangers in the environment, identifying behavioral characteristics in children, and guiding parents on child development. Due to these roles, nurses must educate caregivers and children to prevent accidents (Gündüz & Aytekin, 2015). In a study conducted by Alrimawil et al. (2019), it was determined that the majority of mothers had positive attitudes toward preventing home accidents, but they stated that mothers could not prevent home accidents due to general living conditions due to socioeconomic factors. Similarly, in their study, Whitehead and Owens (2012) found that although the majority of parents stated that they could identify potential accident risks for their children and that they thought injuries were preventable, they had perceptions about the inevitability of injuries due to the characteristics of their children. For parents to change their perceptions, it is necessary to emphasize and support that home accidents can be prevented with small changes in the house. Situations that are risk factors for home accidents and are not noticed by the family should be determined together with the family; In this way, the family's awareness should be increased, and the learning should be permanent. Situations that may cause home accidents should be explained together with the cause-effect relationship. The consequences that may be seen when risk factors are not intervened in should be addressed (Altundağ & Körükçü, 2023).

Home visits are of great importance to prevent home accidents and to take protective measures. Nurses have the opportunity to make observations about the family and home during home visits. By reporting home accident risks, they can alert the necessary units to reduce risks and cooperate with other members of the healthcare team. In this way, the nurse can fulfill the role of an active observer (Laux Kaiser & Rector, 2014). Various videos can be watched to prevent home accidents. Studies have shown that the training given to families regarding home accidents increases both their level of knowledge and their awareness of these accidents (Alrimawil et al., 2019; Bayram et al., 2019; Riberio et al., 2019).

The best way to prevent home accidents is by conducting studies that determine the risks related to home accidents. The aim is to develop forms of education that eliminate the harms of factors related to family and environment and to contribute to organizing a safe environment (Bhatta et al., 2020; Satır and Ulupınar, 2023). Nurses should be encouraged to plan training in light of evidence-based practices and participate in legal regulations to prevent home accidents and identify risk factors (Elmas et al., 2020).

Conclusion

Home accidents are among the priority issues of public health because they are preventable. Accidents are often caused by parents' carelessness, but sometimes they may be related to the child's behavior. It includes prevention of childhood accidents, protection of children, and education of caregivers. Nurses should educate children, families, teachers, and society to prevent accidents in different age groups. Home security should be evaluated during home visits and training should be provided during visits. Nurses should provide guidance and counseling to parents and other caregivers about the physical and cognitive development characteristics of children according to their age group, protective measures for possible home accidents that may occur in childhood, and first aid in case of accidents. Being careful about the risks that may arise at home, taking safety precautions, and keeping children under surveillance will contribute to reducing the risk of home accidents.

References

Abbassinia, M., Barati, M., & Afshari, M. (2019). Effectiveness of interventions in the prevention of home injuries among children under 5 years of age: A systematic review. *Arch Trauma Res*, *8*, 190-197. https://doi.org/10.1177/2158244018824483.

Ahmedov, Y., & Ortabağ, T. (2023). Determination of the frequency of admission of children aged 0-6 years to the emergency department due to a home accident and the first aid practices of their parents. *JEUNF*, *39*(3), 315-323 https://doi.org/10.53490/egehemsire.1060875.

Alrimawil, I., Watson, M. C., Hall, C., & Saifan, A. R. (2019). Preventing unintentional injuries to children under 5 in their homes: Palestinian Mothers' Perspectives. *SAGE Open*, *9*(1), 1-11. https://doi.org/10.1177/215824401882448.

Altundağ, S., & Körükçü, Ö. (2023). Risk reduction education to prevent preschool children's home accidents: A pilot study. *Disaster Medicine and Public Health Preparedness*, 17, 115. https://doi.org/10.1017/dmp.2022.20.

American Burn Association (2019). National Burn Repository 2019 Update, Report of data from 2009–2018 ameriburn.site-ym.com https://ameriburn.site-ym.com/store/ViewProduct.aspx?id=14191872.

Anton-Pacheco, J. L., Martin-Alelu, R., López, M., Morante, R., Merino-Mateo, L., Barrero, S., ... & Luna-Paredes, M. C. (2021). Foreign body aspiration in children: Treatment timing and related complications. *International Journal of Pediatric Otorhinolaryngology*, *144*, 110690. https://doi.org/10.1016/j.ijporl.2021.110690.

Banks T. L. (2014). Still drowning in segregation: Limits of law in post–civil rights America. *Law Inequality*, *32*(2), 215-255.

Bayram, T., Ilgin, C., Kulbay, H., Tozakoglu, B., Karaduman, I., Colak, B. C., & Save, D. (2019). The factors associated with mothers' preventive measures against home accidents: A descriptive study from Istanbul, Turkey. *Clinical and Experimental Health Sciences, 9*(2), 151-156. https://doi.org/10.33808/clinexphealthsci.564220.

Bhatta, S., Mytton, J., & Deave, T. (2020). Environmental change interventions to prevent unintentional home injuries among children in low-and middle-income countries: A systematic review and meta-analysis. *Child: care, health and development*, *46*(5), 537-551. https://doi.org/10.1111/cch.12772.

Büyük, E. T. & Seferoğlu, E. G. (2020). Mothers' identification of safety measures associated with children's home accidents. *Journal of Samsun Health Sciences*, *5*(2), 201-206. https://doi.org/10.47115/jshs.793194.

Canturk, N., Esiyok, B., Ozkara, E., Canturk, G., Ozata A. B., & Yavuz, M. F. (2007). Medi colegal child deaths in Istanbul: Data from the Morgue Department. *Pediatr Int, 49*(1), 88-93. https://doi.org/10.1111/j.1442-200X.2007.02298.x.

Çapık, C., & Parlak Gürol, A. (2014). Effect of education on mothers' capability of identification of safety precautions of home accidents. *Kafkas J Med Sci*, *4*(3), 87–94. https://doi.org/10.5505/kjms.2014.65365.

Chaudhary, S., Figuero, J., Shaikh, S., Mays, E. W., Bayakly, R., Javed, M., Smith, M.L., Moran, T.P., Rupp, J., & Nieb, S. (2018). Pediatric falls ages 0-4: understanding demographics, mechanisms, and injury severities. *Inj Epidemiol*, *5*(1), 78-87. https://doi.org/10.1186/s40621-018-0147-x.

Çiçek, B., Şahin, H., & Erkal, S. (2022). Examination of safety measures against home accidents of parents with children aged 0-6 years: The Covid-19 Pandemic. Istanbul Commerce University *Journal of Social Sciences*, *21*(43), 212-230. https://doi.org/10.46928/iticusbe.1053663.

DeGeorge, K. C., Neltner, C. E., & Neltner, B. T. (2020). Prevention of unintentional childhood injury. *American Family Physician, 102*(7), 411-417. https://www.aafp.org/afp/2020/1001/p411-s1.html.

Dereci, S., Koca, T., Serdaroğlu, F., & Akçam, M. (2015). Foreign body ingestion in children. *Turkish Archives of Pediatrics, 50*(4), 234-240. https://doi.org/10.5152/TurkPediatriArs.2015.3164.

Doğan, Z. (2019) Çocukluk Çağında Sık Görülen Kazalar ve Zehirlenmeler. In D. Aydın, Y. A. Aba (Eds.), *Anne ve Çocuk Sağlığı* (pp. 479-486). Istanbul Tıp Kitabevi.

Elmas, E. G., Durna, Z., Akın, S. (2020). Assessment of knowledge and attitudes of mothers with children about first aid practices for home accidents and security precautions. *JAREN*, *6*(2), 267-279. https://doi.org/10.5222/jaren.2020.38258.

Emeksiz, S., & Perk, O. (2020). Childhood intoxications: Are we aware of the danger? *Turkish Journal of Pediatric Disease*, *14*, 465-470. https://doi.org/10.12956/tchd.585124.

Esen, O., Güven, M., Yıldırım, A., Turgut, H. T., Tiryaki, Ç., Yazicioglu, M. B., Haksal, M. C., Çiftçi, A., & Esen, H. K. (2021). Epidemiology of burn injuries in the Burn Center. *Southern Clinics of Istanbul Eurasia, 32*(4), 360-365. https://doi.org/10.14744/scie.2021.93270.

Fidancı, İ., Derinöz, O., & Tokgöz, A. (2021). Cases admitted to Pediatric Emergency Department due to trauma related to fall. *Pediatric Practice and Research*, *9*(1), 5-10. https://doi.org/10.21765/pprjournal.874688.

Gosain, A., DiPietro, L. A. (2004). Aging and wound healing. *World J Surg, 28*, 321-326. https://doi.org/10.1007/s00268-003-7397-6.

Gummin, D. D., Mowry, J. B., Spyker, D. A., Brooks, D. E., Fraser, M. O., & Banner, W. (2017). 2016 Annual Report of The American Association of Poison Control Centers' National Poison Data System (NPDS): 34th Annual Report. *Clinical Toxicology*, *55*(10), 1072-1254. https://doi.org/10.1080/15563650.2017.1388087.

Gündüz, G., Aytekin, A. (2015). Attitudes of mothers towards protecting their children from home accidents and the affecting factors. *İzmir Journal of Behcet Uz Children's Hospital, 5*(3), 184-192. https://doi.org/10.5222/buchd.2015.184.

Gür, K., & Kılınç, E. (2023). Çocukluk Çağı İstemsiz Yaralanmalar ve Korunma. In A. B. Temel (Ed.), Sağlığı Koruma ve Geliştirme 3 Risk Grupları, *Yaşam Ortamları ve Hastalıklardan Korunma* (pp. 861-884). Ema Tıp Kitabevi.

Javaid, A. A., Johnson, E., Hollén, L., & Kemp, A. M. (2021). Influence of agents and mechanisms of injury on anatomical burn locations in children < 5 years old with a scald. *Archives of Disease in Childhood, 106*(11), 1111-1117. https://doi.org/10.1136/archdischild-2020-320710.

Jeschke, M. G., van Baar, M. E., Choudhry, M. A., Chung, K. K., Gibran, N. S., & Logsetty, S. (2020). Burn injury. *Nature reviews Disease primers*, *6*(11), 1-25. https://doi.org/10.1038/s41572-020-0145-5.

Kawalec, A., & Pawlas, K. (2020). Home environment and burns in children. *Burns Open*, *4*(4), 167-175. https://doi.org/10.1016/j.burnso.2020.05.006.

Kayıran, D., Sönmez, M., & Nazik, F. (2022). Determining families' awareness of home accidents and for preschoolers. *Journal of Education in Health Sciences*, *5*(1), 21-30.

Kırcı, G., Öztürk, D. U., Özer, E., Bölükbaşı, H. S., Çakır, H., & Özer, E. (2023). Evaluation of Intoxication Case Application to the Child Emergency Department Between 2016-2021. *The Bulletin of Legal Medicine*, *28*(1), 66-73. https://doi.org/10.17986/blm.1638.

Kim, I. A., Shapiro, N., & Bhattacharyya, N. (2015). The national cost burden of bronchial foreign body aspiration in children. *Laryngoscope*, *125*, 1221–1224. https://doi.org/10.1002/lary.25002.

Kipiki, P. E., Chussi, D., Shija, P., Kimwaga, F., Sadiq, A., & Mlay, K. (2023). Button battery ingestion: A serious pitfall of diagnosis of ingested foreign bodies in children from resource-limited settings–A case report. *International Journal of Surgery Case Reports*, *109*, 108593. https://doi.org/10.1016/j.ijscr.2023.108593.

Kurt, F. Y., Çalbayram, N., Oğul, T., & Aldemir, F. (2022). The frequency of home accidents in 0-6 years old children and the investigation of the safety measures taken by mothers for home accidents: Example of the pandemic period. *Journal of Infant, Child and Adolescent Health*, *2*(3), 177-188.

Küçük, F., & Balcı, S. (2011). Characteristics of children between 1-6 ages who drink corrosive substances and the first applications of families. *Journal of Anatolia Nursing and Health Sciences*, *14*(3), 32-39.

Laux Kaiser, K., & Rector, C. (2014). *Community & Public Health Nursing. Maternal–Child Health: Working with Perinatal, Infant, Toddler, and Preschool Clients.* (8th ed.). Wolters Kluwer Health | Lippincott Williams & Wilkins.

Liu, W. H., Lok, J., Lau, M. S., Hung, Y. W., Wong, C. W. Y., & Tse, W. L. (2015). Mechanism and epidemiology of paediatric finger injuries at Prince of Wales Hospital in Hong Kong. *Hong Kong Med J*, *21*, 237-242.

Mytton, J., Ingram, J., Manns, S., Stevens, T., Mulvaney, C., Blair, P., Powel, J., Potter, B., Towner, E., Emond, A., Deave, Thomas, J., Kendrick, D., & Stewart-Brown, S. (2014). The feasibility of using a parenting programme for the prevention of unintentional home injuries in the under-fives: A cluster randomised controlled trial. *Health Technology Assessment*, *18*(3), 1- 184. https://doi.org/10.3310/hta18030.

Nageh, H. M., El-Raouf, A., Samar, E. L., El-Mouty, A., & Samia, M. (2020). Mothers' knowledge and subjective practice toward most common domestic injuries among under-five children. *Mansoura Nursing Journal*, *7*(1), 19-35. https://doi.org/10.21608/mnj.2020.175751.

Orton, E., Whitehead, J., Mhizha-Murira, J., Clarkson, M., Watson, M. C., Mulvaney, C. A., Staniforth, J. U., Bhuchar, M., & Kendrick, D. (2016). School-based education programmes for the prevention of unintentional injuries in children and young people. *Cochrane database of systematic reviews*, *12* (CD0102), 1-109. https://doi.org/10.1002/14651858.CD010246.pub2.

Özkaya, N., Alğan, S., & Akkaya, H. (2014). Assessment and defining the treatment of the patients with burns. *Ankara Med J.*, *14*(4), 170-175. https://doi.org/10.17098/amj.10837.

Patchala, A., Phanindra, D., & Jagannath, R. D. (2020). A Study on Prevalence of Domestic Accidents in A Rural Community. *International Journal of Advanced Community Medicine*, *3*(2), 53-58. https://doi.org/10.33545/comed.2020.v3.i2a.166.

Pathak, A., Agarwal, N., Mehra, L., Mathur, A., & Diwan, V. (2020). Incidence, Risk and Protective Factors for Unintentional, Nonfatal, Fall-Related Injuries at Home: A Community-Based Household Survey from Ujjain, India. *Pediatric Health, Medicine and Therapeutics*, *11*, 65–72. http://doi.org/10.2147/PHMT.S242173.

Piffer, S., Demonti, S., Rampani, C., Giustini, M. & Pitidis, A. (202). Home Accidents in the Province of Trento, Ten Years of Observations Regarding Admissions to the Emergency and First Aid Department. *Ann Ing*, *33*(2), 152–162. https://doi.org/10.7416/ai.2021.2421.

Price, K., Lee, K. C., Woolley, K. E., Falk, H., Peck, M., Lilford, R., & Moiemen, N. (2021). Burn injury prevention in low-and middle-income countries: Scoping systematic review. *Burns & Trauma, 9*, tkab037. https://doi.org/10.1093/burnst/tkab037.

Ribeiro, M. G. C., Paula, A. B. R., Bezerra, M. A. R., Rocha, S. S. D., Avelino, F. V. S. D., & Gouveia, M.T.D.O. (2019). Social determinants of health associated with childhood accidents at home: An integrative review. *Revista brasileira de enfermagem*, *72*, 265-276. https://doi.org/10.1590/0034-7167-2017-0641.

Rumhi, A. A, Awisi, H. A, Buwaiqi, M. A., Rabaani, S. (2020), "Home accidents among children: A retrospective study at a tertiary care center in Oman," *Oman Medical Journal*, *35*(1). https://doi.org/10.5001/omj.2020.03.

Sabea, M. T. M., El-Maksoud, M. M. A. & Hegazy, A. E. S. (2019). Educational program for information caregivers about home accident prevention. *Academic Journal of Nursing and Health Education*, *8*(1), 16-33.

Satir, G., & Ulupinar, S. (2023). Impact of domestic accidents training given to parents with mentally disabled children. *Acıbadem University Health Sciences Journal (AUHSJ), 14*(2), 279-286. https://doi.org/10.31067/acusaglik.1162789.

Schwebel, D. C., Evans, W. D., Hoeffler, S. E., Marlenga, B. L., Nguyen, S. P., Jovanov, E., & Sheares, B. J. (2017). Unintentional child poisoning risk: A review of causal factors and prevention studies. *Children's Health Care*, *46*(2), 109-130. https://doi.org/10.1080/02739615.2015.1124775.

Silva, E. C. S., Fernandes, M. Y. F., Nascimento, Sá M. C., Souza, L. M., Araújo Gordon, S. A., Jesus Costa, A.C. P., Araújo, T. S., Silva Carvalho, Q. G., Maia, C. C., Gomes Machado, A. L., Amaral Gubert, F. A. Silva, L. A., & Cunha Vieira, N. F. (2016). The effect of educational intervention regarding the knowledge of mothers on prevention of accidents in childhood. *The Open Nursing Journal*, *10*, 113-121. https://doi.org/10.2174/1874434601610010113.

Soori, H., Khodakarim, S. (2016). Child unintentional injury prevention in Eastern Mediterranean Region. *International Journal of Critical Illness and Injury Science*, *6*(1), 33-39. DOI: https://doi.org/10.4103/2229-5151.177366.

Sutherland, J., & Bowen, L. (2023). Ingestion of foreign bodies and caustic substances in children. *BJA education, 23*(1), 2. https://doi.org/10.1016/j.bjae.2022.09.003.

Şentepe, T., & Kahriman, İ. (2022). Examination of safety measures against home accidents of mothers with 1-6 years age group children presenting to emergency service according to some variables. *Gümüşhane University Journal of Health Sciences*, *11*(3), 1211-1220. https://doi.org/10.37989/gumussagbil.1135908.

Tobin, J. M., Ramos, W. D., Pu, Y., Wernicki, P. G., Quan, L., & Rosano, J. W. (2017). Bystander CPR is associated with improved neurologically favourable survival in cardiac arrest following drowning. *Resuscitation, 115*, 39-43. https://doi.org/10.1016/j.resuscitation.2017.04.004.

Väli, M., Lang, K., Soonets, R., Talumäe, M., & Grjibovski, A. M. (2007). Childhood deaths from external causes in Estonia, 2001-2005. *BMC Public Health*, *7*, 158. 8 doi:10.1186/1471-2458-7-158. https://doi.org/10.1186/1471-2458-7-158.

Villar, M. I. M., Brais, L., Diaz, J. R. &Garcia, S. L. (2021). Infancia protegida ante ahogamiento acuatico. In A. S. J. Hernandes, J. C. Munoz, M. V. Arboleda, E. M. R. Pereita, & M. A. M. Sanchez (Eds.), *Construyenda juntos una escueala para la vida* (pp. 1554–1560). Dykinson.

Watson, M. C., & Errington, G. (2016). Preventing unintentional injuries in children: Successful approaches. *Paediatrics and Child Health 26*(5), 194-199, 2016.

Whitehead, E., & Owens, D. (2012). Parental perceptions of unintentional injury risks to children. *International Journal of Health Promotion and Education*, *50*, 20-27.

WHO (2021). Drowning. Access: 22.03.2024 https://www.who.int/news-room/fact-sheets/detail/drowning.

WHO (2018). Injuries. Injuries in the Western Pacific. Access: 22.03.2024 https://www.who.int/westernpacific/health-topics/injuries.

WHO (2014). Global report on drowning: Preventing a leading killer. Access: 24.03.2024 https://www.who.int/publications/i/item/global-report-on-drowning-preventing-a-leading-killer.

Yorulmaz, D., & Hisar, F. (2020). Safety measures taken by mothers of 0-6-year-old children towards home accidents in rural areas. *Health and Society*, *3*, 103-109.

Chapter 21

Evidence-Based Nursing Practices Involving Yoga in Children

Pelin Gökoğlu Gürer*, MSc

Department of Nursing, Faculty of Health Sciences, Halic University, Istanbul, Türkiye

Abstract

Yoga, which is among the complementary and alternative treatment methods that have become popular in health services in recent years, has also become one of the evidence-based care practices in the field of child health and diseases.

Adopting the holistic approach inherent in nursing care, yoga is a holistic practice that includes physical postures, breathing exercises, and meditation. Many evidence-based studies support the various benefits of yoga for both mental and physical health. Studies have shown that yoga reduces symptoms such as stress-anxiety and depression, improves flexibility and balance, increases strength and endurance, relieves pain, improves heart health (lowering blood pressure, cholesterol levels, and heart rate) improves breathing (pranayama). It is envisaged that it will become a part of nursing care with increasing evidence-based practices and supported research in different areas such as improvement in sleep quality and cognitive functions and development of support mechanisms in the process of chronic disease.

For the child to have healthy development, he/she must make holistic progress in all areas of development. This approach makes yoga a valuable practice to improve holistic health in children.

In this section, we will discuss yoga practices, which are among the evidence-based nursing practices, and complementary and alternative treatment methods in child health, which can be among the independent roles of the nurse, which supports medical treatment in nursing care.

Keywords: yoga, evidence-based practice, children, nursing, pediatric healthcare

---

* Corresponding Author's Email: pelingokoglu@halic.edu.tr.

In: Evidence-Based Care Practices in Pediatric Nursing
Editors: Feyza Küçük and Serap Özdemir
ISBN: 979-8-89530-304-7

Introduction

Yoga, which is a physical and mental practice, is used for different purposes in Eastern and Western cultures. In Eastern culture, yoga is practiced as a philosophy of life in the form of Patanjali's philosophical system, Raja Yoga, and Classical Yoga (De Michelis, 2008), while in Western culture, yoga is known as an activity practiced by individuals with a certain ailment to be treated or by those who want to do sports to improve performance (Singleton et al., 2013). In Turkey, similar to the United States, it is seen to be practiced based on physical exercise and health.

Yoga, which has taken its place among complementary and alternative treatment methods that have become popular in health services in recent years, is traditionally accepted as a practice by adults. However, it has been included in nursing care for children of all ages and has become one of the evidence-based care practices in the field of pediatric health and diseases.

Yoga is a practice based on mind-body unity that includes pranayama, which provides voluntary control of the breath, asana, which has several postures, meditation, which provides voluntary concentration on thoughts, and repeated verbal expressions. This unity of mind and body is in harmony with the philosophy of a holistic approach to nursing care. Many evidence-based studies support the various benefits of yoga for both mental and physical health. Studies show that yoga reduces symptoms such as stress-anxiety and depression, improves flexibility, and balance, increases strength and endurance, alleviates pain, improves heart health (decreases blood pressure, cholesterol levels, and heart rate), improves breathing (pranayama), improves sleep quality and cognitive functions in the chronic disease process, and improves support mechanisms.

For children to grow up healthy, they need to make holistic progress in all areas of their development. This approach makes yoga a valuable practice to improve holistic health in children.

In this chapter, we discuss evidence-based nursing practices, including yoga in children, and summarizes the scope of the subject and its relevance to pediatric health services, we will also discuss yoga practice among evidence-based nursing practices that support medical treatment in nursing care and can be among the independent roles of the nurse.

Evidence-Based Nursing Practices Involving Yoga in Children

Yoga Concept

Yoga is a comprehensive system of physical, mental, and spiritual practices originating in ancient India. The word "yoga" is derived from the Sanskrit root "yuj," which means "to unite or yoke together."

Yoga is the spiritual discipline of the body, mind, and spirit working in harmony. It takes the individual holistically in life and adapts to the whole of life. For this reason, it should be a way of life as a protective and healing source for a healthy life (Basavaraddi, 2015). Today, individuals identify yoga only with asana, which is a physical practice, but asana is only one of the tools used to heal the individual. Only three of the sutras include asanas, the rest of the sutras mention other yoga components such as conscious breathing, meditation, lifestyle, dietary changes, and the use of visualization and sound (Desikachar, 2005). In yoga philosophy, the mind and body are prepared for meditation and spiritual development through physical postures and breathing exercises (Collins, 1998).

The positive effects of yoga cover all aspects of physical, mental, and emotional health. For this reason, regular yoga practices reduce anxiety and depression, increase mental clarity, and bring the individual to emotional balance. It also supports inner growth by increasing self-awareness (Bussing et al., 2012; Neumark-Sztainer et al., 2020). According to Patanjali, known as the "Father of Yoga", "what limits the thought process and calms the mind" is referred to as yoga (Iyengar, 1993). Furthermore, he stated that there are eight stages of yoga. These are,

1. *Yama:* describes the social ethical rules in yoga practice and supports the application of moral values to the individual to live in harmony with society.
2. *Niyama:* supports the individual in adopting the principles of self-discipline and self-regulation to take responsibility for oneself.
3. *Asana:* promotes development on a physical level, aiming to increase the health and flexibility of the body.
4. *Pranayama*: aims to calm the mind and increase spiritual awareness by balancing energy through breath control.
5. *Pratyahara:* supports inner focus by withdrawing one's attention from the external world.
6. *Dharana:* aims to improve mental focus and increase the concentration skills of the individual.
7. *Dhyana*: is the meditation stage in which the individual's mind calms down, finds inner peace, and increases awareness.
8. *Samadhi*: describes the individual's state of unity, wholeness, and harmony, and is the highest stage of yoga practice.

Doing the eight stages mentioned above in order will improve the physical, mental, and spiritual health of the individual, enable him/her to find inner balance, and support him/her in understanding the philosophy of life (Bodur, 2020).

The components of yoga are postures (asanas), breath control, and meditation (Tamilselvi and Mala, 2016). Asanas are yoga-specific movements that improve balance and flexibility. Pranayamas are various practices in which the individual focuses on body awareness by providing breath control. Meditation is a mental process in which the individual can consciously focus on his/her thoughts.

Yoga includes different types and practices according to needs, preferences, and goals. Accordingly, some types of yoga are Hatha yoga, Karma yoga, Jinana, Bhakti, Raja, Karma, Kundalini, Pregnant, and Children's yoga.

Child Yoga

It is a type of yoga designed for children to increase their concentration and body awareness while supporting their physical, mental, and emotional development, to develop flexibility-balance skills, and support them in adopting a healthy lifestyle (Özgün et al., 2020).

Preparations before yoga practice (Bodur, 2020):

1. *Preparation of the Soul and Body*: Before starting to practice yoga, it is necessary to calm the mind and relax the body by breathing deeply in silence for a few minutes. Thus, the children will be mentally and physically ready.
2. *Creating a comfortable environment*: A calm, comfortable, clean, and organized environment in which yoga is practiced calms the child's mind and helps them focus. Yoga can be practiced in a quiet room or in a quiet corner of nature.
3. *Selection of appropriate clothing*: It is important to choose flexible and breathable clothes that can move comfortably during yoga practice.
4. *Providing adequate space and equipment*: A sufficient space where the body can lie down, hands can be easily placed on the floor, and the floor should be supported by using equipment such as a yoga mat.
5. *Application of correct breathing techniques*: Using correct breathing techniques during yoga practice is important for calming the mind and relaxing the body. Correct breathing techniques will be achieved through deep and conscious breathing.
6. *Warmth and hydration*: Before starting a yoga practice, you should avoid prolonged exposure to the sun and pay attention to the ambient temperature. Yoga practices should be interrupted in cases such as illness.
7. *Nutritional status*: Eating a light meal before yoga practice or having a snack about 2-3 hours before the meal will keep the body energy in balance.

Children's yoga is pedagogically divided into two groups. The first group refers to children between the ages of 2-7 (Bayraktar, 2021; Bodur, 2020; Radiant Child Yoga, 2022), while the second group refers to children between the ages of 8-18 (Bayraktar, 2021; Radiant Child Yoga, 2022). Accordingly, yoga should be planned for 15-20 minutes for children aged three to four, 30-35 minutes for children aged five to six, 40-45 minutes for children aged seven to nine, and 50-55 minutes for children aged ten to twelve (Bodur, 2018). Yoga practices for children include asanas combined with various games, singing, storytelling-listening, and creative movements (McGonigal, 2006). Children's yoga practices cover the third and seventh stages of the eight stages of yoga. These stages are asana, pranayama, prathyhara, dharana, and dhyana. Practices that will ensure the assimilation of the yama and niyamas in the first two steps also include children's yoga (Bayraktar, 2021). This practice flow includes warm-up movements, breathing techniques, special asanas and games, partner work, deep relaxation, and meditation steps.

1. *Warming up:* Warm-up exercises are performed with the children to get their bodies moving. For example, arm and leg movements, circular movements, or light jogging.

2. *Breathing Techniques*: Children can be taught simple breathing techniques such as deep breathing, nose breathing, and mouth breathing. This practice helps children understand their breathing and relax.
3. *Asanas:* Children can be shown various yoga postures (asanas) to help them develop flexibility, strength, and balance. For example, dog pose, tree pose, and snake pose should be simple and appropriate for children.
4. *Games and Stories*: Using games and stories in children's yoga classes, imitating the movements of an animal, and associating yoga postures with a story to attract children's interest.
5. *Closing:* At the end of the practice, the children are allowed to relax and unwind in the "Shavasana" position.

The application of different educational materials and teaching methods in children's yoga and the demonstration of yoga postures accompanied by fairy tales will enable children to practice yoga more effectively and discover their inner balance more effectively.

Children's yoga is a special form of yoga designed for children by exploring movements, breath, and awareness, making yoga engaging and age-appropriate. In doing so, the practitioner combines traditional yoga techniques with fun elements such as storytelling, games, and music.

Research

The history of yoga practice goes back much further than nursing. Nurses can use yoga practices as evidence-based interventions to help patients manage their symptoms, alleviate undesirable effects of treatment, minimize stress and anxiety, achieve better health, and be part of an integrated care plan. The oldest sources containing nursing and yoga in literature date back to the XXI century. It seems to have emerged at the beginning of the century. The first studies on yoga were in the field of psychiatry and were considered studies in which the stress-reducing and meditative effects were actively used (Richardson, 2001; Domingues, 2018; Adaiçi and Çıray, 2023).

Yoga is one of the complementary health approaches for which the National Institute of Health's National Center for Complementary and Integrative Health (2013) provided information, education, and research support in previous years. Its therapeutic properties have been used all over the world for centuries (Aydın and Özgen, 2018). Nowadays, yoga has become more interesting as a mind-body technique therapy with increasing popularity and importance (Cooley and Grant, 2006; Fouladbakhsh and Stommel, 2010). There is increasing evidence in studies supporting the effectiveness of yoga (Bower et al., 2011; Carlson and Bultz, 2008).

Although there are many studies related to yoga practices and nursing, there are not enough studies on different types of yoga with children of different age groups. Yoga practices can be used in healthy child-adolescent or chronically ill child-adolescent groups.

We will examine yoga practices and their effects on children and adolescents of different age groups in recent years.

Studies show that yoga practice, which aims to develop a holistic personality in children's social lives, positively affects the child's social relations with peers, harmony, and school-course relations, thanks to physical, social, mental, and meditation techniques. The Integrative Oncology Clinical Practice Guideline Association also recommends yoga to improve quality of life, anxiety, mood disorder, and depressive symptoms (Lyman et al., 2018, Palmer et al., 2020). Manjunath and Telles (2005) stated that yoga practice (including postures, regular breathing, relaxation techniques, and meditation) in school children increases social adaptation, improves the ability to plan and execute cognitive tasks, and has positive effects on well-being. In a study conducted in India, it was determined that children diagnosed with attention deficit and hyperactivity disorder increased their social harmony with their peers, quality of life, interest in school lessons, and academic success after yoga and meditation practices (Yadav et al., 2012). Studies conducted in recent years have stated that yoga positively affects adolescent development and health and has many spiritual and physical benefits for adolescents (Frank et al., 2017, Felver et al., 2015, Noogle et al., 2012, Felver et al., 2020). In addition to this information, it has been observed that yoga has a positive effect on the psychological problems adolescents have to deal with. This effect is thought to be the regulation of breathing through muscle relaxation in yoga practice and the reduction of stress through the benefits of meditation (Frank et al., 2014, Singh, 2018). In the review examining the relationship between quality of life and level of physical activity in healthy children and adolescents, it was concluded that the sedentary lifestyle of children and adolescents due to the recent increasing technological developments reduces their social relationships and causes a decrease in the quality of life of children and adolescents as a whole. It has been stated that yoga practice is recommended (Berjemo et al., 2017).

Yoga practice, especially pranayama, reduces the pressure on the hypothalamic-pituitary-adrenal (HPA) axis and sympathetic nervous system, minimizes sensitivity to stress triggers, and ensures mental well-being. This has effects on physiological markers of stress, such as reduction in the salivary gland, cortisol, blood sugar, blood pressure, heart rate, inflammation levels, and contributing to an overall relaxation response (Ross, 2001). Re et al., in their study, reported that yoga practices applied to adolescents had a decreasing effect on stress levels related to illness and hospitalization. In various studies examining the effect of yoga practice on adolescents, it has been revealed that it has positive results on adolescents' stress, anxiety, and psychological resilience and in coping with stress (Khalsa Butzer, 2016; Sarkissian et al., 2018; Singh, 2018). Furthermore, other studies have found that yoga has positive effects on adolescents' stress, anxiety, and psychological resilience. It has been found that it reduces aggression and increases awareness in addition to feelings of calmness and relaxation (Singh, 2018, Velásquez et al., 2015). In studies examining anxiety, depression, and self-esteem, yoga practice in adolescents has also been found to have a positive effect (Tejvani et al., 2016; Janjhua et al., 2020). In the randomized controlled study conducted by Fishbein et al. (2016), in adolescents, it was concluded that there was a decrease in anger in adolescents after yoga practice.

It has been observed that yoga practices regulate endocrine function along with hormone production, and it has been observed that the cortisol level in the body decreases and the melatonin level increases after yoga practice, and as a result, it is thought that it will affect the improvement of sleep quality (Evans et al., 2009). It has been stated that regular yoga practice improves the time it takes to fall asleep and total sleeping hours and helps wake up rested in the morning (Manjunath et al., Oksal Güneş, 2021).

Studies have been conducted showing the positive effects of yoga practice in children and adolescents with various chronic diseases. However, it does not have the level of evidence to support alternative medical treatment. Jacobs (2014) in his study with children receiving chemotherapy; It has been found that yoga practice reduces the cortisol level in saliva, plasma renin level, and urine level, which positively affects the autonomic nervous systems, but it has been emphasized that more studies are needed to prove the issue of symptom management. Govardhan et al. (2019), in their study of children receiving radiotherapy and chemotherapy; A decrease in children's pain intensity and fatigue, an increase in their appetite, and an improvement in their sleep quality were observed. Narasingharao et al. (2017), in their study on children with autism spectrum disorder, an improvement in their sleep quality was achieved as a result of uninterrupted sleep at the end of the yoga applied. Koenig et al. (2012) noted that it had a significant effect on classroom behavior in children with autism spectrum disorder when done in a classroom-based daily routine. Culver et al. (2015) concluded that yoga practice is effective in the treatment of traumatic stress disorders. It is thought that yoga practices contribute to the regulation of breathing physiologically and regulate the autonomic system that provides respiratory system control by changing neurotransmitters (Önder, 2019). Studies have shown that breathing exercises and yoga/pranayama in the treatment of childhood asthma improve asthma control and anxiety depression parameters (Das et al., 2019, Lack et al., 2020). It has been determined that the individual who practices regular pranayama in yoga contributes by increasing his awareness of his own breathing, affecting pulmonary, autonomic, and neurocognitive functions in the body, and regulating biochemical and metabolic activities (Ilter and Ovayolu, 2021; Kupershmidt and Barnable, 2019). However, it was not recommended because the data-evidence level was not sufficient.

In studies that have used yoga in school settings, it has been shown to benefit children and adolescents on issues such as anger management, sleep patterns, and obesity. Thanks to children's yoga, they will be able to learn how to react to various situations and how to calm themselves (Radiant Child Yoga, 2022, Bayındır, 2022). Bernstein et al. (2014), in their study on weight control and obesity, stated that yoga practice has positive effects that help reduce food intake. Dairy et al. (2021), in their review study examining yoga practice for obesity and weight management in children and adolescents, pointed out that the effects of yoga interventions were low but significant. When yoga practice was examined in children with hemophilia, it was concluded that their quality of life increased and school absenteeism decreased (Beheshtipoor et al., 2015).

When we examine the literature on yoga applied to preschool-age children, it focuses on studies conducted with healthy children. It is emphasized that yoga supports the acquisition of emotional regulation skills in this age group (Özyayla, 2023). In their study, Stapp and Wolff (2019) examined the benefits of yoga practices from the perspective of 3-5-year-old children and concluded that yoga is a practice that supports children's physical, cognitive, and social development. In their study where Jarraya et al. (2019) evaluated the effects of yoga practice on the cognitive performance, visual-motor coordination, inattention, and hyperactivity behaviors of 5-year-old children, they concluded that it could be a holistic exercise and an effective exercise activity in kindergarten that can increase children's learning-related functions.

Conclusion

Yoga practice for children of different age groups is a holistic practice that we examined and is a low-cost, supportive treatment method. When existing studies are examined, it is seen that yoga has positive effects on body and mind health. This should include supporting yoga practices in children, increasing their applicability by health professionals and educators, and improving the awareness of parents and children about yoga.

The effects of yoga programs on children become more evident when applied regularly and systematically. However, studies on the risks of yoga practice or groups in which it is at risk are not sufficient. Additionally, there are no evidence-based results to recommend a particular type of yoga to a certain age group. In future studies, there is a need for protocols explaining which type of yoga and how yoga practice should be done for children and adolescents. For this reason, in future yoga practices, evidence-level data should be obtained by studying different types of yoga with larger samples according to age groups. Child health is a multidisciplinary field; therefore, educational sciences and health professionals should make plans to introduce yoga practice for children and adolescents into the curriculum at educational levels.

Yoga education should be included in the nursing education curriculum to be applicable in clinics and include yoga in nursing care. Child Health and Diseases nurses should integrate yoga practice with care plans, and plans should be made to create yoga areas where practice can be performed in hospitals. In families with children with chronic diseases, parent-child (partner yoga) yoga should be planned to improve the quality of life and reduce the stress of the caregiver while maintaining family-centered care.

Overall, children's yoga offers a holistic approach to promoting children's physical, mental, and emotional well-being. By providing a safe and nurturing space for exploration and self-discovery, children's yoga enables children to develop lifelong skills for health, happiness, and resilience.

In conclusion, yoga programs designed and implemented based on scientific evidence can support and improve children's physical, mental, and emotional health. It is predicted that yoga practice will increase its popularity as an alternative and complementary treatment by supporting the independent functions of nurses.

References

Adaiçi, M., Çıray, N. (2023). The Effect of Vinyasa Yoga with the Natural Flow of Breath on Nursing Care: Traditional Compilation. *Journal of Traditional Medical Complementary Therapies, 6*(1).

Aydın, D., Özgen, Z. E. (2018). Cocuklarda yoganin etkileri: Sistematik derleme. *In International Conference on Empiricial Economics&Social Science*, 96-103.

Basavaraddi, I. V. (2015). Yoga: Its origin, history and development. *Public Diplomacy*, *1*, 1-5.

Bayındır, N. (2022). Opinions of prospective classroom teachers on the benefits of children's yoga. *Journal of Interdisciplinary Educational Research, 6*(11), 12-21.

Bayraktar, A. (2021). Children's yoga instructor certificate program 2nd module. *Active Person.*

Beheshtipoor, N., Bagheri, S., Hashemi, F., Zare N., Karimi, M. (2015). The effect of yoga on the quality of life in the children and adolescents with haemophilia. *Int J Community Based Nurs Midwifery, 3*(2):150-155.

Belfer, I., Shurtleff, D. (2023). Yoga What do you need to know. *National Institutes of Health National Center for Complementary and Integrative Health.* Available from: https://www.nccih.nih.gov/health/yoga-what-you-need-to-know

Bermejo A, Alvarez B, Martinez V, Garcia H, Torres C, Sanches L. (2017). Association between physical activity, sedentary behavior, and fitness with health related quality of life in healthy children and adolescents. *Medicine Baltimore, 96* (12): 6407.

Bernstein, A. M., Bar, J., Ehrman, J. P., Golubic, M., Roizen, M. F. (2014). Yoga in the management of overweight and obesity. *Am J Lifestyle Med, 8*(1):33-41.

Bodur, B. (2020). Children's yoga. Reading Us.

Bower, J. E., Garet, D., & Sternlieb, B. (2011). Yoga for persistent fatigue in breast cancer survivors: Results of a pilot study. *Evidence-Based Complementary and Alternative Medicine, 2011*(1), 623168.

Büssing, A., Michalsen, A., Khalsa, S. B. S., Telles, S., & Sherman, K. J. (2012). Effects of yoga on mental and physical health: a short summary of reviews. *Evidence-Based Complementary and Alternative Medicine, 2012*(1), 165410.

Carlson, L. E., & Bultz, B. D. (2008). Mind–body interventions in oncology. *Current Treatment Options in Oncology, 9*(2), 127-134.

Collins, C. (1998). Yoga: Intuition, preventive medicine, and treatment. Journal of Obstetric, *Gynecologic, & Neonatal Nursing, 27*(5), 563-568.

Culver, K. A., Whetten, K., Boyd, D. L., O'Donnell, K. (2015). Yoga to Reduce Trauma-Related Distress and Emotional and Behavioral Difficulties Among Children Living in Orphanages in Haiti: A Pilot Study. *J Altern Complement Med., 21*(9), 539-45.

Dai, C., Sharma, M., Chen, C., Yesilyurt, E., Godbey, S. (2021). Yoga as an Alternative Therapy for Weight Management in Child and Adolescent Obesity: A Systematic Review and Implications for Research. *Alternative Ther Health Med, 27*(1), 8-55.

Das, R. R., Sankar, J., Kabra, S. K. (2019). Role of Breathing Exercises and Yoga/Pranayama in Childhood Asthma: A Systematic Review. *Curr Pediatr Rev., 15*(3), 175-83.

De Michelis, E. (2008). A history of modern yoga: Patanjali and Western esotericism. London; Continuum.

Desikachar, K., Bragdon, L., & Bossart, C. (2005). The yoga of healing: Exploring yoga's holistic model for health and well-being. *International Journal of Yoga Therapy, 15*(1), 17-39.

Domingues, R. B. (2018). Modern postural yoga as a mental health promotion tool: A systematic review. *Complement Ther Clin Pract., 31,* 248-55.

Evans, S., Tsao, J., Sternlieb, B. & Zeltzer, L. (2009). Using the Biopsychosocial Model to Understand the Health Benefits of Yoga. *Journal of Complementary and Integrative Medicine, 6*(1). https://doi.org/10.2202/1553-3840.1183

Felver, J., Butzer, B., Olson, K., Smith, I. M., Khalsa, S. (2015). Yoga in Public School Improves Adolescent Mood and Affect. *Contemp School Psychology, 19*(3), 184-192.

Felver, J. C., Razza, R., Morton, M. L., Clawson, A. J., & Mannion, R. (2020). School-based yoga intervention increases adolescent resilience: a pilot trial. *Journal of Child & Adolescent Mental Health, 32*(1), 1-10.

Fishbein, D., Miller, S., Stahl, M. H., Williams, J., Lavery, B., Markovitz, L., Kluckman, M., Mosoriak, G., Johnson, M. (2016). Behavioral and psychophysiological effects of a yoga intervention on high-risk adolescents: a randomized control trial. *Journal of Child and Family Studies, 25,* 518–529.

Fouladbakhsh, J., & Stommel, M. (2010). Gender, Symptom Experience, and Use of Complementary and Alternative Medicine Practices Among Cancer Survivors in the U.S. Cancer Population. *Oncology Nursing Forum,* E7-E15.

Frank, J. L., Bose, B., Clonan, A. S. (2014). Effectiveness of a school-based yoga program on adolescent mental health, stress coping strategies, and attitudes toward violence: findings from a high-risk sample. *Journal of Applied School Psychology, 30,* 29–49.

Frank, J. L., Kohler, K., Peal, A., Bose, B. (2017). Effectiveness of a school-based yoga program on adolescent mental health and school performance: findings from a randomized controlled trial. *Mindfulness, 8,* 544–553.

Fundamentals of children's yoga. (2024,10 March). Access address: https://childrensyoga.com/about-radiant-child/

Iyengar, B. K. S. (1993). *Light on the yoga sutras of Patanjali* (pp. 136). Aquarian/Thorsons.

Govardhan, H. B, Nelson, N., Khaleel, I., Kumar, A., Roy, M., S.J. D, K.R. H, Hegde A, K.R. A., Vasana, H., Merrin, S., Paula, S., Kashyapa, R., Kalyyani, B. (2019). Effect of yoga on the symptomps response in pediatric brain tumor in-patients undergoing chemo and radiotherapy. *Oncology and Radiotherapy, 1*(46), 034-038.

İlter, S. M., Ovayolu, Ö. (2023) Pranayama and Nursing. *Holist Nurs Pract* [Internet], *35*(1):29–33. Available from: https://journals.lww.com/hnpjournal/Fulltext/2021/01000/Pranayama_and_Nursing.5.aspx.

Jacobs, S. S. (2014). Integrative Therapy Use for Management of Side Effects and Toxicities Experienced by Pediatric Oncology Patients. *Children(Basel), 1,* 24-40.

James-Palmer, A., Anderson, E. Z., Zucker, L., Kofman, Y., & Daneault, J. F. (2020). Yoga as an intervention for the reduction of symptoms of anxiety and depression in children and adolescents: A systematic review. *Frontiers in pediatrics, 8,* 78.

Janjhua, Y., Chaudhary, R., Sharmave N., Kumar, K. (2020). A study on the effect of yoga on emotional regulation, self-esteem, and feelings of adolescents. *J Family Med Premium Care, 9*(7), 3381–3386.

Jarraya, S., Wagner, M., Jarraya, M., & Engel, F. A. (2019). 12 weeks of kindergarten-based yoga practice increases visual attention, visual-motor precision and decreases behavior of inattention and hyperactivity in 5-year-old children. *Frontiers in psychology, 10,* 796.

Khalsa, S. B. S., Butzer, B. (2016). Yoga in school settings: a research review. *Ann NY Acad Sci.* 1373:45–55.

Koenig, K. P, Buckley-Reen, A, Garg, S. (2012). Efficacy of the Get Ready to Learn yoga program among children with autism spectrum disorders: a pretest-posttest control group design. *Am J Occup Ther., 66*(5), 538-46.

Kupershmidt, S., Barnable, T. (2019). Definition of a Yoga Breathing (Pranayama) Protocol That Improves Lung Function. *Holist Nurs Pract* [Internet]. *33*(4), 197–203. Available from: https://journals.lww.com/00004650- 201907000-00002.

Lack, S., Brown, R., Kinser, P. A. (2020). An Integrative Review of Yoga and Mindfulness-Based Approaches for Children and Adolescents with Asthma. *Journal of Pediatric Nursing, 52,* 76-81.

Lyman, G. H., Bohlke, K., Cohen, L. (2018). Integrative therapies during and after breast cancer treatment: ASCO endorsement of the SIO clinical practice guideline summary. *Journal Oncology Practice, 14*(8), 49.

Manjunath, N. K., Telles, S. (2005). Influence of Yoga and Ayurveda on self-rated sleep in a geriatric population. *Indian Journal Medicine Research, 121*(5), 683-90.

Mcgonigal, K. (2006). Yoga for kids. *IDEA Fit Journal, 3,* 91-9.

Narasingharao, K, Pradhan, B, Navaneetham, J. (2017). Efficacy of Structured Yoga Intervention for Sleep, Gastrointestinal and Behavior Problems of ASD Children: An Exploratory Study. *Journal of Clinical and Diagnostic Research, 11*(3), 01-06.

Neumark-Sztainer, D., Wall, M. M., Choi, J., Barr-Anderson, D. J., Telke, S., & Mason, S. M. (2020). Exposure to adverse events and associations with stress levels and the practice of yoga: Survey findings from a population-based study of diverse emerging young adults. *The Journal of Alternative and Complementary Medicine, 26*(6), 482-490.

Noogle, J. J., Steiner, N. J., Minami, T., Khalsa, S. B. S. (2012). Benefits of yoga for psychosocial well-being in a US high school curriculum: a preliminary randomized controlled trial. *Journal Dev Behav Pediatr. 33,*193–201.

Önder, Ö. (2019). *365 days of breathing.* Istanbul, Kuraldışı Publishing. 78, 79, 84.

Ozgun, S. Y., Özkul, F. B., Oral, E., & Şemin, M. İ. (2021). The effects of yoga education on the cognitive functions of children in early childhood. *Egitim Ve Bilim-Education And Science.*

Özyayla, E. D. (2023). *The effect of yoga program on five-year-old children's emotional regulation and social skills.* Master's thesis, Ege University, Izmir.

ReP, McConnell J. W, ReidingerG, SchweitR, Hendron, A. (2014). Effects of Yoga on Patientsinan Adolescent Mental Health Hospital and the Relationship Between Those Effects and the Patients Sensory-Processing Patterns. *Journal of Child and Adolescent Psychiatric Nursing, 27*(4), 175-182.

Richardson, J. (2001). Integrating complementary therapies into health care education: a cautious approach. *Journal Clinical Nursing, 10*(6), 793-8.

Rojas-Cooley, M. T., Grant, M. (2006). Complementary and alternative medicine: Oncology nurses' experiences, educational interests, and resources. *Oncology nursing forum, 33*(3), 581-588.

Ross, R. (2001). Alternative and Complementary Treatment in Neurologic Illness, Yoga as a therapeutic modality, In M. I. Weintraub (Ed). *NY: NY, Churchill Livingstone*, 75-92.

Sarkissian, M., Trent, N. L., Huchting, K. and Khalsa, S. B. S. (2018) "Effects of a Kundalini Yoga Program on Elementary and Middle School Students' Stress, Affect, and Resilience," *Journal of Developmental and Behavioral Pediatrics, 39*(3), 210-216.

Singh, K. P. (2018). Effect of yoga on stress and academic performance. *Educational Quest-An International Journal of Education and Applied Social Sciences*, *9*(2), 169-173.

Singleton, M., Goldberg, E. (Eds.). (2013). *Gurus of modern yoga*. Oxford university press. Oxford.

Stapp, A. C., Wolff, K. (2019). Young children's experiences with yoga in an early childhood setting. *Early Child Development and Care, 189*(9), 1397-1410.

Tamilselvi, B., & Mala, V. (2016). Yoga--A Boon to the Adjustment Problems and Behavioural Disorders of Adolescent Students. *Journal on Educational Psychology*, *10*(2), 1-8.

Tejvani, R., Metri, K. G., Agrawal, J, Nagenddra, H. R. (2016). Effect of yoga on anxiety, depression and self-esteem in orphanage residents: a pilot study. *Ayu. Jan-Mar, 37*(1), 22–25.

Velásquez, A. M., López, M. A., Quiñonez, N., & Paba, D. P. (2015). Yoga for the prevention of depression, anxiety, and aggression and the promotion of socio-emotional competencies in school-aged children. *Educational Research and Evaluation*, *21*(5-6), 407-421.

Yadav, R. K., Magan, D., Mehta, N., Sharma, R., & Mahapatra, S. C. (2012). Efficacy of a short-term yoga-based lifestyle intervention in reducing stress and inflammation: preliminary results. *The journal of alternative and complementary medicine*, *18*(7), 662-667.

Chapter 22

Evidence-Based Serious Games in Pediatric Care

Hilal Parlak Sert*, PhD
Denizli Healthcare Vocational School, Pamukkale University, Denizli, Türkiye

Abstract

Children may find hospitalization to be a stressful experience. Children who are hospitalized show high levels of anxiety symptoms. Being away from home and entering a hospital environment causes anxiety and stress for both the child and the child's family. The basis of these fears and concerns is inadequate preparation for hospitalization and the lack of information. Children who are afraid and anxious can be uncooperative when performing clinical procedures. If their fears and concerns are not addressed, these negative emotions can become permanent and can be triggered when they return to the hospital, which can have negative effects on long-term health outcomes. These fears of children need to be reduced. Children state that they will have less fear and anxiety if they are informed about hospital-related procedures. While providing this information, it should be child-centered. Interventions that will reduce children's fear and anxiety during hospitalization include classical methods such as developing books or brochures and having them draw pictures. Although these methods have demonstrated various benefits, computer, and web-based interventions have been shown to be the best way to prepare hospitalized children. Computer and web-based interventions have begun to be used frequently in children in recent years. Especially the fact that children are very interested in digital games, and the increase in child internet users day by day has created a different area for nurses to implement interventions using serious game interventions. The uses of serious game interventions in the field of child health are interventions such as increasing the anxiety, pain, and knowledge level of children who are hospitalized for various reasons.

In this section, it will be described the effects of serious game interventions in the care of hospitalized children.

Keywords: artificial intelligence, children, pediatric care, serious games

* Corresponding Author's Email: hilalsert@pau.edu.tr

In: Evidence-Based Care Practices in Pediatric Nursing
Editors: Feyza Küçük and Serap Özdemir
ISBN: 979-8-89530-304-7

Introduction

Serious games are games designed for learning, not just for fun, with education as their main goal (Abt, 1987; Ingadottir et al., 2017; Matthyssens et al., 2020; Kokol et al., 2020). They are also known as the next generation of video games that offer learning and educational opportunities (Ferrante et al., 2021). Serious games are different from traditional ways of teaching. They are shown to be very valuable interventions as teaching tools because they easily capture the attention of the group to which the method is applied and thus ensure more permanent learning (Barbosa et al., 2011; Abidin et al., 2020; Froome et al., 2020).

Serious games are used in different fields such as economy, education, industry, politics, and the military (Blumberg et al., 2012; Abd Majid et al., 2020). Nowadays, serious games are being used more and more in the field of health. Serious game interventions are considered new and promising approaches (Matthyssens et al., 2020).

Serious gaming interventions have started to be used in the field of child health, as they have positive results on children's increased access to the Internet, increased rates of computer use, increased interest in digital games, learning and motivation gains (Abidin et al., 2020; TUIK 2021). The more time the child spend in serious games, the more knowledge they have about the disease and the better they can manage it (Moosa et al., 2020).

Serious games are used in children with chronic diseases that require hospitalization and in children who undergo surgery. Serious games contribute to improving the health outcomes of children with chronic diseases, reducing the anxiety of children hospitalized for surgery, providing pain control in the post-op period of children undergoing surgery, increasing healthy lifestyle skills by providing behavioral change in children, and many other contributions to child health. In addition to contributing to the field of child health, the use of artificial intelligence is also important because it is appreciated by both parents and children. Children are willing to play the designed serious games (Liszio & Masuch, 2017; Ingen, 2018; Buffel et al., 2019, Eijlers et al., 2019, Kim et al., 2019).

Serious games used in many areas to improve the health and quality of life of pediatric patients, are one of the current interventions that nurses involved in the care of children can use (Rewolinski et al., 2021). In this section, the introduction of the serious game and its use in diseases requiring hospitalization will be explained.

Serious Games

The concept of serious games was first used in the literature in 1970 (Abt, 1987). In general terms, "serious games" refer to games that are not only for fun but are designed for learning, where the main goal is education (Abt, 1987; Ingadottir et al., 2017; Abidin et al., 2020, Matthyssens et al., 2020, Kokol et al., 2020). Video and Web-based games, which are digital versions of serious games, are more widely used (Kokol et al., 2020; Matthyssens et al., 2020).

Serious games have their own purposes. The most important difference that distinguishes the serious game from other computer games is that it has two objectives, explicit and implicit. The explicit goal is the fun inherent in every game, and the implicit goal is to increase skills and abilities and to gain knowledge and experience (Wattanasoontorn et al.,

2013). The aim of serious games is to develop skills or behavioral changes in the user through education rather than entertainment (Abt, 1987; Blumberg et al., 2012; Carlier et al., 2020).

Serious games are different from traditional teaching methods. It easily attracts the attention of the group to which the method is applied. Serious games provide more permanent learning with this feature. With such positive outcomes, serious games have been shown to be very valuable interventions as teaching tools (Barbosa & Silva, 2011; Abidin et al., 2020; Froome et al., 2020). Since serious games have a high impact on teaching and learning, the importance of having educational applications in the game when designing them is emphasized (Ravyse et al., 2017; Lööf et al., 2019; Abidin et al., 2020).

Design of Serious Games

Serious game design needs to balance fun and learning. Serious games should have neither a dominant play mode (distraction from learning) nor a dominant learning mode (removal of entertainment elements) (Ravyse et al., 2017). The player should be excited while playing the game, motivated to keep going, and at the same time achieve the primary goal of learning. The information to be provided while playing the game should be provided without tiring the user too much (Graafland et al., 2012; Abd Majid et al., 2020). Although there are different views on how serious games should be designed, there are no clear principles that have yet been fully articulated (Ravyse et al., 2017).

When designing serious games, the emphasis is on having components. Serious games have four components. The first of these components is that it is a game with rules. The second component is a difficulty. In this component, there should be different levels in the game and there should be a reward or punishment system. The aim of this component is to ensure that the player enjoys the game and is encouraged to finish the game and play it again. The third component is interaction. This component aims to enable the player to interact with the game. The interactions are visual (using interesting pictures in the game), physical (allowing the player to type on the device on which the game is played, using a mouse), and auditory (using interesting sounds in the game). The last component is the goal. A goal is defined as something that the player aims to achieve or accomplish through their efforts while playing the game. When creating a serious game, players should be motivated to keep playing, even to play the game over and over again, in order to achieve the goal of the game. The player who wants to be "good" at the game repeats the information given as they play again and again. Serious games have many advantages over traditional learning methods because they include competitive elements, entertainment aspects, and feedback mechanisms (Graafland, 2012; Wattanasoontorn et al., 2013).

The Use of Serious Games in Healthcare

Serious games are widely used in different fields such as health, education, economy, industry, military, and politics (Blumberg et al., 2012; Abd Majid et al., 2020). Another reason for its increasing use is that the games designed can be played on well-established platforms such as personal computers, game consoles, web browsers, and smartphones, making them more accessible to players (Abd Majid et al., 2020; Carlier et al., 2020). The serious game industry is growing rapidly in academic research fields. As serious games have many advantages in teaching and learning, they are frequently used especially in education and health studies (Matthyssens et al., 2020; D'Agostini et al., 2020).

Nowadays, serious games are being used much more in the field of health. Games designed for health have medical goals (to be user-friendly, simple, and attractive, to inform about treatment and diagnosis, or to rehabilitate), technological goals (to design and develop accessible computer applications), and social goals (to help education and socialization at home and school) (Bartolomé et al., 2011). Serious games in the field of health are mostly designed to increase the player's compliance with medical treatments. Serious games are used to make health education enjoyable and provide information by distancing the hospitalized child from the environment (Abd Majid et al., 2020; Carlier et al., 2020; Piil et al., 2021).

Serious games have an impact on learning gains for adults and children. Those who played serious games reported that they recommended serious games in their feedback and were willing to play again (Barbosa and Silva 2011; Ingadottir et al., 2017; Tan et al., 2017; De Sena et al., 2019; Carlier et al., 2020). This advantage also stems from the fact that serious games target child-centered information (Abidin et al., 2020). For example, serious game intervention is effective in vocabulary learning in children with autism, and the retention of the meanings of words learned through serious games is high. Serious game intervention is also an effective educational tool for children to learn nutrition (Khowaja and Salim 2019; Froome et al., 2020). Serious game interventions are considered new and promising approaches to educate, prepare, and distract children (Matthyssens et al., 2020). Serious game interventions have been used for various purposes in children undergoing surgery, children with diabetes, children with asthma, obese/overweight children, and children with autism.

Serious Game Use in Children Undergoing Surgery

Children experience significant anxiety when they have surgery. They also report pain up to one week after surgery. The higher the level of anxiety in children, the more they report pain in the postoperative period. Therefore, anxiety control is very important in children who will undergo surgery. Non-pharmacologic methods to reduce anxiety levels are frequently preferred by nurses because they are both safe and non-invasive. It is aimed to develop and use a non-pharmacological method to reduce the level of anxiety before anesthesia (Vrancken et al., 2021). The use of serious games, one of the non-pharmacological methods used in this field, is becoming increasingly popular (Matthyssens et al., 2020). The use of serious game intervention is recommended to relieve preoperative anxiety in children hospitalized for the surgical procedure (Kim et al., 2019; Ingadottir, 2022). Children using serious game intervention have lower levels of preoperative anxiety than children undergoing routine clinical hospitalization procedures (Buffel et al., 2019; Kim et al., 2019; Matthyssens et al., 2020).

Non-serious games are used to reduce anxiety levels in children before surgery. These games reduce children's preoperative anxiety levels. In comparison, the preoperative anxiety levels of children using serious game interventions were also lower than those of children playing non-serious games (Matthyssens et al., 2020). The developed serious games also reduce the anxiety levels of parents staying with children who will undergo surgery (Buffel et al., 2019).

Serious game designs are made to increase the level of knowledge of children who will undergo surgery. Providing information on hospitalization through games gives positive results (Vrancken et al., 2021). When they play games designed for this purpose, their knowledge about pain medications and pain management strategies improves. (Ingadóttir et al., 2017). Accordingly, anxiety decreases and there is a significant reduction in postoperative pain (Buffel et al., 2019; Kim et al., 2019; Matthyssens et al., 2020). Serious games have been developed to prepare young children for anesthesia. Developed serious games help to increase the level of knowledge in young children (4-7 age group) (Vrancken et al., 2021).

Serious games developed to contribute to children who will undergo surgery have positive results and are enjoyed by children and parents. Children who play serious games recommend these games to their peers to play (Buffel et al., 2019).

Serious Game Use in Children with Diabetes

According to the World Health Organization (WHO), the risk of diabetes in children is increasing worldwide. Type 1 diabetes in children is a chronic disease. Although the cause is not fully explained, it is currently thought to be the result of a combination of genetic and environmental factors. Today, there is no known way to prevent type 1 diabetes. For this reason, if not managed well, it can cause chronic problems and early death in children over time (WHO, 2022).

In children diagnosed with diabetes, treatment processes begin with lifestyle changes. To cope with the disease more easily, they need to learn how to manage this process appropriately on their own. Children with diabetes need to increase their level of awareness about their disease (Rewolinski et al., 2021). They need to be supported in controlling diabetes. Serious games, which are one of the best ways to teach children to have fun, are frequently used in this field (Moosa et al., 2020; Rewolinski et al., 2021; Nørlev, et al., 2022). The reason why serious games have become popular in diabetes management is that traditional education methods are insufficient compared to game-based approaches (Rewolinski et al., 2021).

Serious games used in diabetes are often designed to provide skills, education, and behavioral improvement for people with diabetes (Asadzandi et al., 2020; Ihsan et al., 2020). Several serious games have been designed to teach diabetes self-management to children with T1 diabetes (Nørlev, et al., 2022). The games designed are games that can be played individually and games that are competed as a team (Nørlev, et al., 2022; Moosa, 2020).

Serious games designed for diabetic children motivate children to learn about the disease, eat healthy foods, move, and control blood sugar (Moosa, 2020). It is seen that serious games designed to regulate the eating behaviors of children with diabetes are effective. Diabetic children who play such games show healthier eating behavior (Alsaleh and Alnanih, 2020). The designed serious games helped children decrease their HbA 1c levels (Moosa, 2020).

Serious games developed to support the treatment of diabetic children have enabled children to get used to insulin injections. children who play the serious game designed for this purpose learn the correct injection site and the correct injection method. Thus, psychological preparation is completed in children. It reduces stress, anxiety, and fear of insulin injection in children (Ebrahimpour et al., 2014).

There are serious games developed for the prevention of diabetes. The aim of the games is to educate about healthy food choices and to prevent diabetes by raising awareness about healthy food choices (Ihsan et al., 2020). Serious games are an effective educational tool to support children in learning about healthy nutrition (Froome et al., 2020; Espinosa-Curiel et al., 2022).

Serious Game Use in Children with Asthma

Asthma is one of the most common chronic diseases in children worldwide. Treatment and effective management of asthma save lives. Asthma is an important non-communicable disease affecting both children and adults and is the most common chronic disease among children. Asthma is one of the most common chronic inflammatory diseases worldwide (Kansen et al., 2020; Castro-Rodriguez and Forno, 2020; WHO, 2023). Asthma affects both adults and children. It is the most common chronic disease among children (WHO, 2023). Asthma is a major cause of morbidity in children (Castro-Rodriguez and Forno, 2020; Pijnenburg and Fleming, 2020). Asthma affected an estimated 262 million people and caused 455,000 deaths in 2019 (WHO, 2023).

When asthma is well controlled, the risk of exacerbations is reduced and quality of life is improved. There are no effective treatments for asthma, but uncontrolled asthma in children is quite common. Children are more likely to be admitted to the hospital with an asthma attack. Reasons for this include children's lack of understanding of asthma triggers and fear due to previous negative experiences. These reasons prevent children from participating in asthma self-management (Sarasmita et al., 2021). Therefore, asthma control in children should be handled more carefully (Kansen et al., 2020). Strategies are needed to prevent exacerbations, preserve lung function, and protect children from the harmful effects of asthma (Pijnenburg and Fleming, 2020).

One of the current strategies to improve the health of children with asthma is digital learning. In children, game-based education is effective in gaining knowledge, developing skills, contributing to self-care, and motivating for disease management (Sarasmita et al., 2021). The current digital approach to the care of children with asthma is serious games. Serious games developed for children with asthma increase children's level of knowledge. At the same time, serious games are a fun way for children with asthma to interact with their peers and parents (Ferrante, 2021). It is suggested that more serious games should be developed for asthma education and self-management in children (Silva-Lavigne et al., 2022). There are serious games developed for asthma in the current literature. Informing children about asthma disease is prioritized. The child whose knowledge increases through play increases self-management in asthma and supports the growth of the child (Sarasmita et al., 2021; Drummond et al., 2017).

Serious Game Use in Overweight/Obese Children

Obesity is defined as abnormal or excessive fat accumulation that adversely affects health. WHO defines obesity as a "non-communicable disease in childhood". Childhood obesity is one of the most serious public health problems of the 21st century. It is known that most of those who are overweight/obese in childhood (OOC) maintain this condition in adulthood. OOC children have high rates of non-communicable diseases such as diabetes and cardiovascular diseases at an early age. Therefore, prevention of childhood obesity is a high priority (WHO, 2020).

Today, different strategies are being developed to prevent OOC in children. One of these is serious games. Serious games have made significant contributions to the fight against childhood obesity. Serious games developed to prevent childhood obesity are categorized into 4 groups. The first of these groups includes games that aim to reduce energy intake. In these games, health education and/or changing children's attitudes toward food are prioritized. Group 2 games, on the other hand, aim to ensure weight control and put nutritional knowledge into practice. It aims to control the child's behavior and calorie intake in an obesogenic environment through self-regulation. Group 3 games include games that aim to increase energy expenditure. Physical activity and exercise are prioritized in the games. In the last group of games, a multidisciplinary approach is aimed. In such games, increasing motivation, healthy eating, coping with stress, and creating behavioral change are prioritized (Belghali et al, 2021). In serious games developed for the prevention of OOC in children, the guidelines actively used by countries are also utilized (Fossariet al., 2023).

Serious games are considered a fun and effective format that can be used in OOC prevention. It can be considered an alternative educational tool that can be used in children's education in this field (Holzmann et al., 2020). In health education provided through serious games, children's health knowledge increases (Dias et al., 2018). Serious games are very effective in developing positive habits in children and providing motivation for obesity treatment (Dias et al., 2021). Some serious games designed in this field are used to raise awareness about balanced calorie intake, nutrition, and healthy lifestyle (Michael et al., 2018). Another important factor for children is the sustainability of the information they learn and the behavioral changes they create. Developed serious games increase children's knowledge about nutrition and coping with stress in a sustainable way (Mack et al., 2020).

Another component of the formation of OOC in childhood is the family. Examples include eating behaviors and unbalanced lifestyle habits of family members. In addition, family support is very important to create behavioral change in children. Weight management practices should motivate both children and families to create behavioral change (Weiland et al., 2022). Therefore, a family-centered approach should be adopted in programs to prevent or treat childhood OAC. It is not easy for parents to adapt to and sustain a new lifestyle. Therefore, effective and engaging strategies are needed. The most current strategies are the use of serious games (Afonso et al., 2020). Parents are included in serious games developed to protect children from obesity/overweight. Parents are willing to play games designed for this purpose. Serious games developed to protect children from oak are effective for parents. With the serious games developed, parents learn which foods are suitable for a healthy diet (Gonçalves et al., 2020).

Serious Game Use in Children with Autism

Autism Spectrum Disorder (ASD) is a neurodevelopmental disorder that starts early in life and continues. Children have symptoms ranging from mild to severe (Lauritsen, 2013). With the increasing prevalence rates of ASD, the issue of helping to treat autistic children has become important. In this regard, serious games seem to make valuable contributions (De Carvalho et al., 2023). In recent years, there has been an increase in serious games designed for autistic children. Studies offer intervention and evaluation for autistic individuals (Hassan et al., 2021; Chua et al., 2022). It is known that children affected by Autism Spectrum Disorder have an increased incidence of obesity. For this reason, serious games are used to prevent obesity and increase the frequency of movement. Serious game allows children with ASD to do activities in the water environment and develop motor skills with a fun approach (De Carolis and Argentieri 2020).

ASD is a disorder characterized by social interaction and communication difficulties (Carlier et al., 2020). In recent years, there has been an increase in the number of serious games designed for social and socio-emotional skills to improve children's quality of life (De Carvalho et al. 2023). Designed serious games have shown positive results in helping to develop social and socio-emotional skills (Hassan et al., 2021).

Serious games were designed to improve daily life activities in children with autism. Positive results were obtained in the serious game aimed at supporting the child's showering skills (Kang, 2019). The serious game developed to help them learn how to ride the bus had positive results and the anxiety felt by children while riding the bus decreased (Simões et al., 2018). Positive feedback was received from the game developed to support them to shop at the grocery store, one of the activities of daily life (Vallefuoco et al., 2022). Another serious game designed to support life skills is to help students understand the concept of money and transfer it to their practical lives (Caria et al., 2018). In addition to these existing games, it is currently recommended to design serious games that aim to develop different skills in children with ASD (De Carvalho et al., 2023).

Conclusion

The serious game has many contributions to child health. Serious game interventions yield positive results in children with chronic diseases and children preparing for surgery. Serious game interventions reduce children's anxiety in children with chronic diseases who are hospitalized (Parlak Sert, 2023; Keehn et al., 2013; Wijnhoven et al., 2015; Carlier et al., 2020).

Serious games are interactive, engaging, and provide permanent learning and consequently facilitate behavior change (Froome et al., 2020). Because serious games have these advantages, they are used to gain self-care competence in children with chronic diseases. In studies conducted in various countries around the world, it has been concluded that it has a motivating effect on behavior change to gain the necessary competence for self-care in children with chronic diseases such as hemodialysis, diabetes, asthma, attention deficit, hyperactivity disorder, and strengthening children's coping behaviors with the disease they have (Bul et al., 2018; Santana et al., 2020; Sarasmita et al., 2021). It also has positive contributions to children with developmental disabilities and children with speech-hearing-vision problems. The development of self-management behaviors in children makes it easier to cope with the disease and also contributes to the growth and the development of children (Sarasmita et al., 2021).

Serious game intervention is recommended to be used by health professionals working in this field due to its contributions to the field of child health (Jin & Kim, 2019). The awareness of health professionals working in the field of child health should be increased. The contribution to child health should be made by conducting more different studies in this field (for example, involving parents or children with different diseases/age groups).

References

Abd Majid, E. S., Garcia, J. A., Nordin, A. I., Raffe, W. L. (2020). Staying motivated during difficult times: a snapshot of serious games for paediatric cancer patients. *IEEE Transactions on Games, 12*(4), 367-375. https://doi.org/10.1109/TG.2020.3039974.

Abidin, S. R. Z., Noor, S. F. M., Sahari, N., & Talib, N. H. A. (2020). Serious game development-a miraculous literacy tool for halus students. In 2020 *5th IEEE International Conference on Recent Advances and Innovations in Engineering (ICRAIE)* (pp. 1-6). IEEE. https://doi.org/10.1109/ICRAIE51050. 2020.9358278.

Abt, C. C. (1987). *Serious Games.* University press of America, New York.

Afonso, L., Rodrigues, R., Reis, E., Miller, K., Castro, J., Parente, N., ... & Torres, S. (2020). Fammeal: A gamified mobile application for parents and children to help healthcare centers treat childhood obesity. *IEEE Transactions on Games, 12*(4), 351-360. https://doi.org/10.1109/TG.2020.3015804.

Alsaleh, N., & Alnanih, R. (2020). Gamification-based behavioral change in children with diabetes mellitus. *Procedia Computer Science, 170,* 442-449. https://doi.org/10.1016/j.procs.2020.03.087.

Asadzandi, S., Sedghi, S., Bigdeli, S., & Sanjari, M. (2020). A systematized review on diabetes gamification. *Medical Journal of the Islamic Republic of Iran, 34,* 168. https://doi.org/10.47176/mjiri.34.168.

Barbosa, A.F. & Silva, F.G. (2011). Serious Games: design and development of OxyBlood. In *Proceedings of the 8th International Conference on Advances in Computer Entertainment Technology, Article15,* 1-8. https://doi.org/10.1145/2071423.207144. 2

Bartolomé, N. A., Zorrilla, A. M., Zapirain, B. G. (2011). Can game-based therapies be trusted? Is game-based education effective? A systematic review of the Serious Games for health and education. In *2011 16th international conference on computer games. Louisville,* KY, USA https://doi.org/10.1109/ CGAMES.2011.600035.

Belghali, M., Statsenko, Y., & Al-Za'abi, A. (2021). Improving serious games to tackle childhood obesity. *Frontiers in Psychology, 12,* 657289. https://doi.org/10.3389/fpsyg.2021.657289.

Blumberg, F. C., Almonte, D. E., Anthony, J. S. ve Hashimoto, N. (2012). Serious games: what are they? what do they do? why should we play them. *The Oxford Handbook of Media Psychology*, 334–351. https://doi.org/10.1093/oxfordhb/9780195398809.013.0019.

Buffel, C., Van Aalst, J., Bangels, A., Toelen, J., Allegaert, K., Verschueren, S. ve Stichele G. V. (2019). A web-based serious game for health to reduce perioperative anxiety and pain in children (CliniPup): pilot randomized controlled trial. *JMIR Serious Games, 7*(2), Article12431. https://doi.org/10.2196/12431.

Bul, K. C., Doove, L. L., Franken, I. H., Oord, S. V. D., Kato, P. M., & Maras, A. (2018). A serious game for children with Attention Deficit Hyperactivity Disorder: Who benefits the most?. *PloS one, 13*(3), e0193681. https://doi.org/10.1371/journal.pone.0193681.

Caria, S., Paternò, F., Santoro, C., & Semucci, V. (2018). The design of web games for helping young high-functioning autistics in learning how to manage money. *Mobile Networks and Applications, 23*(6), 1735-1748. https://doi.org/10.1007/s11036-018-1069-0.

Carlier, S., Van der Paelt, S., Ongenae, F., De Backere, F., & De Turck, F. (2020). Empowering children with ASD and their parents: Design of a serious game for anxiety and stress reduction. *Sensors, 20*(4), 966. https://doi.org/10.3390/s20040966.

Castro-Rodriguez, J. A., & Forno, E. (2020). Asthma and COVID-19 in children: a systematic review and call for data. *Pediatric pulmonology, 55*(9), 2412-2418. https://doi.org/10.1002/ppul.24909.

Chua, Y. W., Lu, S. C., Anzulewicz, A., Sobota, K., Tachtatzis, C., Andonovic, I., ... & Delafield-Butt, J. (2022). Developmental differences in the prospective organisation of goal-directed movement between children with autism and typically developing children: A smart tablet serious game study. *Developmental Science, 25*(3), e13195. https://doi.org/10.1111/desc.13195.

D'Agostini, M. M., Aredes, N. D. A., Campbell, S. H. ve Fonseca, L. M. M. (2020). Serious Game e-Baby Família: an educational technology for premature infant care. *Revista Brasileira de Enfermagem, 73(*4), 1- 8. https://doi.org/10.1590/0034-7167-2019-0116.

De Carolis, B., & Argentieri, D. (2020). iBall to Swim: A Serious Game for children with Autism Spectrum Disorder. In *Proceedings of the International Conference on Advanced Visual Interfaces* (pp. 1-5). https://doi.org/10.1145/3399715.3399917.

De Carvalho, A. P., Braz, C. S., dos Santos, S. M., Ferreira, R. A., & Prates, R. O. (2023). Serious Games for Children with Autism Spectrum Disorder: A Systematic Literature Review. *International Journal of Human–Computer Interaction,* 1-28. https://doi.org/10.1080/10447318.2023.2194051.

De Sena, D. P., Fabrício, D. D., da Silva, V. D., Bodanese, L. C. ve Franco, A. R. (2019). Comparative evaluation of video-based on-line course versus serious game for training medical students in cardiopulmonary resuscitation: a randomised trial. *PloS one, 14*(4), Article0214722. https://doi.org/ 10.1371/journal.pone.0214722.

Dias, J. D., Domingues, A. N., Tibes, C. M., Zem-Mascarenhas, S. H., & Fonseca, L. M. M. (2018). Serious games como estratégia educativa para controle da obesidade infantil: revisão sistemática da literatura. *Revista Latino-Americana de Enfermagem, 26*, e3036. https://doi.org/10.1590/1518-8345.2509.3036.

Dias, J. D., Tibes-Cherman, C. M., Aragão, R. B., Tourinho Filho, H., Zem-Mascarenhas, S. H., & Fonseca, L. M. M. (2021). Serious game assessment in a child obesity tackling program. *Acta Paulista de Enfermagem, 34,* eAPE001045. https://doi.org/10.37689/acta-ape/2021AO001045.

Drummond, D., Monnier, D., Tesnière, A., & Hadchouel, A. (2017). A systematic review of serious games in asthma education. *Pediatric Allergy and Immunology, 28*(3), 257-265. https://doi.org/10.1111/pai.12690.

Ebrahimpour, F., Najafi, M., & Sadeghi, N. (2014). The design and development of a computer game on insulin injection. *Electronic physician, 6*(2), 845. https://doi.org/10.14661/2014.845-855.

Eijlers, R., Dierckx, B., Staals, L. M., Berghmans, J. M., van der Schroeff M. P., Strabbing, E. M., Wijnen, R. M. H., Hillegers M. H. J., Legerstee J. S. ve Utens E. M. W. J. (2019). Virtual reality exposure before elective day care surgery to reduce anxiety and pain in children: a randomised controlled trial. *Eur J Anaesthesiol, 36*(10), 728-737. https://doi.org/10.1097/EJA.0000000000001059.

Espinosa-Curiel, I. E., Pozas-Bogarin, E. E., Hernández-Arvizu, M., Navarro-Jiménez, M. E., Delgado-Pérez, E. E., Martínez-Miranda, J., & Pérez-Espinosa, H. (2022). HelperFriend, a serious game for promoting healthy lifestyle behaviors in children: design and pilot study. *JMIR Serious Games, 10*(2), e33412. https://doi.org/10.2196/33412.

Ferrante, G., Licari, A., Marseglia, G. L., & La Grutta, S. (2021). Digital health interventions in children with asthma. *Clinical & Experimental Allergy, 51*(2), 212-220. https://doi.org/10.1111/cea.13793.

Fossari, L. D. S. C., da Cruz, T. M. P., Mezadri, T., & Grillo, L. P. (2023). Desenvolvimento e validação de um serious game como ferramenta de educação de hábitos alimentares saudáveis em escolares. *Revista Tecnologias Educacionais em Rede (ReTER),* e5-1. https://doi.org/10.5902/2675995071626.

Froome, H. M., Townson, C., Rhodes, S., Franco-Arellano, B., LeSage, A., Savaglio, R., ... & Arcand, J. (2020). The effectiveness of the foodbot factory mobile serious game on increasing nutrition knowledge in children. *Nutrients, 12*(11), 3413. https://doi.org/10.3390/nu12113413.

Gonçalves, F., Carvalho, V., Matos, D., & Soares, F. (2020). Development of a serious game to fight childhood obesity:"barty". In *2020 IEEE Global Engineering Education Conference (EDUCON),* 1641-1646. IEEE. https://doi.org/10.1109/EDUCON45650.2020.9125408.

Graafland, M., Schraagen, J. M. ve Schijven, M. P. (2012). Systematic review of serious games for medical education and surgical skills training. *Br J Surg, 99*(10), 1322-1330. https://doi.org/10.1002/bjs.8819.

Hassan, A., Pinkwart, N., & Shafi, M. (2021). Serious games to improve social and emotional intelligence in children with autism. *Entertainment Computing, 38*. https://doi.org/10.1016/j.entcom.2021.100417.

Holzmann, S. L., Schaefer, H., Groh, G., Plecher, D. A., Klinker, G., Schauberger, G., ... & Holzapfel, C. (2020). Effects of the Digital Game "Fit, Food, Fun" on Nutritional Knowledge: A Pilot Study among German Children and Adolescents. *Proceedings of the Nutrition Society, 79*(OCE2). https://doi.org/10.1017/S0029665120004747.

Ihsan, S. N., Kadir, T. A. A., Benedict, R., & Abdullah, A. R. (2020). Preventive self-care serious games for diabetes: A game design. In *IOP Conference Series: Materials Science and Engineering, 769*(1). https://doi.org/10.1088/1757-899X/769/1/012058.

Ingadottir, B., Laitonen, E., Stefansdottir, A., Sigurdardottir, A. O., Brynjolfsdottir, B., Parisod, H., Nyman, J., Gunnarsdottir, K., Jónsdóttir, K., Salanterä, S. ve Pakarinen, A. (2022). Developing a Health Game to Prepare Preschool Children for Anesthesia: Formative Study Using a Child-Centered Approach. *JMIR Serious Games, 10*(1), Article31471. https://doi.org/10.2196/31471.

Ingadóttir, B., Zoëga, S., Blöndal, K., Thue, D., Thylen, I., & Jaarsmaa, T. (2017). The potential use of a serious game to help patients learn about post-operative pain management–An evaluation study. *Scandinavian Journal of Pain, 16*(1), 186-186. https://doi.org/10.1016/j.sjpain.2017.04.061.

Ingen, D. (2018). AIRplay: designing a game for children with asthma to support self-management [Bachelor's thesis, University of Twente]. https://purl.utwente.nl/essays/75604.

Jin, M. L., ve Kim, J. E. (2019). Usability Test of Serious Game Robot App for Hospitalized Children. *Journal of the Korea Academia-Industrial cooperation Society, 20*(2), 228-234. https://doi.org/10.13065/jksdh.20190043.

Kang, Y. S., & Chang, Y. J. (2019). Using game technology to teach six elementary school children with autism to take a shower independently. *Developmental neurorehabilitation, 22*(5), 329-337. https://doi.org/10.1080/17518423.2018.1501778.

Kansen, H. M., Le, T. M., Uiterwaal, C. S., van Ewijk, B. E., Balemans, W. A., Gorissen, D. M., ... & van Erp, F. C. (2020). Prevalence and predictors of uncontrolled asthma in children referred for asthma and other atopic diseases. *Journal of asthma and allergy,* 67-75 https://doi.org/10.2147/JAA.S231907.

Keehn, R. H. M., Lincoln, A. J., Brown, M. Z. ve Chavira, D. A. (2013). The Coping Cat program for children with anxiety and autism spectrum disorder: A pilot randomized controlled trial. *Journal of autism and developmental disorders, 43*(1), 57-67. https://doi.org/10.1007/s10803-012-1541-9.

Khowaja, K. ve Salim, S. S. (2019). Serious game for children with autism to learn vocabulary: An experimental evaluation. *International journal of human–computer interaction, 35*(1), 1-26. https://doi.org/10.1080/10447318.2017.1420006.

Kim, J., Chiesa, N., Raazi, M. ve Wright, K. D. (2019). A systematic review of technology-based preoperative preparation interventions for child and parent anxiety. *Canadian Journal of Anesthesia/Journal canadien d'anesthésie, 66*(8), 966-986. https://doi.org/10.1007/s12630-019-01387-8.

Kokol, P., Vošner, H. B., Završnik, J., Vermeulen, J., Shohieb, S. ve Peinemann, F. (2020). Serious game-based intervention for children with developmental disabilities. *Current pediatric reviews, 16*(1), 26-32. https://doi.org/10.2174/1573396315666190808115238.

Lauritsen, M. B. (2013). Autism spectrum disorders. *European child & adolescent psychiatry, 22*, 37-42. https://doi.org/10.1007/s00787-012-0359-5.

Liszio S. & Masuch M. (2017) Virtual Reality MRI: Playful Reduction of Children's Anxiety in MRI Exams. [Oral presentation]. *Conference on Interaction Design and Children. Stanford,* CA, USA. https://doi.org/10.1145/3078072.3079713.

Lööf, G., Andersson-Papadogiannakis, N. ve Silén, C. (2019). Children's Use of and Experiences With a Web-Based Perioperative Preparation Program: Directed Content Analysis. *JMIR Perioperative Medicine, 1*(2), 1-15. https://doi.org/10.2196/13565.

Mack, I., Reiband, N., Etges, C., Eichhorn, S., Schaeffeler, N., Zurstiege, G., ... & Zipfel, S. (2020). The kids obesity prevention program: cluster randomized controlled trial to evaluate a serious game for the prevention and treatment of childhood obesity. *Journal of medical Internet research, 22*(4), e15725. https://doi.org/10.2196/15725.

Matthyssens, L. E., Vanhulle, A., Seldenslach, L., Vander Stichele, G., Coppens, M. Ve Van Hoecke, E. (2020). A pilot study of the effectiveness of a serious game CliniPup® on perioperative anxiety and pain in children. *Journal of pediatric surgery,* 55(2), 304-311. https://doi.org/10.1016/j.jpedsurg.2019.10.031.

Michael, S., Katrakazas, P., Petronoulou, O., Anastasiou, A., Iliopoulou, D., & Koutsouris, D. D. (2018, October). Nutritionbuddy: a childhood obesity serious game. In *2018 Second World Conference on Smart Trends in Systems, Security and Sustainability (WorldS4)* (pp. 5-8). IEEE. https://doi.org/10.1109/ WorldS4.2018.8611473.

Moosa, A. M., Al-Maadeed, N., Saleh, M., Al-Maadeed, S. A., & Aljaam, J. M. (2020). Designing a mobile serious game for raising awareness of diabetic children. *IEEE Access, 8,* 222876-222889. https://doi.org/ 10.1109/ACCESS.2020.3043840.

Nørlev, J., Sondrup, K., Derosche, C., Hejlesen, O., & Hangaard, S. (2022). Game mechanisms in serious games that teach children with type 1 diabetes how to self-manage: a systematic scoping review. *Journal of Diabetes Science and Technology, 16*(5), 1253-1269. https://doi.org/10.1177/19322968211018236.

Parlak Sert, H. (2023). The effect of serious game on the level of anxiety, fear, knowledge of hospitalized children and level of anxiety in their parents. [Doctoral thesis, University of Pamukkale]. https://gcris.pau.edu.tr/handle/11499/55447.

Piil, K., Gyldenvang, H. H., Møller, J. K., Kjoelsen, T., Juul, J. ve Pappot, H. (2021). Electronic Games for Facilitating Social Interaction Between Parents With Cancer and Their Children During Hospitalization: Interdisciplinary Game Development. *JMIR Serious Games, 9*(1), Article16029. https://doi.org/ 10.2196/16029.

Pijnenburg, M. W., & Fleming, L. (2020). Advances in understanding and reducing the burden of severe asthma in children. *The Lancet Respiratory Medicine, 8*(10), 1032-1044.

Ravyse, W. S., Seugnet Blignaut, A., Leendertz, V. ve Woolner, A. (2017). Success factors for serious games to enhance learning: a systematic review. *Virtual Reality, 21,* 31-58. https://doi.org/10.1007/s10055-016-0298-4.

Rewolinski, J. A., Kelemen, A., & Liang, Y. (2021). Type I diabetes self-management with game-based interventions for pediatric and adolescent patients. CIN: Computers, Informatics, *Nursing, 39*(2), 78-88. https://doi.org/10.1097/CIN.0000000000000646.

Santana, C. C. D. A. P., Freitas, A. T. V. D. S., Barreto, G. O., De Avelar, I. S., Mazaro-Costa, R., Bueno, G. N., Riberio D. C., Silva G. D. ve Naghettini, A. V. (2020). Serious game on a smartphone for adolescents undergoing hemodialysis: Development and evaluation. *JMIR Serious Games, 8*(3), Article17979. https://doi.org/10.2196/17979.

Sarasmita, M. A., Larasanty, L. P. F., Kuo, L. N., Cheng, K. J., & Chen, H. Y. (2021). A computer-based interactive narrative and a serious game for children with asthma: development and content validity analysis. *Journal of Medical Internet Research, 23*(9), e28796. https://doi.org/10.2196/28796.

Silva-Lavigne, N., Valderrama, A., Pelaez, S., Bransi, M., Balli, F., Gervais, Y., ... & Tse, S. M. (2022). Acceptability of Serious Games in Pediatric Asthma Education and Self-management: Pilot Study. *JMIR Pediatrics and Parenting, 5*(2), e33389. https://doi.org/10.2196/33389.

Simões, M., Bernardes, M., Barros, F., & Castelo-Branco, M. (2018). Virtual travel training for autism spectrum disorder: proof-of-concept interventional study. *JMIR serious games, 6*(1), e8428. https://doi.org/10.2196/games.8428.

Tan, A. J. Q., Lee, C. C. S., Lin, P. Y., Cooper, S., Lau, L. S. T., Chua, W. L. ve Liaw, S. Y. (2017). Designing and evaluating the effectiveness of a serious game for safe administration of blood transfusion: A randomized controlled trial. *Nurse education today, 55,* 38-44. https://doi.org/10.1016/j.nedt.2017.04.027.

TUIK, (2021). Information Technology Usage Research in Children, 2021. Access: February 01, 2024. https://data.tuik.gov.tr/Bulten/Index?p=Cocuklarda-Bilisim-Teknolojileri-Kullanim-Arastirmasi-2021-41132.

Vallefuoco, E., Bravaccio, C., Gison, G., Pecchia, L., Pepino, A.(2022). “Personalized Training via Serious Game to Improve Daily Living Skills in Pediatric Patients With Autism Spectrum Disorder,” in *IEEE*

Journal of Biomedical and Health Informatics, 26,(7), 3312-3322, July 2022, https://doi.org/10.1109/JBHI.2022.3155367.

Vrancken, J., De Gryse, L., & Spooren, A. I. (2021). HospiAvontuur: development of a serious game to help young children and their parents during the preparation for an admission at the hospital for elective surgery. *Behaviour & Information Technology, 40*(2), 134-145. https://doi.org/10.1080/0144929X.2019.1673821.

Wattanasoontorn, V., Boada, I., García, R. ve Sbert, M. (2013). Serious games for health. *Entertainment Computing, 4*(4), 231-247. https://doi.org/10.1016/j.entcom.2013.09.002.

Weiland, A., Reiband, N., Schäffeler, N., Zurstiege, G., Giel, K. E., Zipfel, S., & Mack, I. (2022). A Serious Game for the Prevention of Obesity in School Children–Impact of Parent's Involvement: A Randomized Controlled Trial. *Life, 12*(6), 779 https://doi.org/10.3390/life12060779.

WHO. (2020). Noncommunicable diseases: Childhood overweight and obesity. 19 October 2020. Access: February 10, 2024. https://www.who.int/news-room/questions-and-answers/item/noncommunicable-diseases-childhood-overweight-and-obesity.

WHO. (2022). Diabetes: Risks for children. Access: February 02, 2024. https://www.who.int/news-room/questions-and-answers/item/diabetes-risks-for-children.

WHO. (2023). Asthma 4 May 2023. Access: February 20, 2024. https://www.who.int/news-room/fact-sheets/detail/asthma.

Wijnhoven, L. A., Creemers, D. H., Engels, R. C. ve Granic, I. (2015). The effect of the video game Mindlight on anxiety symptoms in children with an Autism Spectrum Disorder. *BMC psychiatry, 15*(1), 1-9. https://doi.org/10.1186/s12888-015-0522-x.

Chapter 23

Evidence-Based Nursing Practices in Wearable Technologies in Children

Aylin Akca Sumengen[1,*], PhD
and Damla Ozcevik Subasi[2], PhD
[1]Capstone College of Nursing, The University of Alabama, Alabama, USA
[2]Ozsubasi Architecture and Engineering Company, Aydın, Türkiye

Abstract

In recent years, science and technology have rapidly advanced, leading to exciting developments in the healthcare industry. Wearable technology products are a prime example of these developments, with many adapting to the healthcare field. While some of these products focus on disease prevention and maintaining good health, such as physical activity tracking devices for weight control, others are being developed for patient and disease management purposes. Although most of these systems are used by adults, different approaches are required for pediatric patients. While many of these products are still in the prototyping and development phase, extensive research is required to evaluate their clinical impact. However, it is believed that these technologies can significantly improve the quality of life of pediatric patients and their families, while also reducing care costs. In addition to disease-preventive and health-improving applications, there are also smartwatches used for disease management, such as epilepsy monitoring, pathological lung sound detection in children with asthma, and early warning systems for epilepsy attacks. Despite promising research results, there are still questions regarding the use of wearable technologies in pediatric patients. The adaptation, development, and improvement of technologies using artificial intelligence require continuous data collection and processing, which raises new ethical and legal concerns regarding privacy and the processing of personal data. In this section, although there are exciting and rapid developments, there is limited evidence on the use of wearable technologies in pediatric nursing. The clinical use of wearable technologies in long-term health monitoring should be investigated in various socioeconomic and sociocultural segments. Given the need for different approaches depending on the developmental period in pediatric nursing, more clinical evidence is necessary.

* Corresponding Author's Email: aakcasumengen@ua.edu.

In: Evidence-Based Care Practices in Pediatric Nursing
Editors: Feyza Küçük and Serap Özdemir
ISBN: 979-8-89530-304-7

Keywords: nursing practices, wearable technologies, children

Introduction

The use of wearable technologies in health care has increased in recent years. Izmailova et al. (2018) defined wearable technologies as sensors and software applications that are compatible with the body, can be integrated into the body, and can receive health data remotely so that the patient does not need to come to the hospital. According to the definition of Sezgin (2019), wearable technologies are generally defined as networked systems that can be integrated into the human body in different ways. In other words, literature defines technologies as wearable computers, products that communicate with devices that users can use frequently in their daily lives and make daily life easier. These products can be watches, bracelets, necklaces, headphones, glasses, and even smart optical lenses (Ercan & Timur, 2020; Sezgin, 2019). The use of wearable technologies by consumers is seen as a modern technological revolution (Ferreira et al., 2021). Wright and Keith (2014) described wearable technologies simply as wearable computers placed within different accessories or daily used products. In recent years, the daily use of these technologies has increased significantly. Pedometers and smartwatches are the best examples of the frequently used wearable technologies (Nieroda et al., 2018).

The popularity of wearable technologies is increasing rapidly. For example, between 2014 and 2017 alone, the total revenue of fitness and activity tracker devices increased from 5 billion to 20 billion US dollars (Edward et al., 2020; Fitness Trackers Statistics and Facts, 2019). The best example of the increasing use of wearable technologies is the Apple Watch. It was stated that the Apple Watch, first released in 2015, sold up to 31 million units by 2019 (Mawston, 2020). Globally, it is estimated that the total market share of wearable technologies in 2022 is 61.30 billion dollars and will increase rapidly until 2030 with a growth share of 14.6% (Market Analysis Report, 2021). Another source reported that the use of this technology will increase rapidly, and more than 150 billion euros will be consumed annually by 2028 (Hayward et al., 2018). The use of wearable technologies in health has increased much faster after the COVID-19 pandemic (Ometov et al., 2021). The pandemic has been a wake-up call for the entire healthcare system, revealing that during epidemic times, sensitive populations can be monitored remotely without having to leave the house, and this can be included in routine care. It has been stated that individuals of all age groups, especially those with chronic diseases such as asthma, diabetes, and cardiovascular diseases, benefit significantly from wearable technologies and that this is now a necessity (Greiwe & Nyenhuis, 2020; Iqbal et al., 2021).

Nurses, who can keep up with this rapid development of technology and are the supporters of the most significant change, are pioneers every day in many areas, such as increasing people's quality of life and symptom management or preventing chronic diseases (Wilson, 2017). In nursing, this technology supports areas such as patient posture monitoring (Bootsman et al., 2019), activity and nutrition levels monitoring (Sempionatto et al., 2021), as well as clinical decision-making (Wilson, 2017). Acampora et al. (2013) stated in their study that wearable technologies are very diverse in health. These are summarized as sensor networks that can make physiological measurements, physical activity tracking devices, sensors that warn against falls, motivating applications that support healthy living, applications that analyze emotions and improve mental health and can be used at all ages.

Family-centered collaborative care is undoubtedly of vital importance for pediatric patients. Wearable technologies have become a necessity in standard care, especially for preventing pediatric diseases, symptom monitoring, and disease management. To give just one example in this section, it has been stated that symptom monitoring is complex for child patients because age-related developmental milestones are different, and they have difficulty expressing their symptoms (Irwin et al., 2012). For this reason, although parental opinion is frequently taken, it has been reported that the child's symptoms are underreported, especially in acute diseases. This situation has been explained as the necessity of wearable digital technologies in this age group (Pinheiro et al., 2018; Vaughn et al., 2020; Vaughn et al., 2019).

A Brief History Behind Wearable Technologies and Healthcare

Since wearable technologies do not have a single component, it is impossible to look at their history from a single perspective. It has been stated that these technologies can be traced back to the 13th century (The College of Optometrists, 2015). Roger Bacon, who served as an English priest, first mentioned glasses and corrective lenses in his book Opus Majus (Bacon, 1928). It was stated that a few centuries later, Jean Leurechon, a French mathematician, developed the first hearing aid, which he called the ear trumpet (Heeffer, 2004). In the middle of the 20th century, these wearable products began to acquire electronic mechanisms (Casselman et al., 2017).

Biosensors are the basis of wearable technologies. It was first used in 1960 by Leland C. Clark, the father of biosensors, to detect the oxygen level in the blood. This sensor was used in cardiovascular surgery to measure continuous and real-time oxygen in the operating room and was described as groundbreaking at that time (Heineman & Jensen, 2006). It was stated that the first implantable pacemaker was developed in the same year, that is, in 1960 (Aquilina, 2006). Leland C. Clark developed a glucose detection sensor in 1962, and subsequently, in 1969, Guilbault and Montalvo Jr. announced that they had developed a sensor that could detect urea (Guilbault & Montalvo, 1969). As a continuation of these developments, biosensor development continued rapidly in various fields from 1970 to 1992 (Bhalla et al., 2016). However, the idea of sensors being integrated into the body and being used/worn continuously was first put forward by Edward O Thorp, a mathematics professor at the Massachusetts Institute of Technology (MIT), in the 1960s (Amft & Lukowicz, 2009). Since then, it has attracted the attention of almost all researchers worldwide. In recent years, with the emergence of the Internet, intelligent hardware, big data, and wearable technologies have continued to develop rapidly in many fields, including pediatric nursing (Khan et al., 2016; Lu et al., 2020).

Examples of Wearable Technologies and Areas of Use in Pediatric Nursing

The use of wearable technology in pediatric nursing is highly accepted and found to be very feasible for both nurses and families, but especially for children (Mack et al., 2022). One of the most important reasons for this is that today's children are born into technology. It has been stated that this generation, especially after the 1990s, was called "iGens" or "iGeneration", and it was stated that iGens' compatibility with mobile devices is relatively high, even if they are sick of them (Rosen, 2011). For this reason, it is thought that the use of wearable technology can reduce the symptom management burden of pediatric nurses in both acute and chronic diseases, especially in this group (Jonassaint et al., 2015; Leonard et al., 2017; Vaughn et al., 2019; von Niederhäusern et al., 2017).

Childhood chronic diseases are increasing day by day, affecting many children and families in every aspect. In the 1960s, only 1.8% of children reported a chronic disease that significantly affected their daily lives. It was stated that this rate increased to 8% after the 2010s. This means an increase in childhood chronic diseases by 400% (Van Cleave et al., 2010). It has been stated that there is a rapid increase in asthma, heart diseases, obesity, and neurodevelopmental disorders. Many factors explain the reason for this concerning increase. Furthermore, the quality of life of children and their families is seriously affected compared to their peers without chronic diseases (Blackwell et al., 2019). For families, since having a child with a chronic disease increases their anxiety levels, wearable technologies have been promising for them (Kasparian & Badawy, 2022). Wearable technologies have begun to be tested and researched in various areas of pediatric nursing.

Prevention of Disease and Maintenance of Health

Weight Control and Monitoring

Childhood obesity is a significant health problem that overgrows every year and increases health-related care costs. It has been shown that children who are obese in childhood struggle with obesity and the diseases it causes in adulthood (Sahoo et al., 2015). It is known that obesity is prevented with a good diet and physical activity, endocrine and cardiovascular diseases caused by obesity are minimized, and health costs are similarly reduced (Kumari et al., 2022). To combat this problem, wearable technologies that track physical activity, one of the most up-to-date patient-centered care solutions, have entered rapidly since the 2000s. In particular, smart watches or wristbands can measure minutes of physical activity, track heart rate, and help set goals to increase motivation (Lam et al., 2020; Telama, 2009). In addition, devices that count calories and measure sleep quality have begun to have a significant place in pediatric nurses' childhood obesity care and management (Evenson et al., 2015; Telama, 2009).

Evidence-based application data indicates that wearable technologies are used in the management of childhood obesity, focusing on three main outcomes. It is expressed as body weight, waist circumference, and total body weight (Amanda E. Staiano, 2017; Jauho et al., 2015; Mameli et al., 2018; Pittman, 2020). Wearable technologies are now used as an outcome measurement tool in many studies conducted as randomized controlled trials. An example of studies conducted mainly to measure the effectiveness of programs made/implemented is Amanda E. Staiano (2017) study, which included overweight and obese children between the ages of 8-17. In the 10-week program, which included 105 children between the ages of 8-17, a pedometer/pedometer was used to measure their activity levels. As a result of the study, it was stated that there was a statistically significant decrease in the BMI of the group in which the pedometer was used. Lubans et al. (2016) in another study conducted in Australia, an 18-month follow-up was conducted. The study results indicated no change in the children's BMI. When systematic reviews and meta-analyses that provide evidence-based data are examined, it cannot be said that there is clear evidence. Böhm et al. (2019) stated in their meta-analysis study that more studies are needed to demonstrate the effectiveness of activity-tracking devices.

Fall Identification and Prevention

Wearable technologies that improve health and prevent falls are now quite common. It has been emphasized that this technology, which includes the analysis of human movements as its working logic, is affected by various factors. These have been described as disease-related conditions with physiological, anatomical, environmental, and social effects (Godfrey et al., 2008; Shany et al., 2012). Three stages are specified for the identification and prevention of falls. These are prediction, prevention, and detection (Mozaffari et al., 2019). Although these devices are mainly produced for the elderly and are widely used (Warrington et al., 2021), there are some products that have been developed for pediatric patients.

The best example of wearable devices focused on fall identification and prevention developed for children is the algorithm which developed by Smith and Bagley (2010) for cerebral palsy patients, including a miniature wearable activity meter and a fall assessment monitor. In the development of this device, a total of 50 hours of video recordings of 35 children with cerebral palsy and 51 children with typical development were taken. They reported that the developed algorithm worked with 100% accuracy and could determine trunk rotation. However, they stated that they achieved a sensitivity of 72% to 78% in detecting lower extremity movements. Cory's (2021) thesis study, which included 12-25-month-old children, is a device that helps make sense of the mechanism of the falls, especially falls that are very rarely reported, or rather, they are the most misreported cases of child abuse and neglect. Another study is a wearable device developed by Thelagathoti and Ali (2022) that can detect developmental delays in children. Thelagathoti and Ali (2022) revealed in their study that since the wearable sensors are small, they can be used quite easily in newborns, and the abnormal motor development of the baby can be detected early. From an evidence-based practice perspective, it has been determined that the trials of these devices in children are pretty limited. When an umbrella review (review of systematic reviews) evaluated fall prevention sensors, it was reported that these technologies are low-cost compared to the consequences of falls and are effective regardless of the type of device and the body part where they are placed. However, more studies are needed (Warrington et al., 2021).

Epilepsy Monitoring

Epilepsy has been stated as the most common and severe neurological disease in childhood (Russ et al., 2012). The constant anxiety and fear of having a seizure is an element that significantly reduces the quality of life of children and their parents as a nightmare (Arthurs et al., 2010). It has been emphasized that this problem can be prevented with wearable devices that can determine and predict the risk of seizures. In this way, it has been argued that injuries caused by unexpected seizures can be prevented, and the patient will be able to take a safer position while having a seizure (Patterson et al., 2015).

Various methods for various age groups have developed sensors that perform seizure detection and continue to improve every day. The smart clothing that can be used for newborns is the best example of this. The basic logic used during development is generally to take video recordings and analyze the recorded recording to make predictions from the following possible signals. Chen et al. (2017) demonstrated in their study that their developed sensor could distinguish high-quality signals. When examined in terms of evidence-based practices, very few studies in the literature on this subject have been completed and demonstrated their effectiveness as randomized controlled trials. Rukasha et al. (2020) included 12 research articles with both qualitative and quantitative components in their systematic review and meta-analysis study. They stated that more studies are needed to prove the effectiveness of this technology.

Disease Management

Congenital Heart Disorders

Congenital heart diseases are one of the most common birth malformations, and it has been stated that 8 out of every 1000 births are born with this malformation (Van Der Linde et al., 2011). When the development process of wearable technologies is examined, almost the starting point was the development of devices that can detect heart diseases or monitor the rhythm. Due to its high complexity, it is undeniable that wearable technologies have the potential for solutions in the monitoring and treatment of pediatric heart diseases (Donati et al., 2020). However, although most digital health technologies related to heart diseases are generally first developed for adult patients, it is stated that some specific pathologies can benefit from this technology (Tandon & Ferranti, 2019). The underlying technology generally includes three types of biosensors. These are heart rhythm recognition, heart rate determination, and physical activity tracking sensors (Behere & Janson, 2023).

Some of the sensors developed for heart diseases have received FDA (Food and Drug Administrative) approval, unlike other developing technologies (Behere & Janson, 2023). These are found in the literature as smart watches, smart socks, and special smartphone accessories (Hwang et al., 2019). The most striking of these may be the Owlet smart sock. This smart sock was developed to detect Supraventricular Tachycardia (SVT), the most common arrhythmia in newborns. They reported that this technology was very effective in their study, which they tested in a 37-week premature baby and published as a case report (Young & Flores, 2020). When examined in terms of evidence-based applications, no device with proven clinical suitability that can be used as a monitor for early detection of pediatric heart diseases or a systematic review and meta-analysis study describing this has been found. However, when the literature was examined, Tandon and Ferranti (2019) explained in their study the areas where these devices could potentially be used, specifically in pediatric diseases, as shown in Table 1.

Table 1. Physiological Measurements Collected by Wearable Biosensors and their Potential Clinical Uses for Pediatric Patients

Measurement	Potential Clinical Scenario(s)
SpO_2	Follow-up of cyanotic heart disease with home monitoring
Heart Rate and Rhythm	• Home monitoring to compare before and after starting medication in the follow-up of chronic heart diseases • Follow-up of patients with arrhythmia and monitoring of drug responses • Corrected Tetralogy of Fallot tracking • Long QT drug titration monitoring
Impedance/Volumetry	• Cardiac output follow-up • Pulmonary circulation follow up

Tandon, A., & Ferranti, S. D. (2019). Wearable Biosensors in Pediatric Cardiovascular Disease. Circulation, 140(5), 350-352.

When the literature was examined in terms of evidence-based applications, it was found that artificial intelligence and deep learning technologies have begun to be integrated into wearable technologies. In their systematic review, Sitaula et al. (2023) examined the AI and deep learning technologies developed for neonatal cardiorespiratory system monitoring. They stated that technologies using AI methods are becoming more effective, but there is a need to conduct clinical trials and develop more sensors.

Hematologic Oncologic Disorders

When wearable technologies developed for childhood hematological diseases are examined, it is seen that they are mainly used in the management symptoms (Dias & Paulo Silva Cunha, 2018). Wearable technologies provide the opportunity to monitor hematological diseases and others. However, in these diseases, since immunosuppressive drugs are used in the treatment, the importance of home follow-up goes a few steps further than others (Beauchamp et al., 2020). For example, Haemmerli et al. (2022) measured continuous vital signs in pediatric oncology patients in their study. In their study, which included 20 patients, measured nine body parameters for 14 days and 274 hours. At the end of their study, they reported that their measurements were feasible and acceptable. Ha et al. (2022) stated that in their pilot study, they used a digital health intervention called iBounce to improve the healthcare behaviors of childhood cancer survivors and that they ensured its effectiveness with Fitbit devices, which are also wearable devices. As a result of their pilot study involving 30 patients, they showed that the application was quite effective.

When examined in terms of evidence-based practices, although there are not many randomized controlled trials or systematic review and meta-analysis studies, Ramsey et al. (2020) evaluated eHealth and mHealth applications for pediatric cancer survivors in their systematic review and meta-analysis study. Five of the included studies were evaluated as mHealth applications and stated that they explained wearable technologies in this way. At the end of their studies, it was revealed that wearable technologies caused cancer survivors to experience less emotional distress, better health behaviors, better neurocognitive function, and less anxiety.

Diabetes Mellitus

Childhood diabetes is a common chronic endocrinological disease. It has been stated that the prevalence of type 1 diabetes, which is most common in childhood, is 0.82 per 100 people between the ages of 0-9 and 2.97 between the ages of 10-19 (Imperatore et al., 2018). Diabetes, like other chronic diseases, requires an interdisciplinary approach. These children, who are under the supervision of the child, the family, the pediatric, diabetes and school nurses, the pediatric endocrinologist, and the teachers at school, need to be monitored almost 24 hours a day, seven days a week (Castensoe et al., 2017). Children with diabetes must fulfill three main components to achieve optimal disease control. These are explained as blood sugar monitoring, insulin delivery, and maintaining the balance between the two. Wearable technologies are important at this point (Brew-Sam et al., 2021).

Boucsein et al. (2024) conducted a study in New Zealand. They piloted a study for children's glycemic control was targeted with the newly developed CO-PILOT (Closed Loop In children and youth with Type 1 diabetes and high-risk glycemic control). Another good example could be Gandrud et al. (2018), in their study, argued that remote monitoring will be more effective in reducing costs. This study compared two forms of care: routine care and Intensive Remote Monitoring (IRT) and Conventional Care, which include wearable technologies. As a result of the study in which they used Medtronic Paradise Device, Fitbit (activity tracker), and glucose sensor, they stated that IRT's diabetes outcomes and quality of life were higher than in the other group. When examined in terms of evidence-based applications, according to the systematic review by Brew-Sam et al. (2021), it was determined that wearable technologies are very effective in the management of pediatric diabetes, and more research is needed on their introduction into standard care.

Asthma

Asthma is a chronic inflammatory disease characterized by narrowing the airways, causing symptoms such as respiratory distress, wheezing, chest tightness, and cough. It is a common lung disease affecting 18% of the total population of the world (GINA, 2023). To manage symptoms, it is essential to monitor symptom frequency. Sometimes, children fail to monitor their activity levels or determine the need for inhaler medication and use it at the right time. With correct monitoring, the quality of life of children who receive medication in the right amount and at the right time, which will restrict activity or avoid allergen exposure, will increase, the risk of asthma attacks will decrease, and the need for repeated emergency room visits and intensive care will decrease (Tesse et al., 2018). For this reason, the monitoring of pediatric asthma patients at home with wearable technologies has been evaluated as very promising. When the studies are examined, it is thought that there has been a significant increase in wearable technologies, especially after COVID-19 (Kouis et al., 2021). For example, van der Kamp et al. (2023) included 370 included in their systematic review, which included devices that measure air quality and lung capacity, sleep quality, or other digital health technologies. As a result of these studies, it has been revealed that the applications are promising, especially the studies that monitor medications and include lung function measuring devices, which are more effective. Other examples of these applications can be given: Hosseini et al. (2017) developed a wireless smartwatch for self-management in pediatric asthma van der Kamp et al. (2020), created a wearable home monitoring system in their study, and finally Kouis et al. (2021) developed a wearable sensor for children with asthma to reduce hospital visits during COVID-19.

The Role of Emerging Technologies in Pediatric Nursing Care

Acceptance, Effectiveness, and Efficiency of Wearable Technologies

Wearable technologies are becoming widespread and coming into use at an ever-increasing pace. Health care is a multifactorial process requiring the coordinated work of many disciplines. Keeping up with this developing technology and ensuring the integration of these applications into health care can be even more complicated when this multidisciplinary process is working. Acceptance of technology has been defined as the opposite of rejection and has emerged as a new terminology that includes a person's concerns about using the new technology developed (Krick et al., 2019b; Taherdoost, 2018). Protecting the sensitive and vulnerable population while developing a new ethical product or process is among the most essential duties of pediatric nurses (Penticuff, 1990). Considering all this, wearable technologies in pediatric nursing are developing rapidly, but we are still at the very beginning. When it comes to wearable technology, it is now possible to talk about an extensive range. Users' adaptation to these devices and willingness to use them vary depending on the device, type of use, age, gender, and disease (Talukder et al., 2019). Furthermore, patients and their family's acceptance of this technology varies according to their trust in technology, beliefs, motivations, and privacy concerns (Attig & Franke, 2020).

The Place in Evidence-Based Pediatric Nursing Practice

When considered within the scope of evidence-based practices, it was observed that all studies examined generally developed these technologies only for certain age groups, certain diseases, and specific symptoms (Krick et al., 2019a). Another striking point in the literature review for this book section was the scarcity of multidisciplinary studies. It was observed that most of the published articles were published by researchers from the engineering field. However, it should be noted that pediatric nurses who work one-on-one with patients are the main source of data for these studies. The experiences of pediatric nurses, who can provide accurate data by revealing the cause of the real problem regarding innovative studies, are presented in the Semerci et al. (2024) study. They studied pediatric nurses who had previously tried to bring technology and nursing care together. Pediatric nurses stated that they experienced severe problems in product development. They stated they had difficulty finding a place for themselves within the multidisciplinary team. It has been reported that some nurses fear that their ideas will be stolen by the team that produces the technical knowledge or that they abandon their work before they can get a patent because they experience burnout during the product development process. For this reason, pediatric nurses should be included more in these studies, and nurses who directly communicate with children in product development and use will be able to detect better problems and develop more feasible wearable technologies. Furthermore, because of the literature review conducted within the scope of this section, it was determined that most of the wearable technologies developed and published were first developed based on data collected from adult patients. It has been observed that most of the studies conducted on pediatric patients were published as pilot studies, feasibility studies, or incomplete research protocols (Bortone et al., 2020; Byun et al., 2018; Di Palma et al., 2017; Müller et al., 2018). For this reason, no studies have been found that provide good evidence for the clinical use of these technologies.

Conclusion

In recent years, there have been significant advances in science and technology, which have led to several promising developments in the field of health. Wearable technology products represent a particularly salient example of these developments, with numerous adaptations made for use in the health sector. The utilisation of wearable technologies in the field of healthcare has witnessed a notable surge in recent years, with a concomitant exponential growth in popularity. Nurses are ideally positioned to keep pace with this rapid technological development and are the most important supporters of change. They are at the forefront of many areas of innovation, including improvements in quality of life and symptom management, as well as the prevention of chronic diseases. Wearable technologies are now being tested and researched in several areas within the field of paediatric nursing. Some of these products are designed for disease prevention and health maintenance, such as physical activity trackers for weight control, while others are developed for patient and disease management. In addition to disease prevention and health promotion applications, there are also smartwatches used for disease management, including epilepsy monitoring, pathological lung sound detection in asthmatic children and early warning systems for epilepsy attacks. The use of wearable technologies is becoming increasingly widespread.

References

Acampora, G., Cook, D. J., Rashidi, P., & Vasilakos, A. V. (2013). A Survey on Ambient Intelligence in Health Care. *Proc IEEE Inst Electr Electron Eng*, *101*(12), 2470-2494. https://doi.org/10.1109/jproc.2013.2262913.

Amanda E. Staiano, R. A. B., Daniel S. Hsia, Amber R. Jarrell, Peter T. Katzmarzyk, Savarra Mantzor, Robert L. NewtonJr, and Patrice Tyson. (2017). Step Tracking with Goals Increases Children's Weight Loss in Behavioral Intervention. *Childhood Obesity*, *13*(4), 283-290. https://doi.org/10.1089/chi.2017.0047.

Amft, O., & Lukowicz, P. (2009). From backpacks to smartphones: Past, present, and future of wearable computers. *IEEE Pervasive Computing*, *8*(3), 8-13.

Aquilina, O. (2006). A brief history of cardiac pacing. *Images Paediatr Cardiol*, *8*(2), 17-81.

Arthurs, S., Zaveri, H. P., Frei, M. G., & Osorio, I. (2010). Patient and caregiver perspectives on seizure prediction. *Epilepsy & behavior*, *19*(3), 474-477.

Attig, C., & Franke, T. (2020). Abandonment of personal quantification: A review and empirical study investigating reasons for wearable activity tracking attrition. *Computers in human behavior*, *102*, 223-237.

Bacon, R. (1928). *Opus Majus, Volumes 1 and 2*. University of Pennsylvania Press.

Beauchamp, U. L., Pappot, H., & Holländer-Mieritz, C. (2020). The Use of Wearables in Clinical Trials During Cancer Treatment: Systematic Review. *JMIR Mhealth Uhealth*, *8*(11), e22006. https://doi.org/10.2196/22006.

Behere, S. P., & Janson, C. M. (2023). Smart Wearables in Pediatric Heart Health. *The Journal of Pediatrics*, *253*, 1-7. https://doi.org/10.1016/j.jpeds.2022.08.009.

Bhalla, N., Jolly, P., Formisano, N., & Estrela, P. (2016). Introduction to biosensors. *Essays Biochem*, *60*(1), 1-8. https://doi.org/10.1042/ebc20150001.

Blackwell, C. K., Elliott, A. J., Ganiban, J., Herbstman, J., Hunt, K., Forrest, C. B., & Camargo, C. A. (2019). General health and life satisfaction in children with chronic illness. *Pediatrics*, *143*(6).

Böhm, B., Karwiese, S. D., Böhm, H., & Oberhoffer, R. (2019). Effects of Mobile Health Including Wearable Activity Trackers to Increase Physical Activity Outcomes Among Healthy Children and Adolescents: Systematic Review [Review]. *JMIR Mhealth Uhealth*, *7*(4), e8298. https://doi.org/10.2196/mhealth.8298.

Bootsman, R., Markopoulos, P., Qi, Q., Wang, Q., & Timmermans, A. A. A. (2019). Wearable technology for posture monitoring at the workplace. *International Journal of Human-Computer Studies*, *132*, 99-111. https://doi.org/https://doi.org/10.1016/j.ijhcs.2019.08.003.

Bortone, I., Barsotti, M., Leonardis, D., Crecchi, A., Tozzini, A., Bonfiglio, L., & Frisoli, A. (2020). Immersive Virtual Environments and Wearable Haptic Devices in rehabilitation of children with neuromotor impairments: a single-blind randomized controlled crossover pilot study. *Journal of NeuroEngineering and Rehabilitation*, *17*(1), 144. https://doi.org/10.1186/s12984-020-00771-6.

Boucsein, A., Zhou, Y., Haszard, J. J., Jefferies, C. A., Wiltshire, E. J., Styles, S. E., Crocket, H. R., Galland, B. C., Pasha, M., Petrovski, G., Paul, R. G., de Bock, M. I., & Wheeler, B. J. (2024). Protocol for a prospective, multicenter, parallel-group, open-label randomized controlled trial comparing standard care with Closed lOoP In chiLdren and yOuth with Type 1 diabetes and high-risk glycemic control: the CO-PILOT trial. *Journal of Diabetes & Metabolic Disorders*. https://doi.org/10.1007/s40200-024-01397-4.

Brew-Sam, N., Chhabra, M., Parkinson, A., Hannan, K., Brown, E., Pedley, L., Brown, K., Wright, K., Pedley, E., Nolan, C. J., Phillips, C., Suominen, H., Tricoli, A., & Desborough, J. (2021). Experiences of Young People and Their Caregivers of Using Technology to Manage Type 1 Diabetes Mellitus: Systematic Literature Review and Narrative Synthesis. *JMIR Diabetes*, *6*(1), e20973. https://doi.org/10.2196/20973.

Byun, W., Lau, E. Y., & Brusseau, T. A. (2018). Feasibility and Effectiveness of a Wearable Technology-Based Physical Activity Intervention in Preschoolers: A Pilot Study. *International Journal of Environmental Research and Public Health*, *15*(9), 1821. https://www.mdpi.com/1660-4601/15/9/1821.

Casselman, J., Onopa, N., & Khansa, L. (2017). Wearable healthcare: Lessons from the past and a peek into the future. *Telematics and Informatics*, *34*(7), 1011-1023.

Castensoe, P., Reventlov Husted, G., Teilmann, G., Hommel, E., Olsen, B. S., & Kensing, F. (2017). Designing a Self-Management App for Young People With Type 1 Diabetes: Methodological Challenges, Experiences, and Recommendations. *JMIR Mhealth Uhealth*, *5*(10), e124. https://doi.org/10.2196/
mhealth.8137.

Chen, H., Gu, X., Mei, Z., Xu, K., Yan, K., Lu, C., Wang, L., Shu, F., Xu, Q., Oetomo, S. B., & Chen, W. (2017, 9-12 May 2017). A wearable sensor system for neonatal seizure monitoring. 2017 IEEE 14th International Conference on Wearable and Implantable Body Sensor Networks (BSN).

Cory, D. K. (2021). Biomechanical Characterization of Video-Recorded Short-Distance Falls Involving Children Equipped with a Biometric Device in a Childcare Setting: A Pilot Study.

Di Palma, S., Tonacci, A., Narzisi, A., Domenici, C., Pioggia, G., Muratori, F., & Billeci, L. (2017). Monitoring of autonomic response to sociocognitive tasks during treatment in children with Autism Spectrum Disorders by wearable technologies: A feasibility study. *Computers in Biology and Medicine*, *85*, 143-152. https://doi.org/https://doi.org/10.1016/j.compbiomed.2016.04.001.

Dias, D., & Paulo Silva Cunha, J. (2018). Wearable Health Devices-Vital Sign Monitoring, Systems and Technologies. *Sensors (Basel)*, *18*(8). https://doi.org/10.3390/s18082414.

Donati, M., Panicacci, S., Fanucci, L., Saponara, S., Ait-Ali, L., Dalmiani, S., Festa, P., Mastorci, F., Pingitore, A., Pennè, W., & Celli, A. (2020, 1 June-1 July 2020). Improving care model for congenital heart diseases in paediatric patients using home telemonitoring of vital signs via biomedical sensors. 2020 IEEE International Symposium on Medical Measurements and Applications (MeMeA).

Edward, K.-L., Garvey, L., & Rahman, M. A. (2020). Wearable activity trackers and health awareness: Nursing implications. *International Journal of Nursing Sciences*, *7*(2), 179-183.

Ercan, İ. P., & Timur, Ş. (2020). Changing Terminology of Definition and Design of Wearable Technology Products. *Online Journal of Art and Design*, *8*(3), 90-106.

Evenson, K. R., Goto, M. M., & Furberg, R. D. (2015). Systematic review of the validity and reliability of consumer-wearable activity trackers. *International Journal of Behavioral Nutrition and Physical Activity*, *12*(1), 159. https://doi.org/10.1186/s12966-015-0314-1.

Ferreira, J. J., Fernandes, C. I., Rammal, H. G., & Veiga, P. M. (2021). Wearable technology and consumer interaction: A systematic review and research agenda. *Computers in human behavior*, *118*, 106710.

Fitness Trackers Statistics and Facts. (2019). Retrieved 3/28/2024 from https://www.statista.com/topics/4393/fitness-and-activity-tracker/#topicOverview.

Gandrud, L., Altan, A., Buzinec, P., Hemphill, J., Chatterton, J., Kelley, T., & Vojta, D. (2018). Intensive remote monitoring versus conventional care in type 1 diabetes: A randomized controlled trial. *Pediatric Diabetes*, *19*(6), 1086-1093. https://doi.org/https://doi.org/10.1111/pedi.12654.

GINA. (2023). *Global Strategy for Asthma Management and Prevention*. https://ginasthma.org/wp-content/uploads/2023/07/GINA-2023-Full-report-23_07_06-WMS.pdf.

Godfrey, A., Conway, R., Meagher, D., & ÓLaighin, G. (2008). Direct measurement of human movement by accelerometry. *Medical engineering & physics*, *30*(10), 1364-1386.

Greiwe, J., & Nyenhuis, S. M. (2020). Wearable technology and how this can be implemented into clinical practice. *Current allergy and asthma reports*, *20*, 1-10.

Guilbault, G. G., & Montalvo, J. G., Jr. (1969). Urea-specific enzyme electrode. *Journal of the American Chemical Society*, *91*(8), 2164-2165. https://doi.org/10.1021/ja01036a083.

Ha, L., Wakefield, C. E., Mizrahi, D., Diaz, C., Cohn, R. J., Signorelli, C., Yacef, K., & Simar, D. (2022). A Digital Educational Intervention With Wearable Activity Trackers to Support Health Behaviors Among Childhood Cancer Survivors: Pilot Feasibility and Acceptability Study [Original Paper]. *JMIR Cancer*, *8*(3), e38367. https://doi.org/10.2196/38367.

Haemmerli, M., Ammann, R. A., Roessler, J., Koenig, C., & Brack, E. (2022). Vital signs in pediatric oncology patients assessed by continuous recording with a wearable device, NCT04134429. *Scientific Data*, *9*(1), 89. https://doi.org/10.1038/s41597-022-01182-z.

Hayward, J., Pugh, D., & Chansin, G. (2018). Wearable sensors 2018–2028: Technologies, markets & players. *ed: IDTechEx Cambridge, UK*.

Heeffer, A. (2004). Récréations Mathématiques (1624): A study on its authorship, sources and influence. In: Centre for Logic and Philosophy of Science.

Heineman, W. R., & Jensen, W. B. (2006). Leland C. Clark Jr. (1918–2005). *Biosensors and Bioelectronics*, *21*(8), 1403-1404. https://doi.org/https://doi.org/10.1016/j.bios.2005.12.005.

Hosseini, A., Buonocore, C. M., Hashemzadeh, S., Hojaiji, H., Kalantarian, H., Sideris, C., Bui, A. A., King, C. E., & Sarrafzadeh, M. (2017). Feasibility of a secure wireless sensing smartwatch application for the self-management of pediatric asthma. *Sensors*, *17*(8), 1780.

Hwang, J., Kim, J., Choi, K.-J., Cho, M. S., Nam, G.-B., & Kim, Y.-H. (2019). Assessing accuracy of wrist-worn wearable devices in measurement of paroxysmal supraventricular tachycardia heart rate. *Korean circulation journal*, *49*(5), 437.

Imperatore, G., Mayer-Davis, E. J., Orchard, T. J., & Zhong, V. W. (2018). Prevalence and Incidence of Type 1 Diabetes Among Children and Adults in the United States and Comparison With Non-U.S. Countries. In C. C. Cowie, S. S. Casagrande, A. Menke, M. A. Cissell, M. S. Eberhardt, J. B. Meigs, E. W. Gregg, W. C. Knowler, E. Barrett-Connor, D. J. Becker, F. L. Brancati, E. J. Boyko, W. H. Herman, B. V. Howard, K. M. V. Narayan, M. Rewers, & J. E. Fradkin (Eds.), *Diabetes in America*. National Institute of Diabetes and Digestive and Kidney Diseases (US).

Iqbal, S. M. A., Mahgoub, I., Du, E., Leavitt, M. A., & Asghar, W. (2021). Advances in healthcare wearable devices. *npj Flexible Electronics*, *5*(1), 9. https://doi.org/10.1038/s41528-021-00107-x.

Irwin, D. E., Gross, H. E., Stucky, B. D., Thissen, D., DeWitt, E. M., Lai, J. S., Amtmann, D., Khastou, L., Varni, J. W., & DeWalt, D. A. (2012). Development of six PROMIS pediatrics proxy-report item banks. *Health and quality of life outcomes*, *10*, 1-13.

Izmailova, E. S., Wagner, J. A., & Perakslis, E. D. (2018). Wearable devices in clinical trials: hype and hypothesis. *Clinical Pharmacology & Therapeutics*, *104*(1), 42-52.

Jauho, A.-M., Pyky, R., Ahola, R., Kangas, M., Virtanen, P., Korpelainen, R., & Jämsä, T. (2015). Effect of wrist-worn activity monitor feedback on physical activity behavior: A randomized controlled trial in

Finnish young men. *Preventive Medicine Reports*, *2*, 628-634. https://doi.org/https://doi.org/10.1016/j.pmedr.2015.07.005.

Jonassaint, C. R., Shah, N., Jonassaint, J., & De Castro, L. (2015). Usability and feasibility of an mHealth intervention for monitoring and managing pain symptoms in sickle cell disease: the Sickle Cell Disease Mobile Application to Record Symptoms via Technology (SMART). *Hemoglobin*, *39*(3), 162-168.

Kasparian, A. M., & Badawy, S. M. (2022). Utility of Fitbit devices among children and adolescents with chronic health conditions: a scoping review. *Mhealth*, *8*, 26. https://doi.org/10.21037/mhealth-21-28.

Khan, Y., Ostfeld, A. E., Lochner, C. M., Pierre, A., & Arias, A. C. (2016). Monitoring of vital signs with flexible and wearable medical devices. *Advanced materials*, *28*(22), 4373-4395.

Kouis, P., Michanikou, A., Anagnostopoulou, P., Galanakis, E., Michaelidou, E., Dimitriou, H., Matthaiou, A. M., Kinni, P., Achilleos, S., Zacharatos, H., Papatheodorou, S. I., Koutrakis, P., Nikolopoulos, G. K., & Yiallouros, P. K. (2021). Use of wearable sensors to assess compliance of asthmatic children in response to lockdown measures for the COVID-19 epidemic. *Scientific Reports*, *11*(1), 5895. https://doi.org/
10.1038/s41598-021-85358-4.

Krick, T., Huter, K., Domhoff, D., Schmidt, A., Rothgang, H., & Wolf-Ostermann, K. (2019a). Digital technology and nursing care: a scoping review on acceptance, effectiveness and efficiency studies of informal and formal care technologies. *BMC Health Services Research*, *19*, 1-15.

Krick, T., Huter, K., Domhoff, D., Schmidt, A., Rothgang, H., & Wolf-Ostermann, K. (2019b). Digital technology and nursing care: a scoping review on acceptance, effectiveness and efficiency studies of informal and formal care technologies. *BMC Health Services Research*, *19*(1), 400. https://doi.org/10.1186/s12913-019-4238-3.

Kumari, S., Shukla, S., & Acharya, S. (2022). Childhood Obesity: Prevalence and Prevention in Modern Society. *Cureus*, *14*(11), e31640. https://doi.org/10.7759/cureus.31640.

Lam, C., Milne-Ives, M., Van Velthoven, M. H., & Meinert, E. (2020). Internet of Things-Enabled Technologies for Weight Management in Children and Adolescents: Protocol for a Systematic Review. *JMIR Res Protoc*, *9*(3), e16930. https://doi.org/10.2196/16930.

Leonard, S., Anderson, L. M., Jonassaint, J., Jonassaint, C., & Shah, N. (2017). Utilizing a novel mobile health "selfie" application to improve compliance to iron chelation in pediatric patients receiving chronic transfusions. *Journal of Pediatric Hematology/Oncology*, *39*(3), 223-229.

Lu, L., Zhang, J., Xie, Y., Gao, F., Xu, S., Wu, X., & Ye, Z. (2020). Wearable health devices in health care: narrative systematic review. *JMIR mHealth and uHealth*, *8*(11), e18907.

Lubans, D. R., Smith, J. J., Plotnikoff, R. C., Dally, K. A., Okely, A. D., Salmon, J., & Morgan, P. J. (2016). Assessing the sustained impact of a school-based obesity prevention program for adolescent boys: the ATLAS cluster randomized controlled trial. *International Journal of Behavioral Nutrition and Physical Activity*, *13*(1), 92. https://doi.org/10.1186/s12966-016-0420-8 .

Mack, I., Juchler, N., Rey, S., Hirsch, S., Hoelz, B., Eckstein, J., & Bielicki, J. (2022). Wearable Technologies for Pediatric Patients with Surgical Infections-More than Counting Steps? *Biosensors (Basel)*, *12*(8). https://doi.org/10.3390/bios12080634.

Mameli, C., Brunetti, D., Colombo, V., Bedogni, G., Schneider, L., Penagini, F., Borsani, B., & Zuccotti, G. V. (2018). Combined use of a wristband and a smartphone to reduce body weight in obese children: randomized controlled trial. *Pediatric Obesity*, *13*(2), 81-87. https://doi.org/https://doi.org/10.1111/ijpo.12201.

Market Analysis Report. (2021). *Wearable Technology Market Size, Share & Trends Analysis Report By Product (Head & Eyewear, Wristwear), By Application (Consumer Electronics, Healthcare), By Region (Asia Pacific, Europe), and Segment Forecasts, 2023 - 2030*. G. V. Research. https://www.grandviewresearch.com/industry-analysis/wearable-technology-market.

Mawston, N. (2020). Strategy analytics: Apple Watch outsells entire Swiss watch industry in 2019. February 5, 2020. In.

Mozaffari, N., Rezazadeh, J., Farahbakhsh, R., Yazdani, S., & Sandrasegaran, K. (2019). Practical fall detection based on IoT technologies: A survey. *Internet of Things*, *8*, 100124. https://doi.org/https://doi.org/10.1016/j.iot.2019.100124.

Müller, J., Hoch, A. M., Zoller, V., & Oberhoffer, R. (2018). Feasibility of Physical Activity Assessment with Wearable Devices in Children Aged 4–10 Years—A Pilot Study [Original Research]. *Frontiers in pediatrics*, *6*. https://doi.org/10.3389/fped.2018.00005.

Nieroda, M. E., Mrad, M., & Solomon, M. R. (2018). How do consumers think about hybrid products? Computer wearables have an identity problem. *Journal of Business Research*, *89*, 159-170.

Ometov, A., Shubina, V., Klus, L., Skibińska, J., Saafi, S., Pascacio, P., Flueratoru, L., Gaibor, D. Q., Chukhno, N., Chukhno, O., Ali, A., Channa, A., Svertoka, E., Qaim, W. B., Casanova-Marqués, R., Holcer, S., Torres-Sospedra, J., Casteleyn, S., Ruggeri, G., . . . Lohan, E. S. (2021). A Survey on Wearable Technology: History, State-of-the-Art and Current Challenges. *Computer Networks*, *193*, 108074. https://doi.org/https://doi.org/10.1016/j.comnet.2021.108074.

Patterson, A. L., Mudigoudar, B., Fulton, S., McGregor, A., Poppel, K. V., Wheless, M. C., Brooks, L., & Wheless, J. W. (2015). SmartWatch by SmartMonitor: Assessment of Seizure Detection Efficacy for Various Seizure Types in Children, a Large Prospective Single-Center Study. *Pediatric Neurology*, *53*(4), 309-311. https://doi.org/https://doi.org/10.1016/j.pediatrneurol.2015.07.002.

Penticuff, J. H. (1990). Ethics in pediatric nursing: advocacy and the child's "determining self". *Issues Compr Pediatr Nurs*, *13*(3), 221-229. https://doi.org/10.3109/01460869009009037.

Pinheiro, L. C., McFatrich, M., Lucas, N., Walker, J. S., Withycombe, J. S., Hinds, P. S., Sung, L., Tomlinson, D., Freyer, D. R., & Mack, J. W. (2018). Child and adolescent self-report symptom measurement in pediatric oncology research: a systematic literature review. *Quality of life research*, *27*, 291-319.

Pittman, A. F. (2020). Effect of a School-Based Activity Tracker, Companion Social Website, and Text Messaging Intervention on Exercise, Fitness, and Physical Activity Self-Efficacy of Middle School Students. *The Journal of School Nursing*, *36*(2), 112-120. https://doi.org/10.1177/1059840518791223.

Ramsey, W. A., Heidelberg, R. E., Gilbert, A. M., Heneghan, M. B., Badawy, S. M., & Alberts, N. M. (2020). eHealth and mHealth interventions in pediatric cancer: a systematic review of interventions across the cancer continuum. *Psycho-oncology*, *29*(1), 17-37.

Rosen, L. (2011). Teaching the iGeneration.

Rukasha, T., I Woolley, S., Kyriacou, T., & Collins, T. (2020). Evaluation of wearable electronics for epilepsy: A systematic review. *Electronics*, *9*(6), 968.

Russ, S. A., Larson, K., & Halfon, N. (2012). A national profile of childhood epilepsy and seizure disorder. *Pediatrics*, *129*(2), 256-264.

Sahoo, K., Sahoo, B., Choudhury, A. K., Sofi, N. Y., Kumar, R., & Bhadoria, A. S. (2015). Childhood obesity: causes and consequences. *J Family Med Prim Care*, *4*(2), 187-192. https://doi.org/10.4103/2249-4863.154628.

Semerci, R., Ekim, A., & Ocakçı, A. F. (2024). Challenges experienced by pediatric nurses in the process of developing innovative products: A qualitative study. *Journal of Pediatric Nursing*, *75*, e28-e33. https://doi.org/https://doi.org/10.1016/j.pedn.2023.12.016.

Sempionatto, J. R., Montiel, V. R.-V., Vargas, E., Teymourian, H., & Wang, J. (2021). Wearable and mobile sensors for personalized nutrition. *ACS sensors*, *6*(5), 1745-1760.

Sezgin, S. (2019). Eğitimde giyilebilir teknolojiler: fırsatlar ve eğilimler. *Mehmet Akif Ersoy Üniversitesi Eğitim Fakültesi Dergisi*, *1*(40).

Shany, T., Redmond, S. J., Narayanan, M. R., & Lovell, N. H. (2012). Sensors-Based Wearable Systems for Monitoring of Human Movement and Falls. *IEEE Sensors Journal*, *12*(3), 658-670. https://doi.org/10.1109/JSEN.2011.2146246.

Sitaula, C., Grooby, E., Kwok, T. n. C., Sharkey, D., Marzbanrad, F., & Malhotra, A. (2023). Artificial intelligence-driven wearable technologies for neonatal cardiorespiratory monitoring. Part 2: artificial intelligence. *Pediatric Research*, *93*(2), 426-436. https://doi.org/10.1038/s41390-022-02417-w.

Smith, W. D., & Bagley, A. (2010). A miniature, wearable activity/fall monitor to assess the efficacy of mobility therapy for children with cerebral palsy during everyday living. *Annu Int Conf IEEE Eng Med Biol Soc*, *2010*, 5030-5033. https://doi.org/10.1109/iembs.2010.5627079.

Taherdoost, H. (2018). A review of technology acceptance and adoption models and theories. *Procedia Manufacturing*, *22*, 960-967. https://doi.org/https://doi.org/10.1016/j.promfg.2018.03.137.

Talukder, M. S., Chiong, R., Bao, Y., & Hayat Malik, B. (2019). Acceptance and use predictors of fitness wearable technology and intention to recommend: An empirical study. *Industrial Management & Data Systems*, *119*(1), 170-188.

Tandon, A., & Ferranti, S. D. d. (2019). Wearable Biosensors in Pediatric Cardiovascular Disease. *Circulation*, *140*(5), 350-352. https://doi.org/doi:10.1161/CIRCULATIONAHA.119.038483.

Telama, R. (2009). Tracking of physical activity from childhood to adulthood: a review. *Obes Facts*, *2*(3), 187-195. https://doi.org/10.1159/000222244.

Tesse, R., Borrelli, G., Mongelli, G., Mastrorilli, V., & Cardinale, F. (2018). Treating pediatric asthma according guidelines. *Frontiers in pediatrics*, *6*, 234.

The College of Optometrists. (2015). *The invention of spectacles*. Retrieved 3/18/2024 from http://www.college-optometrists.org/en/college/museyeum/online_exhibitions/spectacles/invention.cfm.

Thelagathoti, R. K., & Ali, H. H. (2022). Quantitative Approaches for Detecting Early Childhood Developmental Disorders using Wireless Sensors and Mobility Data. *International Journal on Advances in Life Sciences*, *14*(1).

Van Cleave, J., Gortmaker, S. L., & Perrin, J. M. (2010). Dynamics of obesity and chronic health conditions among children and youth. *Jama*, *303*(7), 623-630.

Van der Kamp, M. R., Hengeveld, V. S., Brusse-Keizer, M. G. J., Thio, B. J., & Tabak, M. (2023). eHealth Technologies for Monitoring Pediatric Asthma at Home: Scoping Review [Review]. *J Med Internet Res*, *25*, e45896. https://doi.org/10.2196/45896.

Van der Kamp, M. R., Klaver, E. C., Thio, B. J., Driessen, J. M. M., de Jongh, F. H. C., Tabak, M., van der Palen, J., & Hermens, H. J. (2020). WEARCON: wearable home monitoring in children with asthma reveals a strong association with hospital based assessment of asthma control. *BMC Medical Informatics and Decision Making*, *20*(1), 192. https://doi.org/10.1186/s12911-020-01210-1.

Van Der Linde, D., Konings, E. E., Slager, M. A., Witsenburg, M., Helbing, W. A., Takkenberg, J. J., & Roos-Hesselink, J. W. (2011). Birth prevalence of congenital heart disease worldwide: a systematic review and meta-analysis. *Journal of the American College of Cardiology*, *58*(21), 2241-2247.

Vaughn, J., Gollarahalli, S., Shaw, R. J., Docherty, S., Yang, Q., Malhotra, C., Summers-Goeckerman, E., & Shah, N. (2020). Mobile Health Technology for Pediatric Symptom Monitoring: A Feasibility Study. *Nursing Research*, *69*(2). https://journals.lww.com/nursingresearchonline/fulltext/2020/03000/mobile_health_technology_for_pediatric_symptom.8.aspx.

Vaughn, J., Summers-Goeckerman, E., Shaw, R. J., & Shah, N. (2019). A Protocol to Assess Feasibility, Acceptability, and Usability of Mobile Technology for Symptom Management in Pediatric Transplant Patients. *Nursing Research*, *68*(4). https://journals.lww.com/nursingresearchonline/fulltext/2019/07000/a_protocol_to_assess_feasibility,_acceptability,.9.aspx.

von Niederhäusern, B., Saccilotto, R., Schädelin, S., Ziesenitz, V., Benkert, P., Decker, M.-L., Hammann, A., Bielicki, J., Pfister, M., & Pauli-Magnus, C. (2017). Validity of mobile electronic data capture in clinical studies: a pilot study in a pediatric population. *BMC medical research methodology*, *17*, 1-9.

Warrington, D. J., Shortis, E. J., & Whittaker, P. J. (2021). Are wearable devices effective for preventing and detecting falls: an umbrella review (a review of systematic reviews). *BMC public health*, *21*(1), 2091. https://doi.org/10.1186/s12889-021-12169-7.

Wilson, D. (2017). An overview of the application of wearable technology to nursing practice. Nursing forum,

Wright, R., & Keith, L. (2014). Wearable technology: If the tech fits, wear it. *Journal of Electronic Resources in Medical Libraries*, *11*(4), 204-216.

Young, M. L., & Flores, L. (2020). Asymptomatic idiopathic belhassen ventricular tachycardia in a neonate detected using 'smart sock' wearable smartphone-enabled cardiac monitoring [Article]. *American Journal of Case Reports*, *21*, Article e921092. https://doi.org/10.12659/AJCR.921092.

Index

A

acupressure, 182, 183, 187, 198, 201, 205, 206, 210, 212
acupuncture, 99, 101, 102, 103, 182, 183, 187, 194, 198, 201, 205, 206, 207, 212, 214
adolescent, 36, 112, 113, 124, 146, 172, 173, 174, 175, 186, 187, 224, 237, 238, 246, 251, 257, 258, 261, 262, 263, 275, 276, 291, 292
aloe-vera, 33, 35, 36, 37, 38, 77, 85, 182, 185
anxious attachment, 119
aromatherapy, 103, 179, 180, 182, 183, 186, 189, 190, 201, 205, 206, 211, 213
artificial intelligence, 265, 266, 279, 285, 292
asthma, iii, 131, 132, 133, 134, 135, 136, 137, 138, 139, 140, 141, 142, 143, 144, 169, 259, 261, 262, 268, 270, 272, 274, 275, 276, 277, 279, 280, 282, 286, 290, 293
asthma attack, 131, 132, 135, 137, 138, 139, 140, 270, 286
asthma care, 131, 132, 136
asthma triggers, 138, 142, 270
avoidant attachment, 119

B

baby, 13, 14, 16, 17, 18, 19, 21, 24, 25, 26, 27, 28, 29, 30, 31, 32, 33, 34, 43, 44, 53, 56, 57, 58, 59, 61, 62, 63, 64, 65, 67, 70, 75, 77, 78, 79, 80, 82, 83, 84, 88, 89, 95, 96, 97, 98, 99, 100, 106, 107, 109, 117, 118, 119, 120, 121, 122, 123, 124, 125, 126, 127, 128, 130, 231, 232, 247, 274, 283, 284
bathing methods, 13, 14, 15, 16, 17, 18, 21, 24, 25, 26
bathing under running water, 18
body mass index (BMI), 37, 169, 171, 172, 173, 216, 283
breastfeeding, 6, 7, 9, 10, 20, 24, 26, 27, 28, 29, 30, 31, 32, 33, 34, 35, 36, 37, 38, 40, 59, 75, 92, 95, 97, 98, 114, 117, 121, 122, 125, 126, 127, 128, 129, 130, 138, 232, 233, 237
breastfeeding problems, 27, 28, 35, 36, 38
burns, 18, 162, 213, 241, 242, 244, 251
Buzzy, 235, 237, 239, 240

C

care of the umbilicus, 88
childhood obesity, 167, 168, 169, 170, 171, 172, 173, 174, 175, 176, 271, 273, 274, 276, 282, 288, 291, 292
chronic disease, 131, 132, 136, 146, 253, 254, 259, 260, 266, 269, 270, 272, 280, 282, 286, 288
cleansing products, 53, 58, 60, 63
closed-loop technology, 149
colic, 95, 96, 97, 98, 99, 100, 101, 102, 103, 104
congenital heart diseases, 284, 289
continuous glucose monitoring (CGM), 147, 149, 153
cord care, 53, 58, 61, 62, 63, 65, 66, 87, 88, 89, 90, 91, 92, 93, 94
cord clamping, 47, 50, 125
cracked nipples, 27, 36
cradle hold position, 7
creative arts therapy, 205, 207, 212, 213
cryoprotective agents, 181, 221
cryotherapy, 181, 187, 222, 225
cue-based feeding, 2, 3, 4, 10, 11, 12
cut injuries, 245

D

dermis, 14, 54, 55, 56, 58
diabetes management, 145, 146, 147, 148, 149, 150, 153, 269
diaper dermatitis, 57, 58, 64, 65, 67, 68, 69, 70, 71, 72, 73, 74, 75, 76, 77, 78, 80, 82, 83, 84, 85
digestive systems, 7
digital technologies, 149, 281
drowning, 241, 242, 246, 247, 249, 252

E

emotional needs, 118
energy therapies, 191, 192, 193, 194, 195, 197
energy therapy, 191, 197
epidermis, 54, 55, 58, 69, 70, 72, 76, 77, 244
epilepsy, 155, 156, 157, 158, 159, 160, 161, 162, 163, 164, 165, 166, 246, 279, 283, 288, 292

evidence-based care, v, 9, 14, 27, 75, 132, 215, 220, 253, 254
evidence-based nursing, 1, 13, 39, 43, 49, 53, 67, 84, 87, 95, 97, 105, 107, 117, 122, 127, 131, 132, 137, 145, 147, 152, 155, 159, 163, 177, 192, 199, 201, 205, 215, 227, 241, 253, 254, 279
evidence-based nursing practices, 1, 13, 39, 43, 49, 53, 67, 87, 95, 97, 105, 107, 117, 122, 127, 131, 145, 147, 155, 159, 163, 177, 199, 201, 215, 227, 241, 253, 254, 279
evidence-based practice(s), 1, 2, 27, 38, 39, 43, 50, 53, 58, 63, 64, 76, 81, 88, 90, 117, 122, 126, 131, 132, 145, 147, 150, 152, 177, 178, 191, 192, 215, 216, 220, 221, 223, 249, 253, 283, 284, 285, 287

F

fall identification, 283
falls, 1, 2, 17, 21, 88, 162, 241, 242, 243, 244, 250, 281, 283, 289, 292, 293
family-based intervention, 167, 168, 171, 173
flat nipples, 35

G

glutamine, 181, 186, 188, 221, 224, 226

H

hammock positioning, 107, 110, 114
healing touch (HT), 191, 192, 195, 196, 198, 199, 200
healthcare, 8, 19, 22, 38, 62, 66, 87, 96, 97, 100, 122, 123, 132, 137, 138, 139, 147, 152, 163, 168, 171, 172, 173, 174, 194, 195, 199, 204, 212, 226, 227, 228, 229, 230, 234, 236, 242, 244, 248, 265, 267, 273, 279, 280, 281, 285, 288, 289, 290, 291
home accident(s), 241, 242, 243, 244, 245, 248, 249, 250, 251, 252
honey, 33, 36, 181, 182, 186, 187, 189, 222, 223, 224, 225
hyperbilirubinemia, 39, 40, 41, 42, 43, 44, 45, 46, 47, 48, 49, 50, 71
hypnosis, 201, 205, 206, 236, 238, 239
hypodermis, 15, 54, 55, 56
hypoglycemia, 8, 13, 16, 19, 20, 22, 26, 146, 147, 148, 150
hypothermia, 13, 15, 16, 19, 20, 22, 24, 26, 40, 59

I

immersion bathing method, 17, 21
infants, 1, 2, 3, 4, 5, 6, 7, 8, 9, 10, 11, 12, 13, 14, 15, 16, 17, 18, 19, 20, 22, 23, 24, 25, 26, 30, 34, 38, 39, 40, 46, 49, 50, 51, 54, 55, 56, 58, 60, 61, 64, 66, 67, 68, 71, 72, 74, 75, 77, 78, 80, 82, 83, 84, 85, 91, 92, 93, 95, 96, 97, 98, 99, 100, 101, 102, 103, 104, 105, 106, 107, 108, 109, 110, 111, 112, 113, 114, 115, 118, 120, 122, 123, 127, 128, 129, 130, 142, 177, 178, 195, 199, 200, 227, 228, 229, 231, 232, 233, 237, 238, 239, 244
insulin, 145, 146, 147, 148, 149, 151, 269, 274, 286
insulin pumps, 149
intensive care, 1, 2, 6, 9, 11, 13, 14, 15, 23, 56, 113, 125, 130, 186, 187, 191, 193, 225, 231, 239, 286
inverted nipples, 27, 28, 34, 35, 36, 38

K

kangaroo care, 54, 59, 105, 107, 108, 109, 110, 111, 112, 113, 114, 115, 117, 122, 123, 124, 125, 127, 128, 130, 233

L

laser therapy, 187, 222, 223, 224
looped light system, 107

M

manual therapy, 100, 101, 103
massage, 5, 39, 43, 44, 45, 46, 48, 49, 50, 54, 95, 99, 100, 101, 103, 105, 107, 108, 109, 110, 111, 113, 114, 115, 117, 122, 123, 125, 126, 127, 128, 130, 179, 180, 182, 183, 187, 189, 190, 201, 205, 207, 212, 227, 236
maternal attachment, 118, 120, 122, 125, 126, 127, 128, 129, 130
mental health, 12, 103, 118, 126, 150, 175, 261, 262, 281
mobile technology applications, 208
moisturizers, 53, 58, 60, 61, 63, 65, 76
moisturizing products, 58, 60, 63
mother-baby attachment, 109, 117, 118, 120, 121, 122, 123, 124, 125, 126, 127
multidisciplinary approach(es), 159, 167, 168, 170, 173, 174, 182, 194, 271
muscle relaxation, 182, 183, 186, 205, 258
music, 11, 105, 107, 108, 111, 112, 113, 114, 115, 124, 126, 127, 128, 129, 130, 179, 180, 182, 183, 184, 187, 194, 198, 201, 205, 207, 208, 209, 210, 213, 214, 234, 257
music therapy, 11, 105, 107, 108, 111, 112, 113, 114, 115, 124, 126, 127, 128, 129, 180, 183, 184, 187, 194, 198, 207, 214

N

napkin rash, 67
nausea, 177, 178, 179, 182, 183, 186, 187, 188, 189, 190, 192, 195, 196, 201, 202, 203, 204, 205, 206, 207, 208, 209, 210, 211, 212, 213, 214
nausea and vomiting, 177, 182, 183, 186, 187, 189, 201, 202, 203, 204, 205, 206, 207, 208, 209, 210, 211, 212, 213, 214
neonatal intensive care, 1, 2, 3, 5, 6, 8, 9, 11, 12, 14, 15, 16, 17, 21, 22, 23, 24, 25, 26, 53, 57, 64, 65, 84, 90, 105, 106, 107, 112, 113, 114, 115, 122, 124, 126, 128, 129, 230, 231, 238
neonatal intensive care unit (NICE), 2, 3, 5, 6, 8, 9, 11, 12, 14, 15, 16, 17, 21, 23, 24, 25, 26, 53, 60, 64, 65, 68, 77, 82, 84, 90, 94, 105, 106, 107, 108, 110, 112, 113, 114, 115, 122, 124, 126, 128, 129, 159, 161, 165, 170, 171, 174, 175, 230, 231, 238
neonatal nursing, 1, 9, 10, 11, 12, 14, 25, 26, 48, 49, 50, 65, 82, 84, 92, 93, 101, 111, 112, 113, 114, 115, 127, 198, 239, 261
neonatal nursing care, 14, 65
neonatal skin, 14, 15, 19, 25, 26, 54, 57, 58, 60, 61, 63, 64, 65, 66, 77
nest positioning, 107, 110, 112
neurology, 102, 114, 162, 164, 165, 166, 292
newborn, 9, 11, 13, 15, 16, 17, 18, 19, 20, 21, 22, 23, 24, 25, 26, 28, 37, 38, 39, 43, 47, 49, 50, 53, 54, 55, 56, 57, 58, 59, 60, 61, 62, 63, 64, 65, 66, 82, 83, 87, 88, 89, 90, 91, 92, 93, 94, 105, 107, 112, 113, 121, 127, 128, 231, 232, 233, 236, 237
nipple problems, 27, 28, 32, 35, 37
non-nutritive sucking (NNS), 3, 4, 5, 6, 10, 11, 105, 227, 232, 233, 238
non-pharmacological methods, 39, 105, 107, 179, 194, 205, 227, 229, 231, 233, 237, 239, 268
nurse, 3, 4, 7, 9, 16, 21, 38, 57, 115, 117, 136, 137, 142, 143, 144, 161, 166, 200, 206, 215, 230, 242, 248, 253, 254, 276
nursing, v, 1, 9, 10, 11, 12, 13, 14, 18, 22, 23, 25, 26, 27, 28, 29, 30, 31, 32, 34, 36, 37, 39, 43, 49, 50, 53, 59, 64, 65, 66, 67, 81, 82, 83, 84, 85, 87, 88, 92, 93, 95, 97, 101, 103, 105, 107, 108, 112, 113, 114, 115, 117, 122, 127, 128, 131, 140, 141, 142, 143, 144, 145, 147, 150, 152, 153, 155, 159, 161, 162, 163, 164, 165, 166, 167, 175, 177, 178, 186, 187, 188, 189, 190, 191, 192, 194, 195, 196, 197, 198, 199, 200, 201, 204, 205, 206, 208, 209, 210, 211, 212, 213, 214, 224, 225, 226, 228, 230, 234, 237, 238, 239, 240, 241, 248, 251, 252, 253, 254, 257, 260, 261, 262, 263, 276, 279, 280, 287, 288, 289, 291, 292, 293
nursing care, 13, 14, 18, 22, 23, 29, 30, 31, 32, 34, 88, 93, 97, 122, 131, 140, 142, 143, 161, 162, 165, 166, 178, 192, 195, 198, 225, 228, 230, 234, 253, 254, 260, 287, 291
nursing practices, v, 28, 143, 145, 147, 150, 155, 163, 192, 199, 212, 254, 280

O

obesity intervention, 170, 171, 172, 173
obsesity treatment, 168
omphalitis, 62, 88, 89, 90, 91, 93
oral feeding, 1, 2, 3, 4, 5, 6, 7, 8, 9, 10, 11
oral feeding position, 3, 6
oral motor functions, 3, 4
oral motor stimulation, 5, 9
oral mucositis (OM), 177, 178, 179, 180, 181, 182, 185, 186, 187, 188, 189, 202, 215, 216, 217, 218, 220, 221, 222, 223, 224, 225, 226

P

pain, 6, 17, 18, 22, 25, 28, 29, 30, 31, 32, 33, 35, 36, 37, 38, 50, 55, 67, 68, 72, 74, 75, 97, 98, 99, 101, 108, 109, 111, 113, 114, 115, 177, 178, 179, 180, 181, 182, 185, 186, 187, 188, 189, 191, 192, 193, 194, 195, 196, 197, 198, 199, 200, 202, 204, 206, 207, 211, 216, 218, 220, 221, 222, 227, 228, 229, 230, 231, 232, 233, 234, 235, 236, 237, 238, 239, 240, 245, 253, 254, 259, 265, 266, 268, 269, 273, 274, 275, 276, 291
painful nipples, 27, 28
palliative care, 177, 178, 179, 180, 184, 185, 186, 187, 188, 189, 190, 197, 200, 212
parents, 4, 7, 8, 12, 17, 18, 20, 21, 23, 68, 78, 80, 81, 95, 96, 97, 98, 102, 112, 113, 117, 119, 121, 124, 128, 132, 136, 137, 139, 140, 145, 149, 155, 159, 160, 162, 163, 164, 165, 166, 171, 172, 173, 175, 185, 189, 201, 208, 209, 227, 229, 231, 232, 239, 241,242, 247, 248, 249, 250, 252, 260, 266, 269, 270, 271, 273, 274, 276, 277, 283
pediatric, v, 10, 11, 25, 26, 53, 57, 64, 65, 66, 67, 68, 81, 82, 83, 85, 94, 95, 96, 101, 102, 103, 104, 108, 112, 113, 114, 115, 128, 129, 141, 142, 143, 144, 145, 146, 150, 151, 152, 155, 160, 161, 162, 163, 164, 165, 166, 173, 174, 175, 177, 178, 179, 180, 181, 183, 184, 185, 186, 187, 188, 189, 190, 191, 192, 193, 194, 195, 196, 197, 198, 199, 200, 201, 202, 203, 204, 205, 206, 207, 208, 209, 210, 211, 212, 213, 214, 215, 218, 220, 221, 222, 223, 224, 225, 226, 234, 235, 236, 237, 238, 239, 240, 249, 250, 251, 253, 254, 262, 265, 266, 274, 275, 276, 279, 281, 282, 283, 284, 285, 286, 287, 288, 290, 291, 292, 293
pediatric care, 96, 194, 199, 265
pediatric healthcare, 253

pediatric nursing, v, 10, 25, 26, 53, 66, 81, 95, 102, 112, 113, 114, 128, 129, 143, 145, 150, 165, 173, 175, 185, 187, 191, 198, 199, 201, 210, 213, 214, 215, 238, 239, 262, 279, 281, 282, 287, 292
pediatric oncology, 179, 183, 184, 185, 186, 187, 188, 189, 191, 192, 193, 194, 196, 197, 198, 199, 200, 201, 202, 203, 204, 205, 206, 207, 208, 209, 210, 211, 212, 213, 214, 215, 226, 262, 285, 290, 292
perineum care, 62
photobiomodulation, 181, 188
phototherapy, 39, 42, 43, 44, 45, 46, 47, 48, 49, 50, 53, 69
placental transfusion, 47
poisoning, 241, 242, 247, 248, 252
postpartum depression, 38, 117, 123, 125, 126, 127, 128, 129, 130
prebiotics, 39, 45, 48, 95
preterm, 1, 2, 3, 4, 5, 6, 7, 8, 9, 10, 11, 12, 13, 14, 15, 16, 17, 18, 19, 20, 21, 22, 23, 24, 25, 26, 39, 40, 43, 46, 48, 49, 50, 53, 54, 55, 56, 58, 61, 62, 63, 64, 65, 66, 77, 81, 83, 84, 85, 90, 93, 94, 105, 106, 107, 108, 109, 110, 111, 112, 113, 114, 115, 126, 127, 128, 130, 195, 198, 199, 231, 232, 233, 238
preterm bath, 14
preterm birth, 1, 13, 14, 106, 112, 113, 115
preterm oral feeding, 1, 9
probiotics, 30, 31, 39, 45, 48, 49, 50, 51, 95, 98, 101, 102, 103
procedural pain, 107, 110, 111, 113, 180, 186, 187, 198, 199, 227, 228, 229, 230, 231, 232, 233, 234, 235, 236, 237, 238, 239, 240
psychosocial intervention programs, 184, 185
psychosocial problems, 146, 150, 155, 167, 169, 177, 184, 185
psychosocial support, 161, 167

R

reflexology, 39, 43, 45, 48, 49, 50, 99, 100, 101, 102, 183
reiki, 180, 189, 191, 192, 194, 195, 197, 198, 199, 200
respiratory functions, 4, 7, 57, 108, 134

S

secure attachment, 119, 130
seizure, 155, 156, 157, 158, 159, 160, 161, 162, 163, 164, 165, 166, 283, 284, 288, 289, 292
semi-elevated side-lying position, 6, 7, 9
semi-elevated supine position, 7
sensor-enhanced pump therapy, 149
sensory stimulation, 99, 233, 238
serious game, 265, 266, 267, 268, 269, 270, 271, 272, 273, 274, 275, 276, 277
side-lying position, 7, 9, 11
skin barrier, 14, 19, 20, 54, 57, 58, 60, 62, 63, 64, 65, 66, 70, 71, 76, 77, 79, 80, 84
skin development, 14, 19, 57, 60
skin integrity, 23, 53, 56, 57, 58, 59, 60, 61, 62, 68, 79, 83, 84
skincare, 14, 20, 23, 25, 26, 53, 57, 58, 59, 60, 61, 63, 64, 65, 66, 71, 74, 75, 76, 77, 79, 80, 83, 85, 112
skin-to-skin contact, 20, 53, 58, 59, 63, 112, 121, 122, 123, 129, 227, 232, 233
sleep, 77, 95, 96, 97, 99, 100, 105, 106, 107, 108, 109, 110, 111, 112, 113, 114, 115, 128, 136, 137, 158, 169, 187, 196, 198, 209, 211, 243, 247, 253, 254, 258, 259, 262, 282, 286
sleep quality, 107, 108, 110, 111, 128, 187, 253, 254, 258, 259, 282, 286
sleep-wake cycle, 106, 107, 108, 109, 110, 111
smartphone apps, 149
sponge bathing method, 16, 17, 25
swaddling bath method, 18

T

technology-based applications, 179, 184, 208
therapeutic play, 184
therapeutic touch (TT), 117, 179, 180, 191, 192, 195, 196, 198, 199, 200
thermoregulation, 3, 14, 15, 17, 19, 20, 21, 23, 24, 26
tub bathing, 16, 18, 25, 26, 39, 66, 114
type 1 diabetes mellitus (T1DM), 145, 146, 147, 148, 149, 150, 151, 152, 153, 269, 276, 286, 289, 290

U

umbilical cord, 17, 21, 39, 43, 47, 48, 50, 61, 62, 64, 65, 66, 87, 88, 89, 90, 91, 92, 93, 94, 127
umbilical cord care, 21, 62, 64, 65, 66, 87, 88, 89, 90, 91, 92, 93

V

vernix caseosa, 19, 20, 26, 33, 37, 54, 56
vibration, 194, 198, 235, 237, 239, 240
virtual reality (VR), 160, 166, 179, 184, 185, 187, 188, 189, 194, 199, 208, 212, 233, 234, 235, 236, 237, 238, 239, 240, 274, 275, 276
vitamin E, 56, 182, 186, 187, 221, 223, 224, 225
vomiting, 22, 24, 177, 178, 179, 182, 183, 186, 189, 190, 192, 201, 202, 203, 204, 205, 206, 207, 208, 209, 210, 211, 213, 214

W

wearable technologies, 279, 280, 281, 282, 283, 284, 285, 286, 287, 288, 289, 291, 292
weight control, 172, 174, 259, 271, 279, 282, 288
white noise, 99, 100, 103, 105, 107, 108, 109, 111, 113, 114

Y

yoga, 117, 122, 125, 126, 201, 205, 207, 209, 210, 253, 254, 255, 256, 257, 258, 259, 260, 261, 262, 263